HUMAN DEVELOPMENT AND THE THYROID GLAND
Relation to Endemic Cretinism

ADVANCES IN EXPERIMENTAL MEDICINE AND BIOLOGY

Volume 1
THE RETICULOENDOTHELIAL SYSTEM AND ATHEROSCLEROSIS
Edited by N. R. Di Luzio and R. Paoletti • 1967

Volume 2
PHARMACOLOGY OF HORMONAL POLYPEPTIDES AND PROTEINS
Edited by N. Back, L. Martini, and R. Paoletti • 1968

Volume 3
GERM-FREE BIOLOGY: Experimental and Clinical Aspects
Edited by E. A. Mirand and N. Back • 1969

Volume 4
DRUGS AFFECTING LIPID METABOLISM
Edited by W. L. Holmes, L. A. Carlson, and R. Paoletti • 1969

Volume 5
LYMPHATIC TISSUE AND GERMINAL CENTERS IN IMMUNE RESPONSE
Edited by L. Fiore-Donati and M. G. Hanna, Jr. • 1969

Volume 6
RED CELL METABOLISM AND FUNCTION
Edited by George J. Brewer • 1970

Volume 7
SURFACE CHEMISTRY OF BIOLOGICAL SYSTEMS
Edited by Martin Blank • 1970

Volume 8
BRADYKININ AND RELATED KININS: Cardiovascular, Biochemical, and Neural Actions
Edited by F. Sicuteri, M. Rocha e Silva, and N. Back • 1970

Volume 9
SHOCK: Biochemical, Pharmacological, and Clinical Aspects
Edited by A. Bertelli and N. Back • 1970

Volume 10
THE HUMAN TESTIS
Edited by E. Rosemberg and C. A. Paulsen • 1970

Volume 11
MUSCLE METABOLISM DURING EXERCISE
Edited by B. Pernow and B. Saltin • 1971

Volume 12
MORPHOLOGICAL AND FUNCTIONAL ASPECTS OF IMMUNITY
Edited by K. Lindahl-Kiessling, G. Alm, and M. G. Hanna, Jr. • 1971

Volume 13
CHEMISTRY AND BRAIN DEVELOPMENT
Edited by R. Paoletti and A. N. Davison • 1971

Volume 14
MEMBRANE-BOUND ENZYMES
Edited by G. Porcellati and F. di Jeso • 1971

Volume 15
THE RETICULOENDOTHELIAL SYSTEM AND IMMUNE PHENOMENA
Edited by N. R. Di Luzio and K. Flemming • 1971

Volume 16A
THE ARTERY AND THE PROCESS OF ARTERIOSCLEROSIS: Pathogenesis
Edited by Stewart Wolf • 1971

Volume 16B
THE ARTERY AND THE PROCESS OF ARTERIOSCLEROSIS: Measurement and Modification
Edited by Stewart Wolf • 1971

Volume 17
CONTROL OF RENIN SECRETION
Edited by Tatiana A. Assaykeen • 1972

Volume 18
THE DYNAMICS OF MERISTEM CELL POPULATIONS
Edited by Morton W. Miller and Charles C. Kuehnert • 1972

Volume 19
SPHINGOLIPIDS, SPHINGOLIPIDOSES AND ALLIED DISORDERS
Edited by Bruno W. Volk and Stanley M. Aronson • 1972

Volume 20
DRUG ABUSE: Nonmedical Use of Dependence-Producing Drugs
Edited by Simon Btesh • 1972

Volume 21
VASOACTIVE POLYPEPTIDES
Edited by N. Back and F. Sicuteri • 1972

Volume 22
COMPARATIVE PATHOPHYSIOLOGY OF CIRCULATORY DISTURBANCES
Edited by Colin M. Bloor • 1972

Volume 23
THE FUNDAMENTAL MECHANISMS OF SHOCK
Edited by Lerner B. Hinshaw and Barbara G. Cox • 1972

Volume 24
THE VISUAL SYSTEM: Neurophysiology, Biophysics, and Their Clinical Applications
Edited by G. B. Arden • 1972

Volume 25
GLYCOLIPIDS, GLYCOPROTEINS, AND MUCOPOLYSACCHARIDES OF THE NERVOUS SYSTEM
Edited by Vittorio Zambotti, Guido Tettamanti, and Mariagrazia Arrigoni • 1972

Volume 26
PHARMACOLOGICAL CONTROL OF LIPID METABOLISM
Edited by William L. Holmes, Rodolfo Paoletti, and David Kritchevsky • 1972

Volume 27
DRUGS AND FETAL DEVELOPMENT
Edited by M. A. Klingberg, A. Abramovici, and J. Chemke • 1972

Volume 28
HEMOGLOBIN AND RED CELL STRUCTURE AND FUNCTION
Edited by George J. Brewer • 1972

Volume 29
MICROENVIRONMENTAL ASPECTS OF IMMUNITY
Edited by Branislav D. Janković and Katarina Isaković • 1972

Volume 30
HUMAN DEVELOPMENT AND THE THYROID GLAND: Relation to Endemic Cretinism
Edited by J. B. Stanbury and R. L. Kroc • 1972

Volume 31
IMMUNITY IN VIRAL AND RICKETTSIAL DISEASES
Edited by A. Kohn and M. A. Klingberg • 1972

Volume 32
FUNCTIONAL AND STRUCTURAL PROTEINS OF THE NERVOUS SYSTEM
Edited by A. N. Davison, P. Mandel, and I. G. Morgan • 1972

HUMAN DEVELOPMENT AND THE THYROID GLAND
Relation to Endemic Cretinism

Proceedings of a Symposium on Endemic Cretinism held at The Kroc Foundation, Santa Ynez Valley, California, January 24–26, 1972

Edited by
J. B. Stanbury
Unit of Experimental Medicine
Department of Nutrition and Food Science
Massachusetts Institute of Technology
Harvard-MIT School of Health Sciences and Technology
Cambridge, Massachusetts

and
R. L. Kroc
The Kroc Foundation
Santa Ynez Valley
California

PLENUM PRESS • NEW YORK–LONDON • 1972

Library of Congress Catalog Card Number 72-89980
ISBN 0-306-39030-2

A Division of Plenum Publishing Corporation
227 West 17th Street, New York, N. Y. 10011

United Kingdom edition published by Plenum Press, London
A Division of Plenum Publishing Company, Ltd.
Davis House (4th Floor), 8 Scrubs Lane, Harlesden, London,
NW10 6SE, England

Printed in the United States of America

PREFACE

Differentiation of cellular structure and function is the basis for the development of complex organisms; its biochemical foundation is one of the central problems of contemporary biology. More than half a century ago, Gudernatsch demonstrated the role of the thyroid in the metamorphosis of the tadpole into a frog, and showed for the first time that a normal metabolite is indispensable for fulfillment of the scenario of vertebrate maturation. Since then an extensive literature has accumulated which considers the role of the thyroid in animal and especially human development. Nowhere is this role more striking than in cretinism, a term applied to idiocy and physical retardation generally assumed to arise from insufficient thyroid hormone in fetal or neonatal life.

A small group of physicians met at the Institute of Human Biology in Goroka, New Guinea, in January 1971 to consider the nature and prevention of those varieties of cretinism which occur in association with endemic goiter and which are grouped under the term endemic cretinism. Curiously, for centuries this disorder has occupied a distinctive niche under the panoply of mental retardation, and yet it has defied the kind of formal definition which would permit unequivocal ascertainment in individual cases. Indeed, the pathogenesis and even its relationship to the thyroid have remained obscure and controversial. The Goroka meeting was successful in resolving some of the conflicting information regarding the various clinical manifestations of cretinism and in underlining the effectiveness of prophylactic use of iodine in preventing its appearance. The need for additional information from a broader spectrum of medical scientists was apparent. The present monograph, comprising the proceedings of a conference on endemic cretinism and the thyroid in human development, is a direct extension of the Goroka conference.

The symposium was sponsored by The Kroc Foundation and took place January 1972 at their headquarters - the J & R Double Arch Ranch of the Founder, Ray A. Kroc, in the Santa Ynez Valley of California.

The initial papers were concerned with descriptions of endemic cretinism by investigators who have had direct experience with field studies in various parts of the world. Reports were presented from Andean South America, the Himalayas, New Guinea, Switzerland, Italy, and Central Africa. Resolution of some of the seemingly conflicting information was achieved.

The conference then addressed the problems of definition, assessment, and field ascertainment of cretinism. The difficulties caused by cultural and language barriers in the detection of retardation was explored, and the unusual difficulty posed by deafness, a common but not invariable accompaniment of endemic cretinism, was considered. With the clinical patterns of the disease assembled and the experimental approaches identified, an attempt was made to arrive at a formal definition of endemic cretinism which could be operationally adequate and which would permit better communication among investigators.

This was followed by a review of preventive measures. The most important data which have become available in recent years derive from observations made after administration of depot iodized oil. Experience obtained in such programs in New Guinea, Peru, Ecuador and the Zaire Republic were reported. A consensus was reached that the method is feasible, safe, and probably effective, although the small numbers of retardates born in control groups makes this uncertain.

The discussion then turned to the hearing problems in endemic cretinism, with consideration of its embryological, pathological and experimental aspects. This lead naturally into a consideration of the role of thyroid hormone in the development of the central nervous system, and the interactions between the thyroid and environmental factors, such as nutrition, in central nervous system maturation.

The final presentations related to the etiopathogenesis of the developmental abnormalities of endemic cretinism. The relative contributions of maternal and fetal thyroids to embryogenesis were assessed, and toxins from the environment which might act specifically on thyroid function, such as cyanogenic glycosides, were identified. The conference closed with a discussion of the pathophysiology of the thyroid in the clinical variants of endemic cretinism.

The conferees are indebted to Mr. Ray A. Kroc, Chairman and Founder of The Kroc Foundation. Alice (Mrs. Robert L.) Kroc was the gracious hostess for the social occasions of the symposium. Generous financial support for travel and publication were furnished by E. Fougera & Co., the World Health Organization, the Australian-American Educational Foundation, The National Foundation, the Commonwealth Foundation (of London), and The Kroc Foundation. Dr. Peter Amacher has been an invaluable editorial associate.

John Stanbury

Robert L. Kroc

PARTICIPANTS

SYMPOSIUM CHAIRMAN:

J.B. Stanbury, M.D., Unit of Experimental Medicine, Department of Nutrition and Food Science, Massachusetts Institute of Technology,; Harvard-MIT School of Health Sciences and Technology, Cambridge, Massachusetts

PARTICIPANTS:

P. Amacher, Ph.D., Los Angeles, California

R. Balázs, M.D., Medical Research Council Neuropsychiatry Unit, Carshalton, Surrey, England

C. Beckers, M.D., Centre de Médecine Nucléaire et Laboratoire de Pathologie Générale, School of Medicine, University of Louvain, Belgium

I.H. Buttfield, M.D., Monash University, Alfred Hospital, Prahran, Victoria, Australia

A. Costa, M.D., Mauriziano Hospital, Turin, Italy

L.J. DeGroot, M.D., University of Chicago, Chicago, Illinois

F. Delange, M.D., Departments of Pediatrics and Radioisotopes, St. Peter Hospital, University of Brussel, Belgium

J.T. Dunn, M.D., University of Virginia School of Medicine, Charlottesville, Virginia

A.M. Ermans, M.D. Department of Radioisotopes, St. Peter Hospital, University of Brussels, Belgium

R. Fierro-Benitéz, M.D., Departamento de Radioisotopos, Escuela Politecnica Nacional, Quito, Ecuador

L.I. Gardner, M.D. Genetic and Endocrine Unit, Department of Pediatrics, State University of New York, Upstate Medical Center, Syracuse, New York

J.M. Hershman, M.D.,Division of Endocrinology and Metabolism, Department of Medicine, University of Alabama, Birmingham, Alabama

B.S. Hetzel, M.D. Department of Social and Preventive Medicine, Monash University, Alfred Hospital, Melbourne, Australia

R.W. Hornabrook, M.D., Institute of Human Biology, Goroka, Papua, New Guinea

H.K. Ibbertson, M.D., Department of Endocrinology. School of Medicine, Auckland, New Zealand

M.P. Koenig, M.D., The University Medical Clinic, Inselspital, Bern Switzerland

R.L. Kroc, Ph.D.,The Kroc Foundation, Santa Ynez Valley, California

H.D. Mosier, M.D.,University of California at Irvine, Irvine, California

J. Paris, M.D., Santa Monica, California

P.O.D. Pharoah, M.D., Institute of Human Biology, Goroka, Papua, New Guinea

J.A. Pittman, Jr., M.D., Georgetown University School of Medicine and Department of Medicine and Surgery, Veterans Administration, Washington, D.C.

E.A. Pretell, M.D. Departamento de Endocrinologia, Instituto de Investigaciones de la Altura, Lima, Peru

A. Querido, M.D., Department of Medicine, University of Leiden, Holland

N.P. Rosman, M.D., Department of Pediatrics and Neurology, Boston University School of Medicine, Boston City Hospital, Boston, Massachusetts

F.L. Trowbridge, M.D., Center for Disease Control, Atlanta, Georgia

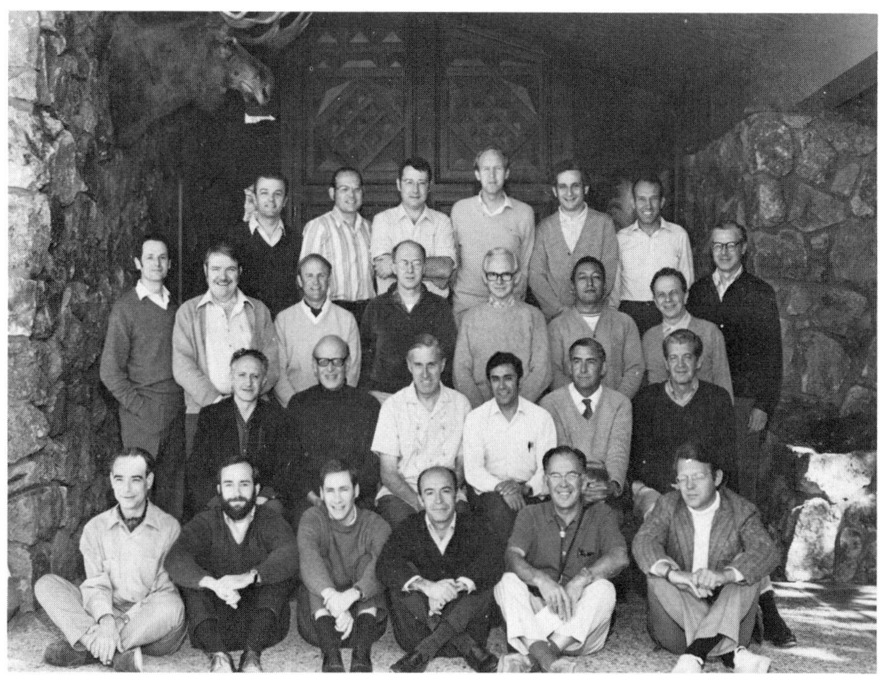

L to R Front Row: Balázs; Trowbridge; Dunn; Paris; Kroc; Amacher.
L to R Second Row: Ermans; Querido; Hetzel; Pretell; Hornabrook; Stanbury.
L to R Third Row: Koenig; Gardner; Ibbertson; Pittman; DeGroot; Fierro-Benítez; Costa; Mosier.
L to R Fourth Row: Beckers, Hershman, Delange, Buttfield, Rosman, Pharoah.

CONTENTS

SECTION 5: THE CENTRAL NERVOUS SYSTEM AND CRETINISM

SECTION 6: ETIOPATHOLOGY OF CRETINISM

SECTION 1
CLINICAL PATTERNS OF CRETINISM

THE CLINICAL PATTERN OF CRETINISM AS SEEN IN HIGHLAND ECUADOR

John B. Stanbury

Unit of Experimental Medicine, Department of Nutrition

and Food Science, Massachusetts Institute of Technology

Cambridge, Massachusetts

When Sir Robert McCarrison described cretinism as he saw it in the Gilgit and Chitral valleys of the Indian Himalayas in the early years of this century, he distinguished two forms of the disease (1). The more common form, which he called the nervous type, was characterized by spasticity, extreme difficulty with gait, and abnormalities of eye movement. The other he termed myxedematous cretins. The latter patients were clinically hypothyroid. Mental retardation, deaf-mutism, and goiter were found in both types, and many patients were described as presenting a combination of these findings.

The patients with severe intellectual retardation who are found in substantial numbers in the villages and farms of Andean Ecuador in close association with severe endemic goiter most closely resemble McCarrison's patients with nervous cretinism (Fig. 1), but the clinical pattern is not uniform (Fig. 2). This communication is a clinical account of these patients drawn from the extensive studies of Fierro-Benítez and his colleagues (2,3, 4) and from personal observations.

EPIDEMIOLOGICAL CONSIDERATIONS

No formal definition or laboratory procedure has been devised which permits precise ascertainment of the endemic cretin. Recognition of the disorder is based on epidemiological considerations, especially the juxtaposition of suspect subjects and severe endemic goiter. These suspect patients are selected because of certain resemblances to those described elsewhere in earlier times who were also found in relationship to severe endemic goiter. Certain characteristics, such as mental deficiency, gait disturbances, goiter, deaf-mutism muscular incoordination, short stature, delayed bone maturation, spotty calcification of the epiphyses, and a demeanor and affect of simple good humor are among the characteristics which tend to identify the endemic cretin. The lack of specificity of most or all of these findings, the fact that patients may present only a few of these, and the realization that many persons in a region of endemic goiter may have only one or two of these findings, or be only intellectually retarded, has made it quite impossible to assign with confidence precise rates of incidence or to correlate cretinism with other aspects of the biosystem in which they reside.

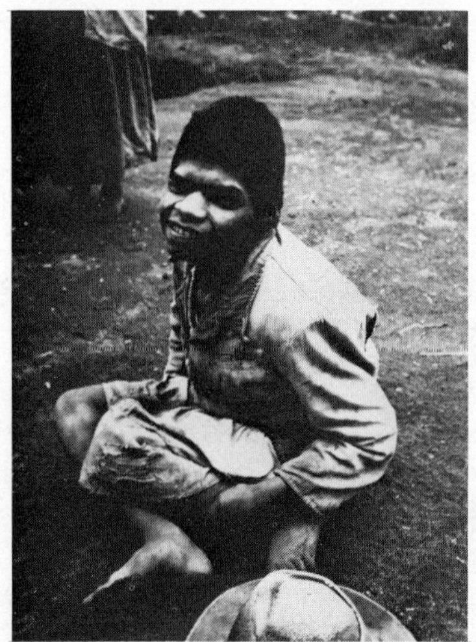

Fig. 1. A typical "nervous" cretin of Andean Ecuador.

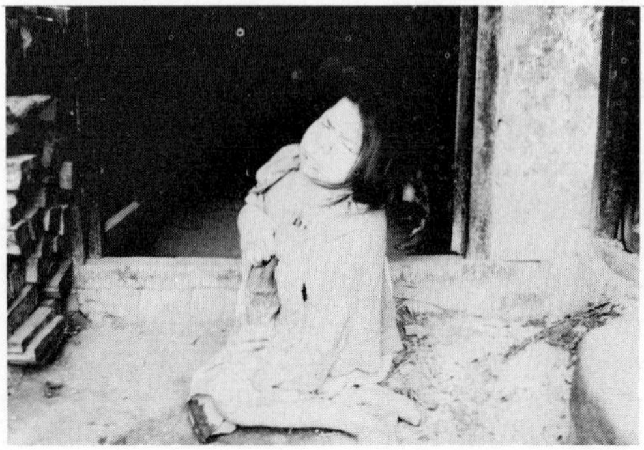

Fig. 2. A "nervous" cretin from Ecuador who has severe neurological signs and clinical evidence of hypothyroidism.

Nevertheless, there can be no doubt that there is an obvious excess of patients who may be called cretins in certain villages of rural Andean Ecuador where goiter is hyperendemic. During the past 15 years Fierro-Benítez and his colleagues have conducted an intensive study of two such villages (2,3,4). These are the communities of Tocachi and La Esperanza, which lie about 60 kilometers north of Quito at an elevation of 10,000 feet. These villages, approximately five kilometers apart, are largely devoted to subsistence agriculture. Sociological surveys have disclosed absence of contact with the outside world, great poverty, limited education, a high incidence of thyroid disease, and a high prevalence of persons with physical and intellectual retardation. Some of these relationships appear in Table 1. The figures in this table correspond to obvious examples of the categories. Modest dimunition in hearing or in intellectual attainment might not be, and undoubtedly was not ascertained frequently because of the difficulties of applying formal testing modalities under field conditions. From the table it may be seen that even neglecting this inadequacy in ascertainment, there is a striking incidence of retardation in the two communities.

*Table 1. Prevalence of certain findings in two villages in Andean Ecuador. (Percent of total population).**

	VILLAGE		
	Tocachi (1,100)**	La Esperanza (2,500)	Source
Infant mortality	43.0	29.0	(3)
Total endemic goiter	54.4	51.0	(2)
Nodular goiter	48.0	34.0	(2)
Mental deficiency and deaf-mutism	7.4	5.5	(2)
Mental deficiency, deaf-mutism, short stature and motor abnormalities	0.8	0.5	(2)

* Adapted from Fierro-Benítez et al.(3).
** Prior to iodized oil prophylaxis program.

A study of the relationship between the cretin and nodular goiter in his family disclosed no correlation. Nevertheless, since nodular goiter exists in unusually high frequency in these communities a relationship might have been easily overlooked. No difference was found in the prevalence of goiter or of thyroid nodules in families with cretins as compared to those without.

A comparison of deaf-mutism, retardation of any kind, or of any other aspect of cretinism in these two villages with others where endemic goiter is not found in Ecuador disclosed a close association of cretinism to the incidence of goiter. Further evidence for a close relationship between endemic retardation has appeared in much diminished frequency following introduction of iodized oil prophylaxis programs. Most of the inhabitants of Tocachi have been injected with iodized oil beginning in 1966, whereas La Esperanza has served as a control group.

Fierro-Benítez and his colleagues have identified a family tendency toward cretinism (3). In 116 families they found 144 cretins. This clearly indicates a familial predisposition, either on a genetic or environmental basis. He has observed normal children and cretins in the same family, several cretins within the same family, cretins born of cretinous mothers, and normal children born of cretinous mothers.

CLINICAL ASPECTS

Since there are no absolute criteria for the selection of a cretin for special study in a particular community any clinical survey must necessarily include an element of bias. Fierro-Benítez et al. selected ten "typical" cretins from Tocachi and La Esperanza for exhaustive observation (4). Some of the results on the ten subjects appear in Table 2. In general, stature was short. The mean height for men in the population at large was 152 cm, and for women 142 cm. In the cretins the height was more than two standard deviations below normal, except for one in whom the height could not accurately be ascertained because of bony deformity. The hair tended to be coarse and dry in most of the subjects, and the tongue was prominent in more than half. All had irregularities of the teeth, including abnormalities in spacing and eruption. Some had thyroids which could not be felt and others had large nodular glands. Eight of the ten had significant impairment of locomotion and one was unable to stand. Seven had a characteristic shuffling gait. Most had an impassive facies, but when amused this gave place to a slow spreading vacuous smile which others have noted as characteristic of the endemic cretin. The bridge of the nose was often depressed and the hairline low. Motor coordination of the upper extremities was frequently limited. Movements were slow. Reflex relaxation time was normal or occasionally impaired. Dry, cool, rough skin may have been related to thyroid state or to the severe climatic conditions and personal hygiene. It may be

*Table 2. Findings in ten "typical" cretins of Andean Ecuador**

No.	Sex	Age	Height (cm)	Goiter	Motor Abnormality	Hearing	Speech
1	F	25	133	++++	++	10%	Severely limited
2	M	20	-	+	+++	10%	Mute
3	F	40	116	+++	++	10%	Mute
4	F	12	101	+	++	30%	Severely limited
5	F	30	130	++++	++	-	Mute
6	M.	20	111	+	+	30%	Mute
7	M	25	118	+	+	-	Mute
8	M	18	130	++	+	-	Mute
9	F	13	123	++	-	10%	Mute
10	F	28	138	++	-	30%	Severely limited

*Adapted from Fierro-Benitez et al. (4).

emphasized that these patients did not present the clinical aspects of myxedema.

Other subjects were found in the community who were obviously retarded but who presented a somewhat different clinical aspect than has been described in the paragraphs above. Deaf-mutism is fairly frequently encountered in La Esperanza and Tocachi. It is seen unaccompanied by short stature, difficulty in walking, or significant motor incoordination, but also accompanied by intellectual deficit and at other times with intellectual deficit which is only apparent on tests of intellectual capability (Fig. 3). All of these subjects, except those with inability to walk, may be employed in the household and farming activities of the community. Occasionally subjects are encountered who are clearly clinically hypothyroid and who in some instances have severe dwarfing (Fig. 4).

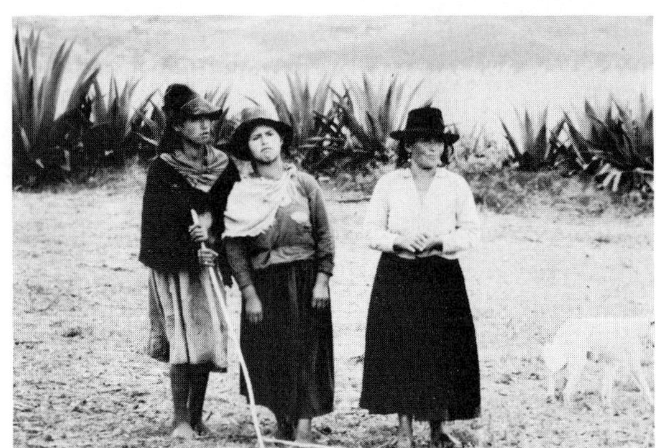

Fig. 3. Two deaf-mutes (left) with their mother. The stature is normal. Both had nodular goiter and were probably mentally retarded.

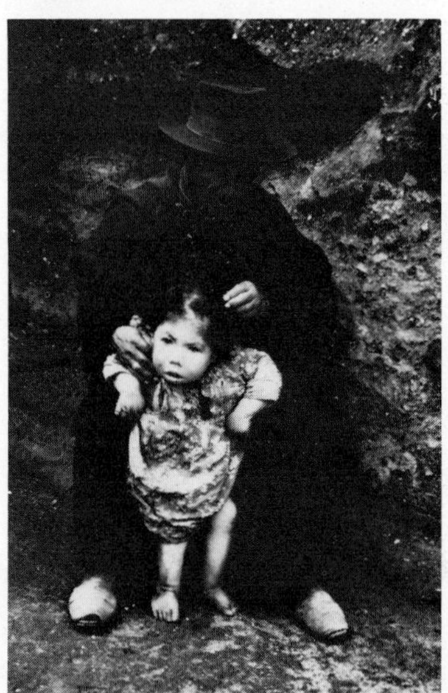

Fig. 4. An Ecuadorean cretin certainly over 15 years of age, with severe dwarfing and clinical myxedema. One sib was similarly affected and three others were cretins, but with much better growth. Patients with this degree of growth retardation are unusual in highland Ecuador.

There is no present information regarding the survival capacity of these retarded subjects. Few are encountered in the community who are in the later decades of life. Some have died in their earlier years while the communities have been under medical surveillance during the past decade and a half. The climate and conditions of living are difficult and the diet is limited. It seems evident that the incidence of newborns who are potential cretins must be considerably higher than those who survive and are actually identified within the population group.

These ten patients displayed a constellation of clinical findings. All had enlarged thyroids, six out of the ten being large enough to be visible without extension of the head. Two had no evidence of neuromotor abnormality. All were severely retarded intellectually. Hearing was impaired in all. Seven were mute and the others made sounds but not intelligible words.

Sexual maturation in cretins of the region is said to be delayed. Among the ten subjects of the study of Fierro-Benítez *et al.*, one aged 12 was somewhat sexually precocious, whereas another age 13 had not yet developed secondary sexual changes. Four other female subjects in this group showed normal secondary sex characteristics. One of these had been pregnant three times and had lactated. Thus, it appeared that for the most part the female cretins could be considered gynecologically normal. In the same villages there were three other cretins who had recently become mothers. One of the children was a typical male cretin, another was mentally deficient, and a third was normal.

While these ten patients described by Fierro-Benítez *et al.* may be accepted as characteristic of severe endemic cretinism, they by no means represent the full spectrum of the disorder. In the community are many patients with normal stature or small stature who have little or no difficulty with motor coordination, but who are obviously severely retarded intellectually, or who are deaf-mute or both, and who are acknowledged by the community as deficient persons (Fig. 5). Fierro-Benítez *et al.* have classified their cretins from these villages into two types, the first with mental deficiency and severe impairment in hearing and speech, and the second with these defects and in addition short stature and motor abnormalities. While it is possible that this classification corresponds to some biological differences amongst patients, it seems more reasonable that they represent varying severity of manifestations.

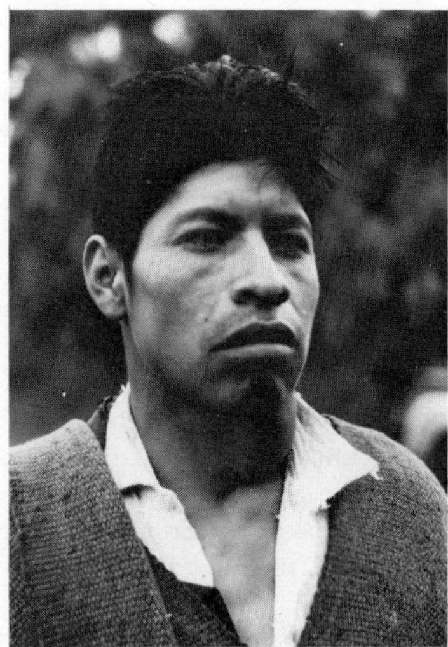

Fig. 5. An Ecuadorean cretin with normal stature, spastic gait, mental deficiency, squint, and a large nodular goiter.

LABORATORY FINDINGS

Roentgenographic examination of the skeleton in the ten cretin subjects of Fierro-Benítez et al. disclosed significant delayed closing of the epiphyses. Five of the ten subjects showed delayed epiphyseal closure in the hands, wrists, and femoral heads. All of these subjects were 18 yr of age or older. In some the changes in the femoral head were entirely similar to those reported from other endemic zones. Changes included increased obliquity of the head of the femur and flattening of the head. An unexplained finding was the presence of mild generalized osteoporosis in most of the bones.

Electrocardiograms in all these subjects were normal. Electroencephalograms in three were normal. The rest showed increased theta activity. Two of these patients had pneumoencephalograms which disclosed microcephaly.

Cholesterol concentration of the plasma varied from 144 to 240 mg per 100 ml. The Achilles reflex relaxation time was elevated moderately in two out of the ten.

Studies of thyroid function appear in Table 3. It may be seen that the mean uptake of radioactive iodine was elevated and that the mean protein bound iodine concentration of the plasma was much lower than normal. The ^{131}I conversion rate was 92 percent on average,

*Table 3. Iodine metabolism and thyroid function in ten "typical" cretins of Andean Ecuador**

	Mean	Range
Total iodine, μg%	4.1	2.8-5.9
PBI, μg%	4.0	2.8-5.3
BEI, μg%	2.9	1.8-5.3
T_4I μg%	2.24	.72-4.15
^{131}I uptake, 24 hrs.	69%	47-87%
$PB^{131}I$, % dose/LT	1.29	.13-4.1
Thyroid clearance rate, ml/min	179 (5 pts)	55-290
Urine iodine, μg/24 hrs	10.4	7.4-25.2

*Adapted from Fierro-Benítez et al. (4).

which is elevated. Kinetic studies disclosed a high maximal uptake value, a high rate of clearance of iodine from the blood and a normal range of renal clearance of iodide. These subjects responded to administration of thyrotrophic hormone by an increased radioactive iodine uptake. In two tested for triiodothyronine suppression the result was positive in one and negative in the other. Thyroid scans in four without palpable enlargement of the thyroid showed diffuse uptake of iodine in the normal position of the thyroid. The others showed irregular distribution throughout the gland area. The kinetic data disclosed high secretion rates for thyroid iodine. This finding indicates release of a large fraction of the thyroid iodine in inorganic form.

Harrison et al. measured the growth hormone response to insulin induced hypoglycemia in 14 cretins from Tocachi and La Esperanza (5). The test was completed satisfactorily in 11 of them, and 10 showed brisk responses which were comparable to those of normal control subjects. Some of these cretins were dwarfed. Plasma hydrocortisone also rose in response to insulin administration.

NEURAL AND INTELLECTUAL ATTAINMENT

Dodge *et al.* (6) undertook a neurological and intellectual appraisal of 28 cretins from Tocachi and La Esperanza. Eleven of these were males with a mean age of 27.2. The mean age of the females was 25.7. Most had large nodular goiters. Psychological tests included those of Gesell, Leiter, and Ayres. All had short stature. It varied from 117 cm to 147 cm. Head circumference was within normal limits in all but two, but the mean was approximately a standard deviation below the expected mean for normal subjects.

All subjects were mentally defective, since this constituted one of the prime criteria of choice for inclusion in this study group. Of the 16 subjects examined by the Leiter test only four scored at the third year level or above. Most failed to complete items normally accomplished by two year old children. Other tests of intellectual capacity gave similar findings.

Twenty-seven of these subjects had impaired hearing and speech. Seventeen appeared to be completely deaf-mute, whereas 10 had some residual hearing. Only one had fairly coherent speech. Twenty-three patients showed impairment in walking. This was evident in a stooped position with slightly flexed knees and a shuffling gait. Two had abductor spasm with scissoring when walking. Three were unable to stand or walk and had marked flexion contractions at the knees. None could walk tandem. Nineteen showed evidence of spasticity. Sustained ankle clonus was found in only one subject. In only two were the tendon reflexes normal. A Babinski or Oppenheim response was demonstrated in nine of these subjects and was questionable in several others, but the Babinski maneuver was difficult to execute in this group of subjects who seldom wore shoes. Thus, it appears that the large majority of these patients had pyramidal tract dysfunction involving predominantly the lower extremities, but it was not possible by neurological assessment to localize precisely the neural lesions.

RETARDED PERSONS NOT TYPICALLY CRETINS

In an economically deprived subsistence agricultural society the intellectual demands placed on the individual may be limited and intellectual deficit may pass unnoticed. Dodge *et al.* described one such patient who was not recognized as being mentally defective by the community (6). She had fine features but somewhat coarse hair and was a deaf-mute. The severity of her mental retardation became evident when she was subjected to formal testing and proved to perform at approximately the five year old level, whereas she was chronologically an adult. This poor performance could not be ascribed to problems in communication since other individuals in the community performed quite normally without verbal clues. This problem was discussed more fully elsewhere in this volume by Trowbridge. While recognizing the difficulties in appraisal of intellectual development across language and cultural barriers, and in patients who may have developed in a severe state of intellectual deprivation, one still has the impression in these villages that there are numerous subjects without any of the other clearly recognizable stigmata of cretinism but who are intellectually slow. The problem remains as to their number and as to their relationship to the prevailing endemic goiter and "typical" endemic cretinism.

RESPONSE TO THYROID MEDICATION

Many of the patients diagnosed as cretins have been treated with thyroid replacement medication. In none has there been clear evidence of intellectual development or improved intellectual performance, but in several, definite acceleration in tooth development and linear growth have occurred with therapy. A more striking finding not heretofore numerically documented has been an improvement in the facies, general appearance, and level of activity of "typical" cretins when treated with thyroid medication. This has occurred in patients who were not originally suspected of being hypothyroid. Their low values for plasma protein bound iodine were attributed to a presumed elevation in triiodothyronine prior to therapy, but it seems probable that the physical changes which occurred over a long period of time during thyroid medication were an indication that their low protein bound iodine values represented more closely their true metabolic state. In this regard it may be useful to note the difficulty in diagnosing hypothyroidism in patients who live in a chronically cold environment with inadequate clothing and who have rough dry skin and thick coarse hair as a result at least in part of limited or absent hygienic facilities.

One child has been observed particularly carefully (7). This male was observed initially at age 12 mo (Fig. 6). At that time he was severely retarded with extremely high plasma levels of thyrotrophic hormone (<200 μU/ml) and low plasma concentration of thyroxine (0.7 μg per 100 ml). Dental eruption and linear growth were retarded, but the conventional signs of infantile cretinism, such as large tongue, umbilical hernia, characteristic facies, dry rough skin and sallow yellow or carotenemic appearance were not present. He has been followed for several years on thyroid medication. His appearance and his growth have improved, but he remains a severely retarded child with permanent neurological deficits.

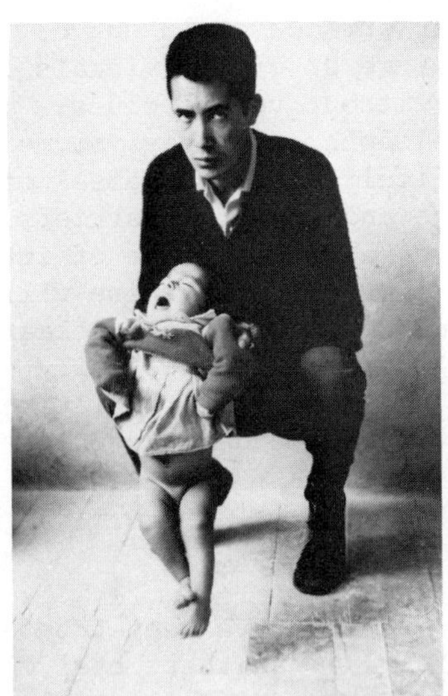

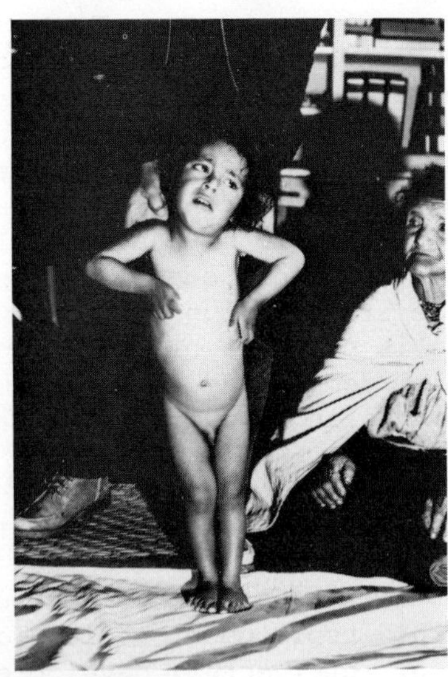

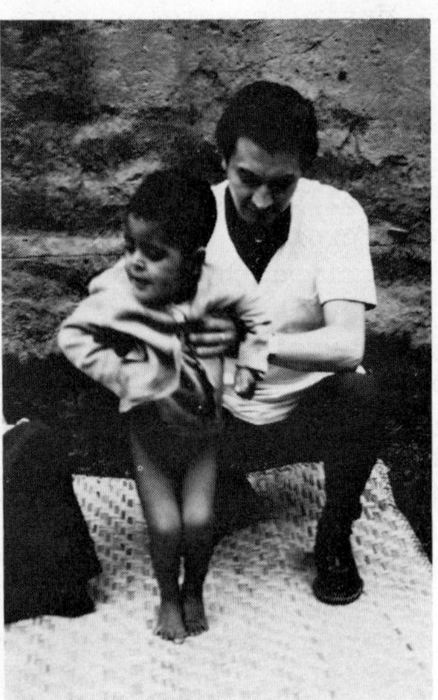

Fig. 6: Ecuadorean cretin. At upper left, age 12 mo. Note scissoring of legs. Slowed attainment of developmental milestones (7). No clinical evidence of hypothyroidism, but T_4 was 0.7 µg% and TSH was>200 µU/ml. At upper right, age 3 yr. Severely retarded, but linear growth and eruption of teeth has occurred following thyroid replacement medication. Lower, age 4 yr. Severely retarded; does not stand or walk.

CLINICAL PATTERNS OF CRETINISM IN INFANCY

A definitive diagnosis of endemic cretinism during infancy has proved to be an extremely difficult undertaking. Fierro-Benítez and his colleagues have made serial examination of all newborn children in Tocachi and La Esperanza for the past several years. A routine battery of tests are applied successively at intervals throughout infancy and childhood. Among those newborns who subsequently proved to be defective there appear to be no definitive sign during the first weeks and early months. Gradually, as tests of motor function and of growth are applied, the evidence for retardation becomes increasingly evident. There is no ready explanation for this difficulty in diagnosing endemic cretinism during the early weeks of postnatal life, whereas the diagnosis can usually be made at birth or shortly thereafter in the sporadic cretin. One might have expected the reverse since the endemic cretin clearly was severely damaged during uterine life, as is evidenced by the frequent occurrence of deafness. Perhaps an answer may be that the sporadic cretin is athyreotic, and because of limited transfer of maternal hormone through the placenta he is born with an element of physical retardation, as evidenced by umbilical hernia and retarded development of certain enzymes such as the bilirubin glucuronide forming system, whereas the endemic cretin with a functioning thyroid in utero may escape these physical changes only to suffer the full impact of severe thyroid deficiency during the early postnatal months. This still leaves unaccounted the deafness of the endemic cretin. Perhaps this is a function of iodine *per se*, as has been suggested by Pharoah (8), rather than a function of thyroid hormone.

COMMENT

Persons with physical attributes closely resembling those described in northern Italy and in Switzerland several generations ago and illustrated in many old textbooks may be found in high frequency at the present time in isolated communities and farming districts of Andean Ecuador. Evidence that their condition is related to thyroid disease, is their geographical association with the severe endemic goiter of those regions, the frequent presence of large goiters in these affected persons, and abnormalities of thyroid function which may be disclosed by appropriate laboratory tests. Evidence for a role for iodine deficiency in the pathogensis of this disorder is its disappearance in the community among persons born after the introduction of iodized oil prophylaxis. This occurred in Switzerland, and more recently its disappearance has been documented in New Guinea, and there is evidence for its disappearance in central Africa and in Ecuador (cf. elsewhere in this volume).

In the same communities are found many patients who do not fit the classic pattern of cretinism but who may have short stature or deaf-mutism or neurological signs, or who may have mental retardation without other physical findings. The problem remains as to the relationship of these patients to the more classic form of endemic cretinism. The evidence up to the present time seems to suggest that there is a continuum of deficits related to endemic goiter which extends from mild intellectual retardation at one end of the spectrum to the severest mental defect coupled with deficits in growth and development at the other. Some of these patients may be hypothyroid at the time of examination. Others may have achieved an euthyroid state through compensatory growth of the thyroid.

Attempts have been made to classify cretinism into several types. While it is puzzling that in some communities, as in the northern regions of the Zaire Republic, the large majority of retarded persons associated with endemic goiter conform most closely to McCarrison's original description of "myxedematous" cretinism, and in Andean Ecuador, the majority of identifiable endemic cretins conform more closely to McCarrison's "nervous" cretinism, examples of both types may be found in both regions, just as they were according to McCarrison's original description in the foothills of the Himalayas. The influences which cause a predominance of one variant of endemic cretinism in one region and another elsewhere remain to be determined. These differences should not be allowed to obscure the concept that thyroid deficiency is the primary disorder responsible for the appearance of endemic cretinism and that it may be corrected by a supply of iodide through appropriate channels to the population at risk.

SUMMARY

Endemic goiter may be found in many rural agrarian communities of Andean Ecuador. When endemic goiter is severe in these regions, endemic cretinism in its classic forms is found in a substantial percentage of the population. In addition to these patients who conform to classic descriptions there are many other members of the community who are deaf-mute, clinically hypothyroid, or who have intellectual retardation or some combination of these findings. Thus, in Andean Ecuador the majority of cretins appear to conform to McCarrison's original description of "nervous" cretinism, but there are others who fit his description of "myxedematous" cretinism and others who fall between. Furthermore, there are many subjects in these communities whose mild or moderate mental retardation or deaf-mutism may be attributed to the same cause or causes which are responsible for the classic form of the disease.

ACKNOWLEDGEMENTS

Supported by USPHS Grant #AM 10992.

REFERENCES

1. McCarrison, R.: Observations on endemic cretinism in the Chitral and Gilgit valleys. Lancet 2:1275-1280, 1908.

2. Fierro-Benítez, R.; Penafiel, W.; DeGroot, L.J. and Ramirez,I.: Endemic goiter and endemic cretinism in the Andean region. New Engl. J. Med. 280:296-302, 1969.

3. Fierro-Benítez, R.: Ramirez, I.; Estrella, E.; Jaramillo, C.; Díaz, D. and Urresta, J.: Iodized oil in the prevention of endemic goiter and associated defects in the Andean region of Ecuador. I. Program design, effects on goiter prevalence, thyroid function, and iodine excretion. In: Endemic Goiter. Report of the meeting of the PAHO Scientific Group on Research in Endemic Goiter held in Mexico, 1968. (J.B. Stanbury, ed.), Scientific Publication No. 193, Washington, 1969. pp. 306-340.

4. Fierro-Benítez, R.; Stanbury, J.B.; Querido, A.; DeGroot, L.J.; Alban, R. and Cordova, J.: Endemic cretinism in the Andean region of Ecuador. J. Clin. Endocrinol Metab. 30:228-236, 1970.

5. Harrison, M.R.; Fierro-Benítez, R.; Ramirex, I.; Refetoff, S. and Stanbury, J.B.: Immunoreactive growth hormone in endemic cretins in Ecuador. Lancet 1:936-940, 1968.

6. Dodge, P.R.; Ramirez, I. and Fierro-Benítez, R.: Neurological aspects of endemic cretinism. In: Endemic Goiter. Report of the meeting of the PAHO Scientific Group on Research in Endemic Goiter held in Mexico, 1968. (J.B. Stanbury, ed.), Scientific Publication No. 193, Washington, 1969. pp. 373-377.

7. Stanbury, J.B.; Fierro-Benítez, R.; Estrella, E.; Milutinovic, P.S.; Tellez, M.U. and Refetoff, S.: Endemic goiter with hypothyroidism in three generations. J. Clin. Endocrinol Metab. 29:1596-1600, 1969.

8. Pharoah, P.O.D.: Epidemiological studies of endemic cretinism in the Jimi River Valley in New Guinea. In: Endemic Cretinism (B.S. Hetzel and P.O.D. Pharoah, eds.), Surrey Beatty & Sons, N.S.W., 1971, pp. 109-116.

THE CLINICAL PATTERN OF CRETINISM AS SEEN IN SWITZERLAND

M. P. Koenig

The University Medical Clinic, Inselspital

Bern, Switzerland

For a long time the cretins seen almost everywhere in the Alps were a local curiosity, part of the romantic image of Switzerland as a land of shepherds and peasants. Thus, it is not surprising that the first medically acceptable and unequivocal description of endemic cretins was made by a Swiss physician, the brilliant Felix Platter (1546-1614). In an account of his observations in the Valais, he wrote: "...it is usual that many infants suffer from [innate folly]. Besides, the head is sometimes misshapen; the tongue is huge and swollen; they are dumb; the throat is often goitrous. Thus they present an ugly sight; and sitting in the streets and looking into the sun, and putting little sticks in between their fingers, twisting their bodies in various ways, with their mouths agape they provoke passersby to laughter and astonishment." (1)

Since the description of Platter, many publications by Swiss and foreign authors have been published, adding comments or making new observations about cretins in Switzerland, particularly from the region of the Valais and the canton of Bern (2). In accounts the symptomatology of this condition almost always includes severe oligophrenia, stunted growth, large goiters, and deaf-mutism. Although cretins are in general described as rather gentle, most authors describe them as occasionally becoming agitated when they want something and showing sudden anger. De Quervain and Wegelin (3) and we have confirmed this fact. Like Haller [quoted by Merke (2)], We have been impressed by the longevity of these individuals (Fig. 1).

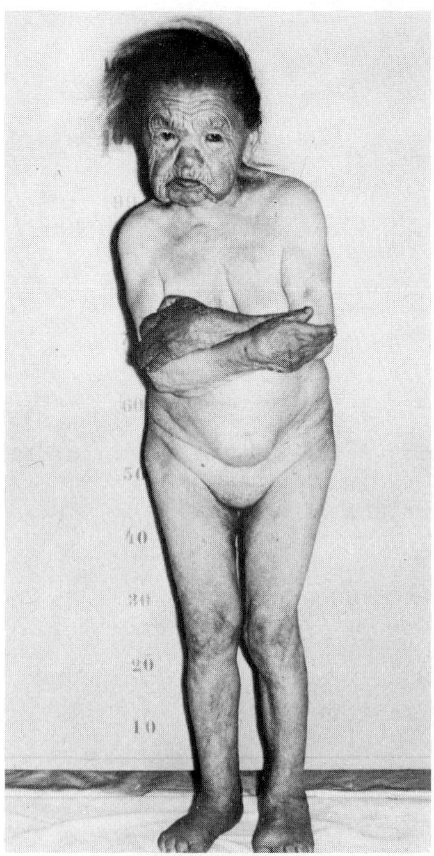

Fig. 1 93 yr old endemic cretin from Canton Bern, Switzerland. Height 113 cm, deaf-mutism, no palpable goiter, clinically mildly hypothyroid, $PB^{127}I$ 4.3 μg%, maximal RAI uptake 64% at 24 hr, cholesterol 248μg%

In Switzerland (as well as in Styria, Austria) a wide spectrum of individual variation in cretinism has been observed by all investigators. If the dwarfed, myxedematous, mostly non-goitrous cretin (frequently with quite a good sense of humor) has always been considered as the most typical representative (Fig. 2), many individuals could be found with only a few findings such as deaf-mutism ("endemic" deaf-mutism), oligophrenia ("endemic" oligophrenia), or only stunted growth. Not many of these have shown more or less severe central nervous system disturbances, mostly some motor incoordination (Fig. 3). But all these neurologically defective individuals are severely oligophrenic. Whether these oligosymptomatic individuals are to be included in the cretinous population or not is a matter of definition (4).

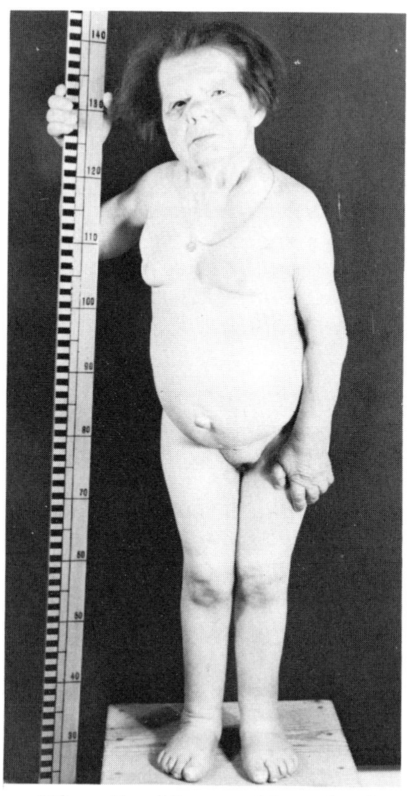

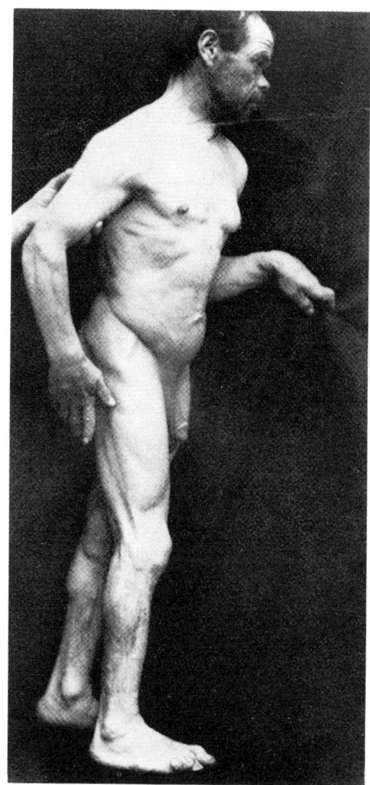

Fig. 2 68 yr old endemic cretin from Canton Zurich, Switzerland. Ht 115 cm, almost entirely deaf, clinically hypothyroid, no palpable thyroid tissue, max. RAI-uptake 10% at 72 hr, $PB^{127}I$ 1.0 µg% (after TSH 2.9 µg%).

Fig. 3 47 yr old endemic cretin from Canton Bern, Switzerland. Small goiter, spastic gait, motor incoordination. From F. de Quervain and C. Wegelin (3).

Most of the reports on endemic cretinism in Switzerland and elsewhere in the world have been critically assessed by de Quervain and Wegelin in their monograph of 1936 *Der endemische kretinismus* (3). Their own observations over a number of years were of several hundred cretins in the age range puberty to old age mainly being cared for in institutions. Younger cretins, from school age on, and in homes for mentally retarded and deaf-mutes, were also studied.

Several statements in that monograph merit attention. They indicated strongly that endemic cretinism is geographically limited to areas with severe endemic goiter. In general terms their description was concerned with mental and somatic retardation, and it was explicitly stated that identifiable congenital or acquired abnormalities, such as consequences of encephalitis, rickets, or other bone diseases, should be excluded. They stressed specifically that two disease entities have confused the issue: congenital thyroid aplasia and acquired juvenile myxedema. The difficulty in defining endemic cretinism was recognized as the lack of uniformity of the disease, both as to mental and somatic manifestations, as well as the fact that the spectrum of symptoms gradually merges with the normal population. This explained to de Quervain and Wegelin why accurate statistics were lacking and suggested that all reports were biased towards a low incidence.

A major distinction was made between cretins with and without goiter. Those without goiter were separated into two entities, described as "early atrophy [Frühatrophie]" and "late atrophy [Spätatrophie]". The cases with early atrophy of the thyroid gland were characterized by stunted growth. Among the patients studied by Swiss authors only seven percent were classified as real dwarfs. Data on hearing and speech were interesting. Earlier studies were quoted which indicated deaf-mutism in 42 percent of the cases and impaired hearing in 32 percent.

It has not been possible in recent years to find any young cretin, i.e. born after 1920, in Switzerland, except those in which "cryptothyroidism [i.e. ectopic thyroid]" or an inborn error of iodine metabolism was the cause of the disease. Thus, endemic cretinism is a vanishing disease in Switzerland, as well as in Austria. The clinical pattern referred to in this paper is largely that of patients over age 50. It is for this reason also that no figure can be given for the prevalence of endemic cretinism for these countries. It should be stressed that endemic goiter and particularly endemic cretinism were diminishing significantly in Switzerland before the introduction of iodine prophylaxis.

SOMATIC DEVELOPMENT

Although our own study has been concentrated on dwarfed, mostly non-goitrous, cretins, in the institutions where most cretins are found in Switzerland today, there is approximately an equal number of nondwarfed, oligophrenic, goitrous individuals, with more or less pronounced hearing defect. All showed more or less normal pubertal development, and the females had all been menstruating during the normal periods of their lives. Yet, in some of the dwarfed cretins examined radiologically, open epiphyses were found. The classic hip disturbance ("cretinous hip"), defective pneumatization of the skull, and increased size of the sella turcica were found in many individuals. As expected, these alterations in the skeleton, apparently directly proportional to deficient thyroid function, could be observed particularly in the dwarfed group, in which a marked disturbance of thyroid function was found. An impressive example of delayed puberty and late growth is shown in Figures 4 and 5.

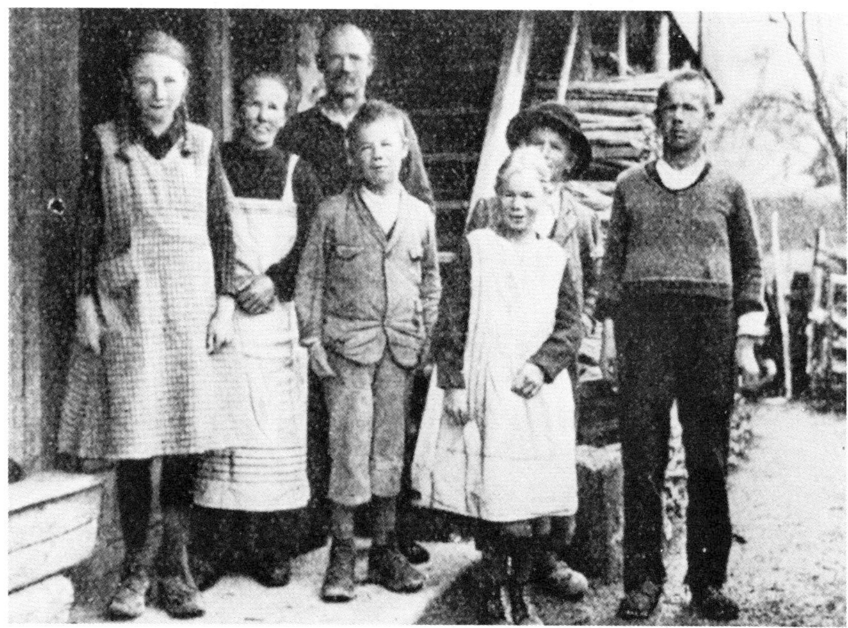

Fig. 4. Sch. family from Blumenstein, Switzerland. The family in 1937 [from Eugster (8)]. The two children in the center are 24 yr old (R.S.) and 19 yr old (F.S.) and have heights of 124 cm and 130 cm respectively. The young man at the extreme right is "cretinoid."

NERVOUS DISTURBANCES

Compared with other endemic goiter areas [e.g. New Guinea,(4)], one gains the impression from de Quervain's description (3), as from our own observations, that the cretins in Switzerland are not as frequently afflicted by severe motor defects. A few individuals with severe muscular spasticity and exaggerated tendon reflexes were seen, mainly in the nondwarfed group. These disturbances were much less frequent in the more intensively studied dwarfed group. In 20 cretins examined with electroencephalography, 10 had a normal rhythm,

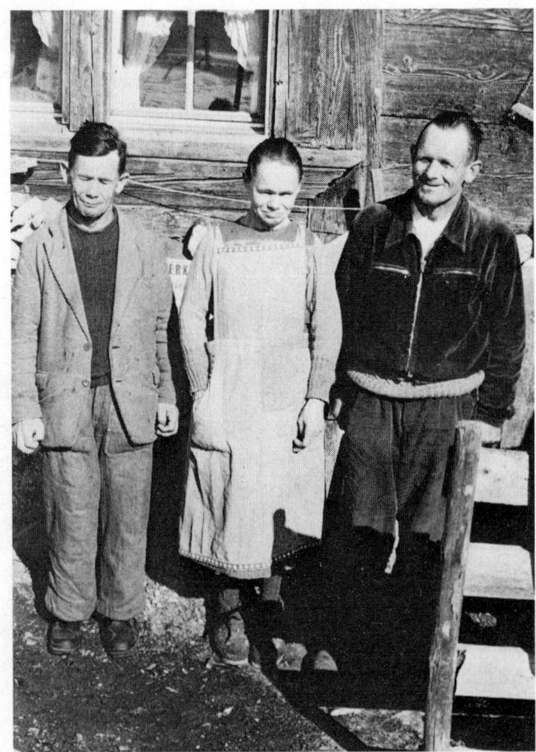

Fig 5 Three siblings from the Sch. family in 1965. The three are clinically euthyroid and have a small nodular goiter. (R.S.)-52 yr old, IQ approx 45, deaf, ht 144 cm, PBI 3.4 µg%. (F.S.)-47 yr old, IQ approx 45, deaf, ht 147 cm, PBI 5.8 µg%. (A.S.)-(not in Fig. 4), 50 yr old, IQ approx 65, moderately deaf, 161 cm, PBI 4.3 µg%. From M. P. Koenig (5).

seven had definitely slowed spontaneous activity (below 8 hz). Our EEG findings were similar to those observed in congenitally hypothyroid patients (5).

THYROID FINDINGS

The pathology of the thyroid glands of Swiss endemic cretins have been examined extensively by Wydler (6). Changes varying from compensating hyperactivity to total inactivity have been found. The results of our thyroid function studies (5) are within normal euthyroid limits or below, except that the radioactive iodine uptake is elevated. This does not mean that the thyroid is intact, nor does it prove that the same results would have been observed earlier in life. As a matter of fact, it is striking to observe entirely clinically euthyroid cretins in whom the clinical picture strongly suggests that in previous years hypothyroidism must have existed (Fig. 4 and 5). In several, clinical hypothyroidism was advanced (Fig. 2).

DEAF-MUTISM

Wydler (6) stressed the fact that among 111 endemic cretins, none had normal hearing, although 25 percent had acceptable hearing. Among the dwarfed patients, one with severe oligophrenia had normal hearing, but that of all the others was impaired. In eight cretins audiograms showed perceptive deafness in all patients and an additional middle ear component in two patients. Great care must be exercised in evaluating monosymptomatic "endemic deaf-mutism"in the Swiss endemic area. In most regions where endemic goiter has been observed, marked inbreeding has been known for a long time. Hanhart (7) has studied familial deaf-mutism, and many of his results and the ones of other Swiss authors have been interpreted repeatedly as representative of "endemic deaf-mutism". The selection for the one or the other group may be extremely difficult if not impossible. The same holds true for the simultaneous occurrence of "endemic deaf-mutism" and Pendred's syndrome.

INCIDENCE OF FACETS OF CRETINISM

Blumenstein (Canton Bern) is one of the villages of Switzerland where a systematic study of the population was carried out - by Eugster in 1937 (8), assisted by de Quervain. His data are probably representative of a severely affected Swiss population when endemic goiter and cretinism were much more frequent than today, (Table 1).

Table 1. Incidence of "defective individuals" in Blumenstein among a population of 963 inhabitants (670 born there)

Impaired hearing	6.0%
Stunted growth	6.0%
"Cretins"	3.5%
Mental retardation	2.0%
Borderline "cretinoid"	1.5%
Deaf-mutism	0.6%

It can be stated that endemic cretinism in Switzerland has shown all or almost all facets of the disease described elsewhere (5). Oligosymptomatic forms are difficult to fit into the larger framework of this disorder and may have been missed. As the question of selection is so eminently important and difficult to answer properly, it is hazardous to make any statement as to the most characteristic feature of the Swiss endemic cretin.

SUMMARY

A brief review of the clinical pattern of endemic cretins in Switzerland, as described by ancient authors and by the classical investigators of the first part of the 20th century, is presented. The author's personal observations of this disease now vanishing from the Swiss scene are added. It is stressed that the clinical spectrum of what is to be included in the term "endemic cretinism" appears to cover, at least in the Swiss type of this anomaly, a wide range of manifestations.

ACKNOWLEDGEMENTS

Figures 3 and 5 reprinted by permission of the publishers, Springer-Verlag.

DISCUSSION BY PARTICIPANTS

QUERIDO: Dr. Koenig, I think everyone knows that we are good friends, so I am allowed to be agressive. You mentioned the reduction of cretinism in Switzerland before iodine prophylaxis was instituted. If you interpret "iodine prophylaxis" as people being forced to eat iodized salt, I immediately agree. But if you suggest, which some people do, that reduction of endemic cretinism is not related to rise of iodine intake, then I disagree for the following reason: If one studies the prevalence of cretinism in relation to iodine intake, it appears that even in areas where only from five to 15 µg is excreted with the urine, only a small percentage of the people are cretins. This means that it is very much a touch-and-go situation. In a family with a succession of normal children, an abnormal child may be born. The situation is apparently that an increase of five µg of iodine intake may change the scene. The burden of proof, therefore, is on anyone who states that endemic cretinism disappears spontaneously to prove that it did not happen through a small increase of intake. The evidence that there is a straight correlation between iodine intake and cretinism is extensive.

KOENIG: May I just repeat this phrase as I said it, "It should be stressed that endemic goiter, and particularly endemic cretinism, were diminishing significantly in Switzerland before the introduction of iodine prophylaxis." By 1922, as you know, Eggenberger and others finally got iodine prophylaxis working on an optional basis, and in the early '30s it became more-or-less generally accepted. I do not say that nothing had changed before that time.

QUERIDO: But not through the social worker bringing proteins to the people.

KOENIG: By many different things. Wespi says that the railroad pushed cretinism away (and brought dental caries). It certainly has changed the food habits of people. While we were doing field studies in Styria, Austria, I was impressed by farmers far away from the highway with food freezers containing seafood. In Austria, when we talked to professional people, they would say, "We have such a bad situation because no iodine prophylaxis is permitted by the constitution of Austria." Yet I was surprised not to find more goiter and especially not to find young cretins. I inquired and found that almost two-thirds of the salt sold to the population is iodized. The physicians do not know that. I agree entirely that iodine prophylaxis on a legal basis is one thing and a change of food habits (and I don't want to say more) is another.

QUERIOD: Then please state that probably changes in food habits have altered the situation. I have met people who say that Dr. Koenig claims that other factors than iodine intake can change the incidence of cretinism.

KOENIG: All right, I will do that. May I add that we have been impressed recently by the high incidence of goiter in medical students. You may be interested to know that we in Switzerland for the last 14 years have been sold a luxury table salt which is uniodized. Sales of this salt, introduced around 1958, have increased from 0.5 million tons in 1958 to 1.6 in 1968. I sent students to ask customers in supermarkets what they were buying and 40 percent of the people replied they did not know whether they were buying iodized or uniodized salt.

ERMANS: I agree partly with the remark of Dr. Querido, but I am afraid he is making an error. If iodine deficiency is clearly associated with all forms of endemic cretinism, I know of no data correlating the severity of the iodine deficiency with the prevalence of cretinism. For instance, there are studies in New Guinea (4) in which the prevalence of goiter and of cretinism have been studied. In the Mulia Valley and in the Tiom valley, where equally severe iodine deficiencies are observed a tremendous difference in the prevalence of both diseases has been reported.

QUERIDO: No, it was below 10 μg in Mulia and on the average above 10 μg, together with normal PBI, in the Tiom valley.

PRETELL: I wish to comment on the data from Ecuador. They have kept as a control group severely iodine-deficient people from La Esperanza. In 272 children born in the last five years, the prevalence of defective children is only three percent, while Dr. Fierro has shown us that the prevalence before was around 10 percent. Something has changed in this environment.

STANBURY: If I may answer for Dr. Fierro, it is very difficult to determine how many defectives have been born in that environment because it is difficult to determine defects in very young children. I do not think that figure you quote is quite fair. It is certainly a minimum figure, but it is not a maximum figure. Would you agree with that Dr. Fierro?

FIERRO: Yes. In Ecuador we did not find a relation between iodine intake and prevalence of endemic goiter and endemic cretinism. For example, in Tocachi the iodine excretion was 17 μg. In Gumbayo village, near Quito, the iodine excretion was 22. In Tocachi the goiter incidence was 54 percent, and cretinism eight percent. In the other village the goiter incidence was 17 percent and incidence of cretinism 0.4 percent. In this village the people have a more varied diet, less biological and social isolation, and a better economic situation. To us, there are many other factors. It is not clear what iodine means in terms of cretinism, perhaps because we do not know what cretinism really is.

STANBURY: If one measures the iodine excretion at a particular time it does not necessarily reflect the mean annual iodine intake. Jorge Maisterrena in Mexico showed marked seasonal variations in iodine excretion. One really needs an integrated measure of iodine excretion, and that is very hard to come by.

DELANGE: I would like to make a point about critical levels which induce goiter and cretinism, in answer to Dr. Querido's comment. I really think that discussion about differences in daily urinary excretion of iodine of five μg is absolute nonsense in terms of the kind of studies we do in the field. You know that the collection of 24 hr urines is subject to a very large error. Nevertheless, our studies in Idjwi show a difference of about five μg per day between the North and the South, and this difference is not significant. In a further stage we have tried to estimate iodine intake by means of a simpler procedure - the measurement of iodine concentration in only one sample. This has no meaning in terms of iodine intake per day, but has meaning as an index of iodine intake if done in large numbers of people and at different periods of the year. Thilly has collected 642 samples and, in a separate study, I have collected 963 samples from 566 patients. The concentration of iodine is exactly the same in the North and in the South and does not vary according to the season. So I really believe that iodine deficiency is the same in both regions investigated. One of these studies is in progress; the other is published (10).

STANBURY: One should not draw the inference that because you found no seasonal variation there is none where cropping might be different. Maisterrena found marked seasonal variations in Mexico.

KOENIG: Why, in the same family, does one find a normal, a subnormal, and a very cretinous child, born one year after the other? On the other hand, in Blumenstein, there are 24 cretins in only six families (out of a population of about 1,000). These families did not live in the same area in the village and were not using the same well. It is a little hard to explain all of that by iodine deficiency alone.

QUERIDO: Would you say that if iodine intake had been normal, these people would have been cretins?

KOENIG: I do not know.

STANBURY: I think everyone would agree that iodine deficiency is not the sole cause of cretinism. There may be contributory genetic or other dietary causes.

PHAROAH: I think there are a number of reasons why a woman has one normal child, then a cretin, then another normal child. It may be that in the meantime she has had a stillbirth or something else making demands on her thyroid and her iodine balance.

IBBERTSON: To get back to the matter of critical iodine need, I think this has to be seen on the background of the functional efficiency of the thyroid gland. What may be adequate intake for one individual may become critical if there has been some intrauterine thyroid damage. We believe that, at least in our area, this is quite a common phenomenon.

REFERENCES

1. Platter, F., quoted by P.F. Cranefield: The discovery of cretinism. Bull,Hist. Med. 16:489-511, 1962.

2. Merke, F.: Geschichte und Ikonographie des endemischen Kropfes und Kretinismus. H. Huber, Bern, 1971.

3. DeQuervain, F. and Wegelin, C.: Der endemische Kretinism. Springer, Berlin, 1936

4. Choufoer, J.C.; Van Rhijn, M. and Querido, A.: Endemic goiter in western New Guinea. II. Clinical picture, incidence and pathogenesis of endemic cretinism. J. Clin. Endocrinol. Metab. 25:385-402, 1965.

5. Koenig, M.P.: Die kongenitale Hypothyreose und der endemische Kretinismus. Springer, Berlin, 1968.

6. Wydler, A.: Die Histologie der Kretininstruma, mit Berücksichtigung der Klinik des Kretinismus und der funktionellen Untersuchung. Mitt. Grenzgeb. Med. Chir. 39:467-542, 1926.

7. Hanhart, E.: Ueber die Bedeutung der Erbforschung von Innzuchtgebieten an Hand von Ergebnissen bei Sippen mit hereditärer Ataxie, Heredo-degenerativem Zwergwuchs and sporadischer Taubstummheit. Schweiz. Med. Wochenschr.54:1143-1151, 1924.

8. Eugster, J.: Zur Erblichkeitsfrage des endemischen Kretinismus. Unterschungen an 204 Kretinen und deren Blutverwandten. Arch. Julius Klaus-Stift. 13: 383, 1938.

9. Steck, A.; Steck, B.; Koenig, M.P. and Studor, H.: Auswirkungen einer verbesserten Jodprophylaxe auf Kropfendemie und Jodstoffwechsel. Schweiz. Med. Wochenschr., in press.

10. Thilly, C.; Delange, F. and Ermans, A.M.: Amer. J. Clin. Nutr. 25:30-40, 1972.

THE CLINICAL PATTERN OF CRETINISM AS SEEN IN NORTHERN ITALY

A. Costa

Mauriziano Hospital, Turin, Italy

The zones where we have studied endemic cretinism are situated in Piedmont (1), Lombardy and Liguria (2). The Piedmontese area is the same as that studied 100 years ago by the Sardinian Commission (3). It lies between 44° and 45° of north latitude, and 7° and 9° east longitude. The climate is continental, with the temperature fluctuating widely over the year (maximum + 35°C., minimum - 15°C); the annual rainfall is 800-1000 mm. Geologically the region consists mostly of tertiary formations (Alpine slopes; hills) and quaternary formations (plains and valleys). The rock structure differs from place to place. Calcareous zones alternate with others poor in calcium but rich in loam and sand; granite and gneiss rocks can be found in certain areas. The countryside is characterized by wooded land, meadows, with a little arable ground including vineyards. The livestock consists of cattle, sheep, goats, pigs, horses, and mules. The way of life is largely pastoral and agricultural, but nearly every village today has some small factories. All the endemic cretins we have examined were born in districts at altitudes between 600 and 5,300 feet above sea-level; none was born in an urban center. A few were born on farms 19-25 miles from Turin, in places neither poor nor isolated, that nowadays are summer vacation resorts.

Data on iodine metabolism and on thyroid pathology of the local population appear in Table 1. The iodine content of the drinking-water (4) and of some local foods, such as milk, eggs, bread and meat of farm animals appear in Table 2. At times an iodine content is lower than in the same foods bought in city markets, but it is subject to variations, so that a significant comparison requires the examination of numerous specimens of the same food.

Table 1. Iodine metabolism and thyroid pathology in Piedmont endemic goiter region (no iodine prophylaxis)

Iodine Content of Water:	Province of Turin: 0.47±0.65 μg per liter
	Province of Cuneo: 1.9±2.05 μg per liter
	Province of Aosta: 0.35±0.28 μg per liter
Daily Urinary Iodine Excretion:	Normal adults (range): 70-140 μg per 24 hr
	Goitrous adults (range): 40-80 μg per 24 hr
School-boys (mean value):	Province of Turin: 40-48 μg per gm creatinine
	Province of Cuneo: 31-39 μg per gm creatinine
	Province of Aosta: 65-76 μg gm creatinine
Prevalence of Goiter Among School Boys:	Province of Turin: 8 percent
	Province of Cuneo: 14.6 percent
	Province of Aosta: 11 percent
Army Rejects Because of Goiter (percent of recruits):	Province of Turin: 1.76
	Province of Cuneo: 1.23
	Province of Aosta: 0.82
	Mean national value: 0.45
Incidence of Endemic Cretinism (indicative value):	0.3 per 1000 inhabitants (a century ago: 1.53-3 per 1000)
Deaf-mutes (normal values: 0.3-0.6 per 1000 inhab):	Province of Turin: 0.71
	Province of Cuneo: 1.6
	Province of Aosta: 1.74
Thyroid Cancer Mortality (per 1000 cases of cancer in general):	6.5 (Mean national value: 4.8)
Thyroiditis:	Seasonal epidemics of granulomatous thyroiditis
Goiter Epidemics:	Have been described in 1899, 1917, 1920, 1940-44
Sudden Appearance of Painful, Hot Nodules:	Small seasonal epidemics

Table 2. Iodine content of fresh foods from Piedmont endemic goiter areas (μg per 100 gm)

From city (Turin) markets	From localities of endemic goiter
White Bread	
1.1; 1.7; 2.2; 4.8	1.1 to 2.5; most frequently less than 2
Whole Cows' Milk	
From private farms: 1.2; 4.6; 7.4, 10	From dairy farms in alpine valleys: 1.1 to 3.7; rarely higher values: 16
From trade (cartons): Mostly 6-7	
Hen Eggs	
White: 10 to 22	1.5 to 18.7
Yolk: 100 to 200 and more	More than 100 in 5 out of 9 samples
Meat	
Chicken: 0.8-1.5	0.8 to 3.4; mean value 2
Veal: 0.68-1.9	1
Rabbit:	0.7; 1.9

In Italy the typical endemic cretin has low stature (5), disproportionate build and ungainly movements. His hands are bulky and unsuitable for seizing and sensitive touching. He is hard of hearing and his speech is limited and labored. He has a childish, fatuous smile (Fig. 1) that testifies to a typical form of idiocy. The smile gives an amusing, sometimes artful, air. Endemic cretins are childish, with none of the liveliness of the normal children, but rather with a solemn wisdom, which springs partly from their awareness of being weaker than and inferior to their fellows. They tend to be humble, shy and obedient. If they are not frightened, these backward yet sensitive and good natured creatures behave towards strangers in a trusting, kindly way. In the less severely afflicted patients, that is those whose intellectual faculties can be evaluated and analyzed, an elementary affectivity and a related

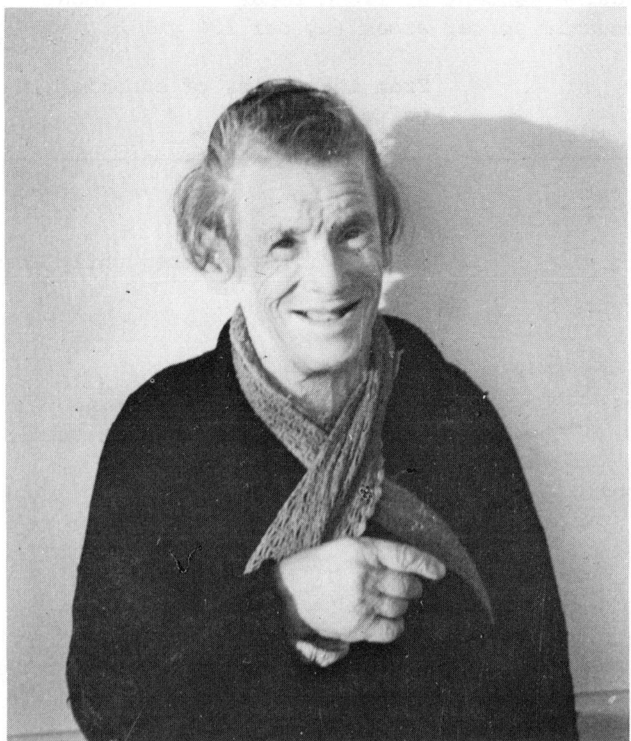

Fig. 1. A goitrous endemic cretin with typical smile.

intuitive faculty of the intellect may be recognized. The majority however, are idiots with an IQ of less than 25.

Endemic cretinism means somatic malformations and mental deficiency, as well as neurological damage (Fig. 2). The neuropathological manifestations most frequently encountered are (6): disturbances of mimicry, characterized by a lack of modulation in facial expression; dystonias in head, trunk and limb posture, heavy camptocormic walking, with the foot resting on the full sole or on the toes, instead of the heel, and awkwardness of gesture due to alterations in automatic and synkinetic motility and regulations of muscular tone (7).

These disturbances form a neuropathological picture which is as typical as the psychopathological one. Together with the perceptive type deafness (8), they enable the patients to be distinguished from the ubiquitous somatopsychically disabled. EEG tracings (9) may be normal or abnormal, and even decidedly abnormal, reminiscent of the pattern associated with brain disease, but differing widely from the EEG pattern of myxedema. In myxedema there is neither such fast background activity nor such marked diffuse paroxysmal activity.

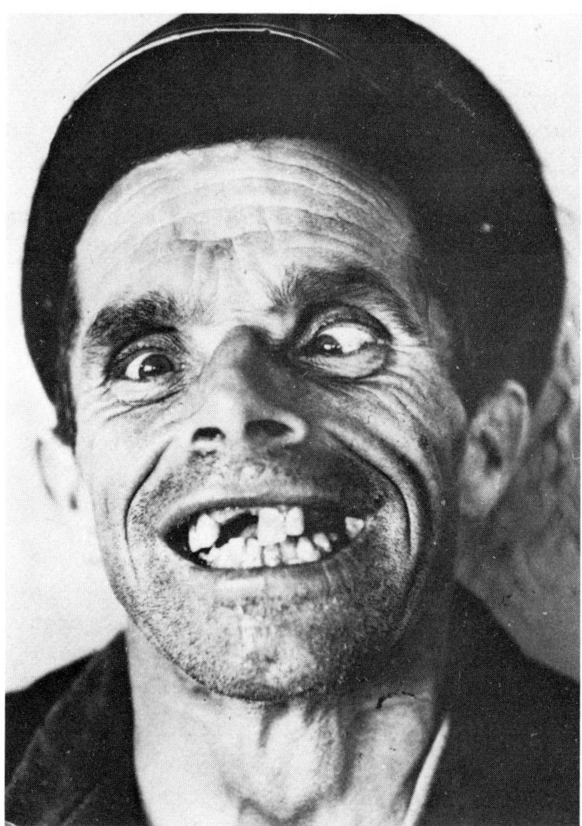

Fig. 2. The grin and the squint of a goitrous endemic cretin.

The prevalent features of the persons we have classified as endemic cretins and separated from ubiquitous idiots are summarized in Table 3. Relevant metabolic data in approximately 100 patients appear in Table 4, with special regard to thyroid function. [For other data see the studies of Vogliazzo _et al._ (10-18)].

The endemic cretin of Northern Italy usually has goiter. As a rule the thyroid shows iodine metabolism which is characteristic of endemic goiter: high uptake, fast conversion rate, and slow discharge. After a tracer dose of labelled iodine we have identified T_4 and T3 in the serum, and in two patients also labelled diiodotryosine. Recently Andreoli _et al._ (19) have demonstrated abnormal iodoproteins in the thyroids of two endemic cretins. The protein-bound iodine concentration values of these patients were 3.4 and 5.2 µg per 100 ml. As disclosed by sedimentation properties these iodoproteins differed from thyroglobulin in certain molecular characteristics; but shared some of the immunochemical properties of the latter.

*Table 3. Features of persons classified as endemic cretins**

Stature: (78 Persons) Male - range 105-174 cm; mean 156 cm
Female - range 102-168 cm; mean 145 cm

Williams' index: 0.99-1.15

Persistence of growth cartilage in adults: In 5 out of 50 persons

Weight: Mostly subnormal

Brachycephaly: In 26 out of 32 persons

Sella Turcica: In most cases hypoplastic

Spheno-occipital (Landzert's) angle: Normal value - 114$\pm$ 5 degrees
In 17 endemic cretins - range 108-148 degrees;
Mean 130.17 degrees

Deforming osteo-chondropathy: Frequent in the elderly

A-B-O blood group: In 77 persons, no relationship between cretinism and A-B-O blood groups has been found

Karyotypes: Normal. In 1 out of 14 persons a XXX syndrome

Hearing: Only 3 out of 37 persons had normal hearing

Vestibular function: Vestibular damage is bilateral; not less frequent than the hearing loss, but not always commensurate with this

ECG: Normal findings

EEG: Mostly abnormal - a fast background with paroxysmal theta activity

* Data from (28,29,30)

*Table 4. Metabolic data - goitrous patients and endemic cretins in Northern Italy**

	ELDERLY NORMAL PERSONS	GOITROUS PATIENTS	ENDEMIC CRETINS (P= number of patients)
^{131}I thyroid 24 hr uptake	39%	50%	(21P) 52%
PBI (μg per 100 ml)	5-8	4.5-7	(85P) 5.61 ± 0.43
BEI			(10P) 80-90% of PBI
Stimulation with TSH	Increase of PBI, increase of BMR, and the fall of serum cholesterol is more pronounced in the endemic cretin than in the normal		
Iodinated aminoacids in serum after a dose of ^{131}I			T_4 and T_3; in two P also iodides & diiodotyrosine
T_4 half-life (days)	7.09 ± 0.43	6.98 ± 1.75	(6P) 7.68 ± 1.08
T_4 degraded daily (μg/24h)	57		(6P) 63
Incidence of myxedema			8 percent of this series
Perchlorate test	Negative	Negative	Sometimes positive in endemic deaf-mute
Conversion ratio	13%	79%	(20P) 83 ± 15.8%
TBG (μg per 100 ml)	25		(24P) 29.4 ± 2.29
BMR		Normal	(49P) $+21.5 \pm 3$
Serum cholesterol (mg/100ml)	150-270	Normal	(81P) 170 ± 12.5
17-ketosteroids (mg/24h) (Drekter's method)	7-20		(24P) 6.8 ± 0.51
11-oxysteroids (mg/24h) (Daughday's method)	3-9		(24P) 1.65 ± 0.25
Stimulation with ACTH	Stimulation of excretion of both 11-oxysteroids and 17-ketosteroids is slight		
Insulin tolerance (10U ipod.) Glycemia after 2h g/l			(10P) 0.51 ± 0.16

*Data from (23,24)

The half-life and the daily degradation rate of thyroxine are the same in the Italian cretins as in normal patients of the same age. Sella volume alterations are not rare (25): frequently the sella is narrow, but it is usually wide in the hypothyroid patients.

Hypothyroidism among endemic cretins in our group was more frequent in the females (Fig. 3).

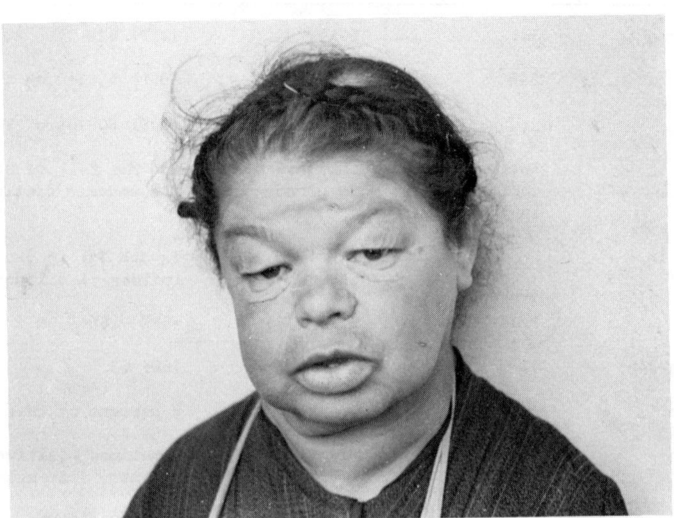

Fig. 3. A goitrous myxedematous endemic cretin.

We have recorded the electrocardiograms in 12 subjects (26) The tracings were almost normal. Bradycardia, low voltage and inversion of the terminal phase associated with hypothyroidism were absent. The thyroid stimulating hormone values by radio-immunoassay were usually normal but high values were found in the hypothyroid patients (Table 5).

Impaired activity of the adrenal cortex has been a frequent finding. Values of growth hormone and of gonadotropin levels by radioimmunoassay have been in the normal range (Table 6), with the exception of the follicle-stimulating hormone values in the postmenopausal women, which are exceedingly low. These data seem to point to lesions of trophic centers and to developmental disorders. The hypothesis has been proposed that endemic cretins who are not hypothyroid in adult life were hypothyroid during early or even intrauterine life. In 1904 Cerletti and Perusini (27) described some cretinous families in the Adda Valley, Lombardy (Fig. 4).

*Table 5. Serum TSH values in the endemic cretin (radioimmunoassay)**

	Number of Patients	PBI (µg per 100ml)	TSH µU/ml
NORMAL		5-8	0.9-2.1
SIMPLE GOITER		4.7	1.64-2.2
HYPERTHYROIDISM		8.5	0-0.7
ENDEMIC CRETINS	4 hypothyroid	2.2	41.7
	24 euthyroid	6.75	1.75

* range or mean value

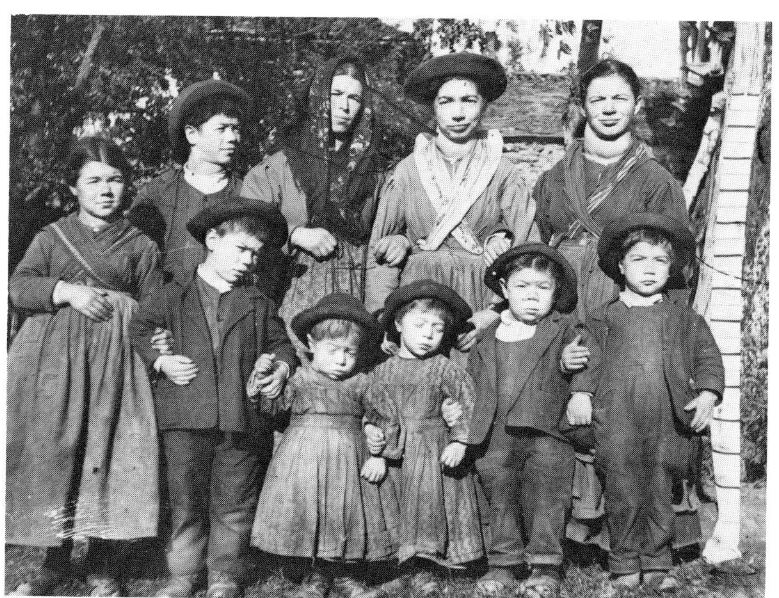

Fig. 4. A cretinous family [from U. Cerletti and G. Perusini (27)]

Table 6. Hypophyseal function in the endemic cretin

	NORMAL VALUES	NUMBER OF ENDEMIC CRETINS EXAMINED	VALUES (Radioimmunoassay)
Sella area	105mm^2	20	54-102mm^2 Larger in the hypothyroid patient
TSH	1.35±0.94 ng/ml	10 euthyroid	2.45±0.34 ng/ml
GH (at rest)	1.61 ng/ml	18	1.87±0.84 ng/ml
FSH			
Males	4.14±2.67 miu/ml	10	10.1±3.6 miu/ml
Antemenopausal females*	(5-28-10)	2	6.6±2.9
Postmenopausal females	88±32.2	3	25.0± 9.6
LH			
Males	13.13±9.11miu/ml	11	15.1±3.4 miu/ml
Antemenopausal females*	(2-35-4)	2	12.2±1.1
Postmenopausal females	47.6±20.3	6	55.9±7.8

*According to the period of the menstrual cycle

By clinical standards only, they judged that a girl and a boy were not only cretinous but hypothyroid, and Dr. Cerletti has permitted us to examine their photographs. We have had an opportunity to examine with Dr. Cerletti these patients 60 yr later (2). Neither was hypothyroid by biochemical standards. The life-span of untreated hypothyroid patients as a rule is not long (28). We have measured some parameters of thyroid function in seven infants born of cretinous mothers with stigmas of mental deficiency and somatic abnormalities (29). Six out of seven showed normal thyroid function (Table 7).

Endemic cretinism is considered not to be a hereditary disease. We have no relationship between endemic cretinism and A-B-O blood groups (30). The chromosome number and morphology were normal in 12 out of 13 subjects; in only one was an extra chromosome found (31). It has been calculated that an XXX syndrome may occur in one in every 300 idiots. Nevertheless, the disease sometimes assumes familial features. We have described two cretinous sisters in a family (Fig. 5) and three brothers in another family, and also an inherited pattern, as in the family Vr., which we found in the Susa valley.

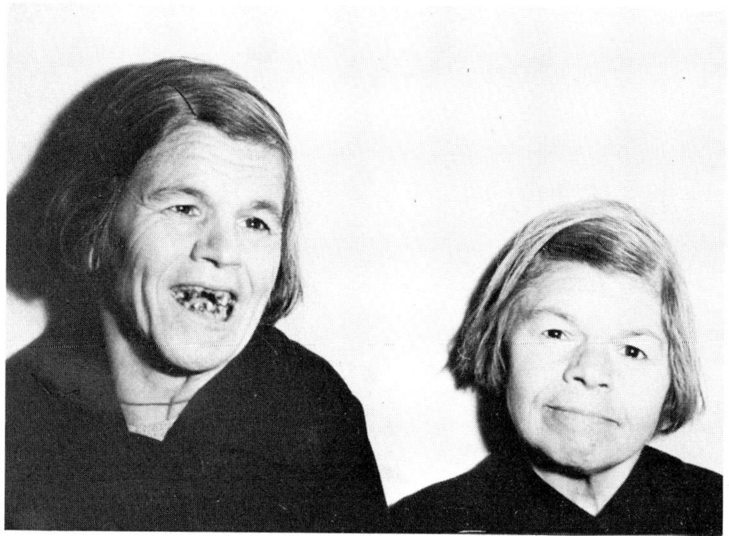

Fig. 5. Two cretinous sisters.

In the latter family cretinism appeared in four generations, passed from the great-grandmother, the grandmother (only 4 ft 8 in tall), the mother (4 ft 10 in tall - the last two both being stupid persons with no signs of hypothyroidism) and to the younger of two daughters, who has been hypothyroid from birth. Her sib is a girl of normal intelligence, but of short stature.

Table 7. Indices of thyroid function in defective children born to endemic cretins

Persons: Sex and age	Clinical conditions	Thyroid ^{131}I-uptake after 6–24 hr	PBI µg per 100 ml	Observations on parents
M.A. M-9 mo.	Psychically and physically defective, cretinoid	48–56	4.9	Born of incestous cretinous parents, mother's PBI: 5.8 µg per 100 ml.
S.M. F-8 mo.	Psychically and physically defective, cretinoid	60–60	5.2	Cretinoid mother from an endemic country
P.M. M-3 mo.	Psychically and physically defective, cretinoid	48–60	6.3	Mother was a poor woman born in an endemic area; her PBI was 7.2 µg per 100 ml
T.M. M-7 mo.	Backward, underdeveloped	36–48	7.9	Mother was an endemic deaf-mute
T.A. M-1 yr	Backward, underdeveloped	66–72		Mother was an endemic cretin
C.G. M-1 yr	Psychically and physically deficient	42–36	5.4	Mother was a dwarf, deaf-mute endemic cretin
B.E. M-2 yr	Stigmata and gait of endemic cretin	23	2.9	Vagabonds from an endemic area

In some areas of endemic goiter in north Italy cases of endemic deaf-mutism intermingled with cases of endemic cretinism (34). Most deaf-mutes have no goiter; their physical and mental development, as well as their thyroid function, is in the normal range (Table 8). Deaf-mutism, endemic cretinism and simple goiter may be observed, either dissociated

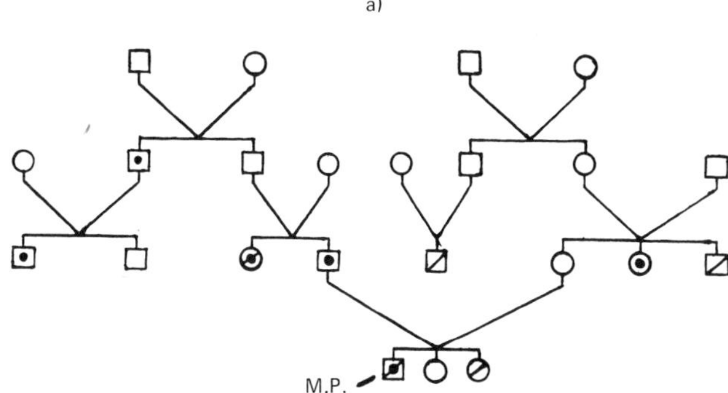

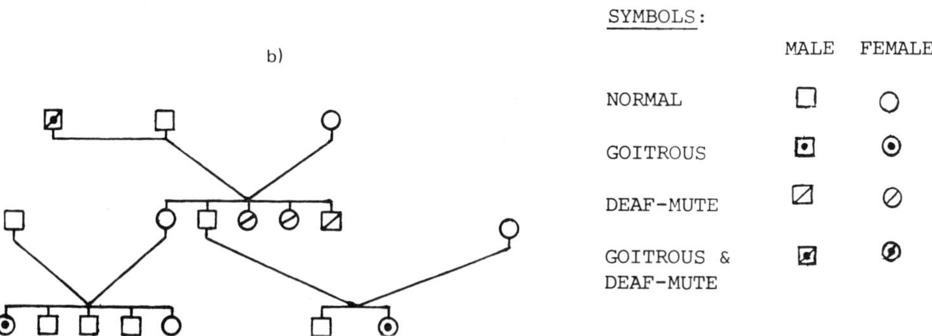

Fig. 6. a) Family tree of M.P., a goitrous, deaf-mute, endemic cretin (from a village 66 miles from Turin).
b) Family tree of Deb. family (from a village 35 miles from Turin).

*Table 8. Comparison of sporadic and endemic deaf-mutes**

	SPORADIC DEAF-MUTES (32 patients)	ENDEMIC DEAF-MUTES (30 patients)
Thyroid gland	Normal	Normal in most cases; sometimes goitrous
Basal metabolism	Normal	Normal
Radioiodine thyroid uptake	Normal	Normal; high in patients with goiter
PBI	In normal range (4.9-8.4 μg per 100 ml)	Normal
Deafness	Deafness of a central and congenital type	Same as in sporadic patients
EEG	In both groups not rarely epileptogenic foci; none of the characteristics of hypothyroidism	
X-ray exam of the cranium and the skeleton	Bone age normal; sometimes signs of cranial hypertension	
Psychometric examination	Never the intellectual and psycho-affective picture of hypothyroidism	

*Data from (32,33)

or associated, in families living in endemic areas. Clinically healthy parents can give birth to deaf-mutes and endemic cretins, alternating with normal and goitrous persons (Fig. 6a). Goiter and deaf-mutism, but possibly not cretinism, can reappear in the second and third generation, even in persons born out of the endemic area (Fig. 6b).

Table 9. Potassium perchlorate test in endemic deaf-mutes (53 patients)

With goiter (42 patients)	Perchlorate test:	positive in 16 patients (38%)
		negative in 26 patients (62%)
Without goiter (11 patients)	Perchlorate test:	postive in 3 patients (27%)
		negative in 8 patients (73%)

In the endemic deaf-mute the perchlorate discharge test not infrequently induces the discharge from the thyroid of previously trapped radioiodine (Table 9). In these patients the disease is similar to, and may even appear the same as, Pendred's syndrome (35). A young goitrous cretinous deaf-mute was operated for a huge goiter. The histological pattern was that of a highly stimulated parenchyma, as Fraser (36) and others have already described in Pendred's syndrome.

At present our position is close to that of Cerletti, a psychiatrist who has devoted his life to these problems: "The question of endemic goiter and cretinism is of paramount importance. . .because of the gravity and the diffusion of these diseases, and because all the researches after their causes have not yet given any definitive result, while they have disclosed the possibility of still unknown factors in human diseases."

SUMMARY

In Northern Italy the endemic cretin usually has low stature, disproportionate build and ungainly movements. His hands are bulky; he is hard of hearing and his speech is limited and labored; he has a childish, fatuous smile that testifies to a typical form of idiocy. Neuropathological manifestations, expecially dystonias and alterations in automatic and synkinetic mobility and regulation of muscular tone, are common.

Most of these patients have goiter. The thyroid displays the iodine metabolism characteristic of endemic goiter, but hypothyroidism is not frequent. The disease may be familial, but it is not genetically determined. It has not yet been proved that iodine deficiency or hypothyroidism is the primary cause of the form of cretinism encountered in Northern Italy.

ACKNOWLEDGEMENTS

These studies derive from the collaboration of the Institute for Endocrine and Metabolic Diseases (Director: Dr. A. Costa) the Service for Nuclear Medicine (Director: Dr. F. Cottino, Mauriziano Hospital, Turin), the 1st medical division of the Civilian Hospital, Alessandria (Director: Dr. M. Mortara), the medical division of the Mauriziano Hospital, Aosta (Former Director, Dr. U. Vogliazzo). The St. Maurice Order, the National Council for Research, and the Public Health Service have supported these researches.

REFERENCES

1. Costa, A.; Cottino F.; Mortara,M. and Vogliazzo,U.: Endemic cretinism in Piedmont. Panminerva Med. 6:250-259, 1964.

2. Cerletti, U.: Costa, A.; Marocco, F.; Masini, A. and Mortara, M.: L'endemia di gozzo oggi e sessanta anni fa. Rilievi nella Valtellina, nella valle del Mera e nella Val Bisagno. Rome, Consiglia Nasionale delle Richerche (Quaderni de la Ricerca Scientifica No. 7), 1963.

3. Relazione della Commissione di S.M.il Re di Sardegna "Studiare il cretinismo". Stamperia Reale, Turin, 1948.

4. Costa, A.; Malvano, R.; Magro, G.; Cottino, F.; Buccini, G.; Ferraris, G.; Mortara, M. and Zoppetti, G.: The relation between goitre prevalence and drinking water iodine concentration - Some observations on iodine estimation techniques. Folia Endocrinol. 19:249-268, 1966.

5. Costa, A.; Massucco-Costa, A. and Mortara, M.: Cretinisme et croissance. VIème Réunion des Endocrinologistes de Langue Française. Masson, Paris, 1961. pp. 83-106.

6. Mortara, M. and Rubino, R.: Cretinismo Endemico. La Malattia-I Suoi Aspetti Neurologici. Rome, Consiglia Nasionale delle Richerche (Quaderni de la Ricerca Scientifica No. 62), 1970. pp. 1-59.

7. Mortara, M. and Fracchia, A.: Funzione vestibolare nel cretinismo endemico. In: Le tireopatie. Vol. 4. Checchini, Turin, 1954. pp. 247-250.

8. Mortara, M. and Fracchia, A.: Ricerche sulla funzione auditiva nel cretinismo endemico. Arch. Med. Interna. IV:177-184, 1952.

9. Costa, A.; Mortara, M.; Cottino, F.; Pellerito, N. and Dall' Acqua, R.: Reserches sur la fonction de la Thyroide, l'electroencéphalographie et la structure du squelette dans le crétinisme endémique. Ann. d'endocrinol.20:237-262, 1959.

10. Vogliazzo, U.; De La Pierre, V.; Borney, G. and Viale, G.: Studi di funzionalita epatica nel cretino endemico. Arch. Sci. Med.105:3,1-11, 1958.

11. Vogliazzo, U.; Borney, G.; De La Pierre, V. and Viale, G.: Di taluni momenti della funzione renale nel cretino endemico. Arch.Sci.Med.105:3,1-11, 1958.

12. Vogliazzo, U.; Borney, G.; De La Pierre V. and Viale, G.: Di taluni momenti della funzione renale nel cretino endemico. Minerva Nefrol. 5:171-175, 1958.

13. Vogliazzo U.; Petronio, L.; Cappelletti, G.A. and De La Pierre, V.: Quadro ematologico periferico e semiologico del midollo osseo nel cretino endemico. Boll. Soc. Medico-Chirurgica di Pavia, 73:901-909, 1959.

14. Vogliazzo, U.; Cappelletti, G.A. and Borney, G.: Ricerche sulla coagulazione del sangue nel cretino endemico. Boll. Soc. Medico-Chirurgica di Pavia. 73:558-568, 1959.

15. Vogliazzo, U; Borney, G. and Gheis, F.: Attività aldolasica ed attività lattocoidrogenasica nel siero di sangue di cretini endemici. Minerva Med.51:1966-1968, 1960.

16. Vogliazzo U.; Viale, G. and Borney, G.: Comportamento delle transaminasi sieriche glutammico-ossalacetica e glutammico-piruvica in un gruppo di cretini endemici. Minerva Med.51: 1719-1721, 1960.

17. Vogliazzo, U.; Borney, G. and De La Pierre V.: La cupremia in un gruppo di cretini endemici. Fol. Endocrinol. 14:104-111, 1961.

18. Borroni, G.; Vogliazzo, U.; Borney, G. and De La Pierre V.: Sulle modificazioni del quadro proteico e lipoproteico nel cretino endemico.: Gazz. Int. Med. e Chirurg. 67:282-291, 1962.

19. Andreoli, M.; Monaco, F.; D'Armiento, M.; Fontana, S.; Scuncio, G. and Salabé, G.B.: Abnormal iodoproteins in human congenital goiter. Hormones 1:209-227, 1970.

20. Costa, A.; Cottino, F.; Ferraris, G.M.; Marchis, E.; Marocco, F.; Mortara, M. and Pietra, R.: Ricerche sulla patogenesi del cretinismo endemico. Medicina Parma 3:455-476, 1953.

21. Costa, A.; Cottino, F.; Ferraris, G.M.; Marocco, F.; Mortara, M.; Martinette, L. and Fregola, G.: Ulteriori contributi allo studio del cretinismo endemico. Medicina Parma 5: 2, 1-20, 1955.

22. Costa, A.; Mortara, M.; Martinetti, L.; Marocco, F.; Ferraris, G.M.; Cottino, F. and Fregola, G.: Raffronti tra cretinismo endemico e cretinismo sporadico. Medicina Parma 5: 2, 1-20, 1955.

23. Vogliazzo, U.; Viale, G.; Scorta, A. and Marchis, E.: Valutazione della funzione tiroidea nel cretinismo endemico. Rassegna Clinico-Scientifica. 28:2,3-13, 1952.

24. Costa, A.;Cottino, F.; Ferraris, G.M.; Fregola, G. and Marocco, F.: Comparison between endemic goiter, cretinism, deaf-mutism and sporadic goiter, cretinism, deaf-mutism. In: Advances in Thyroid Research. Pergamon, London, 1961. pp. 289-293.

25. Ferraris, G.M.; Cottino, F.; Dell'Acqua, R.; Magro, G.; Mortara, M. and Costa, A.: La selle turcique et l'angle de Landzert chez le crétin endémique. Ann. d'Endrocrinol. 28: 739-751, 1967.

26. Mortara, M.: Reperti elettrocardiografici nel cretinismo endemico. Boll. Soc. Medico Chirurgica di Pisa 21:3-8, 1953.

27. Cerletti, U. and Perusini, G.: L'endemia gozzo cretinica nelle famiglie. Tip. Romana Cooperativa. Rome, 1907.

28. Mortara, M.; Ferraris, G.M. and Della Beffa, A.: Senescenza e longevità nel gozzismo e nel cretinismo endemico. Minerva Med. 53:2695-2712, 1962.

29. Costa, A.: Relations between the sporadic and endemic form of cretinism. In: Fortschritte der schildrüsenforschung. Georg Thieme Verlag, Stuttgart, 1962. pp. 20-27.

30. Della Beffa, A.; Mortara, M. and Serra, A.: Gozzismo, cretinismo endemico sordomutismo e gruppi sanguigni del sistema A B O. Fol. Endocrinol. 13:670-680. 1960.

31. Costa, A.; Ferraris, G.M.; Scarzella, A.; Vernon, M.; Volante, G. and Cepellini, R.: Il numero cromosomico in otto casi di cretinismo endemico. Atti A.G.I. 7, 1962.

32. Costa, A.; Ferraris, G.M.; Dall'Acqua, R.; Patrito, G.; Pellerito, N; Pilotti, G. and Zonta, L.: Comparaison entre le sourd-muet des zones d'endemie goitre crétinique et le sourd-muet des zones non endémiques. Ann. d'endocrinol. 21: 791-817, 1960.

33. Costa, A. and Ferraris, G.M.: Surdimutité goitreuse familiale sporadique et surdimutité goitreuse familiale endémique. Ann. d'Endocrinol. 24:23-38, 1963.

34. Costa, A.; Ferraris, G.M.; Patrito, G.; Bo, V. and Lavazza, L.: Il sordomutismo nella endemia piemontese di gozzo. Fol. Endocrinol. 16:151-167, 1963.

35. Ferraris, G.M.; Zoppetti, G.; Bidone, G. and Costa, A.: Sindrome del Pendred ed endemia di gozzo. Fol. Endocrinol. 19:295-312, 1966.

36. Fraser, G.R.; Morgan, M.E. and Trotter, W.R.: Sporadic goitre with congenital deafness (Pendred's Syndrome). In: Advances in Thyroid Research (R. Pitt-Rivers, ed.). Pergamon Press, London, 1961. pp. 19-25.

HIMALAYAN CRETINISM

H. K. Ibbertson, J. M. Tait, M. Pearl, T. Lim,

J. R. McKinnon, M. B. Gill

Department of Endocrinology, School of Medicine

Auckland, New Zealand

The classical studies of McCarrison in the early years of this century in the Gilgit area of Kashmir (1) gave clear evidence of a goiter endemic which ranked in severity with that already recognized in the French Pyrenees and the cantons of Switzerland. The subsequent reduction of goiter and cretinism which characterized these European areas was not, however, reported from the Himalayas. On the contrary, isolated descriptions from climbing expeditions in the Mt. Everest area suggested a continuing endemic of some severity.

The study reported here confirms the continuing occurrence of cretinism and deaf-mutism in the Sherpa population of the Nepalese Himalayas. The pattern of goiter and the accompanying intellectual and physical abnormalities is similar to that described by McCarrison over 50 years ago.

THE SHERPA PEOPLE

The Sherpas studied lived in the Khumbu region of the Nepalese Himalayas, the families having migrated there from Tibet over 200 years ago (Fig. 1). There are about six relatively isolated villages in the area and the total population is around 4,000. The Sherpas are a hardy race of short brown skinned people who eke out a meagre existence on a diet of potatoes, buckwheat and barley, occasionally supplemented by milk, butter and yak meat. Despite the paucity of their diet there is little evidence of protein malnutrition, but acute and chronic infections (including tuberculosis) are common and the infant mortality is high (2).

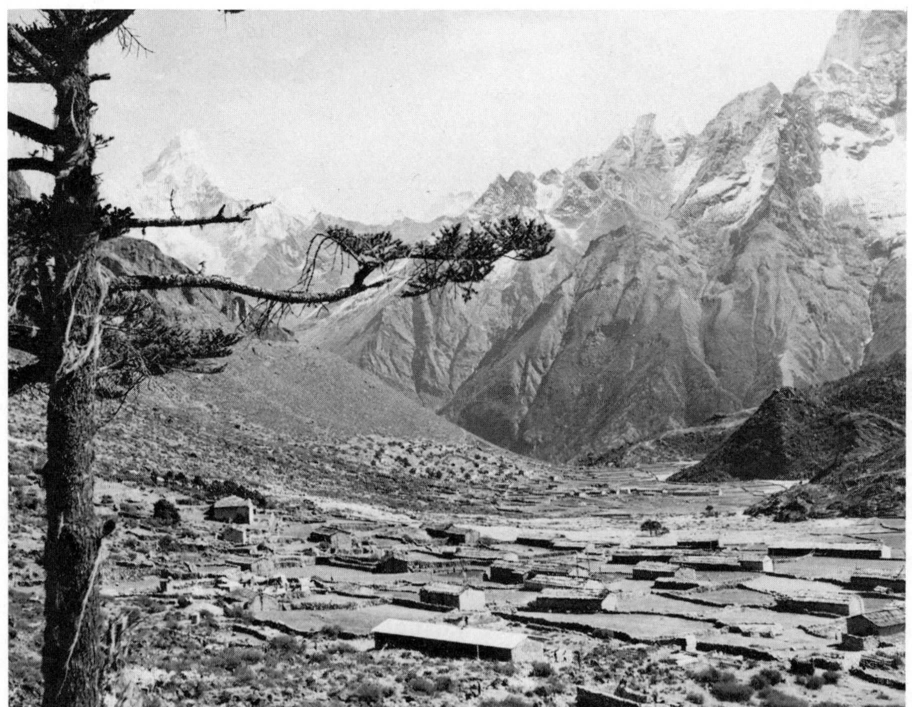

Fig. 1. The tents of the research team (left foreground) amongst Sherpa houses in the village of Kunde in the Khumbu region of the Nepalese Himalayas. Mount Ama Dablam (22,500 ft) is at the head of the valley.

THE RESEARCH PROGRAM

A base camp was established in the village of Kunde (13,000 ft). Sherpas were encouraged to come for assessment and although there was initial reluctance 1,300 were examined, 475 of these in some detail. Goiter was assessed according to the following scheme:

Stage 0 - Impalpable thyroid gland
1 - Readily palpable (<40gm) but not visible
2 - Visible and palpable (<40gm) in position of rest
3 - Clearly visible and palpable (>40gm)
4 - Clearly visible and palpable (>100gm)

Other clinical assessment included measurement of weight, height and body proportions, wrist x-ray, ECG voltage and ankle reflex measurement. Radioiodine studies were performed by methods described elsewhere (3). Approximately 350 blood and urine samples were collected in vacutainers and stored frozen in a mixture of snow and salt for subsequent analysis in New Zealand.

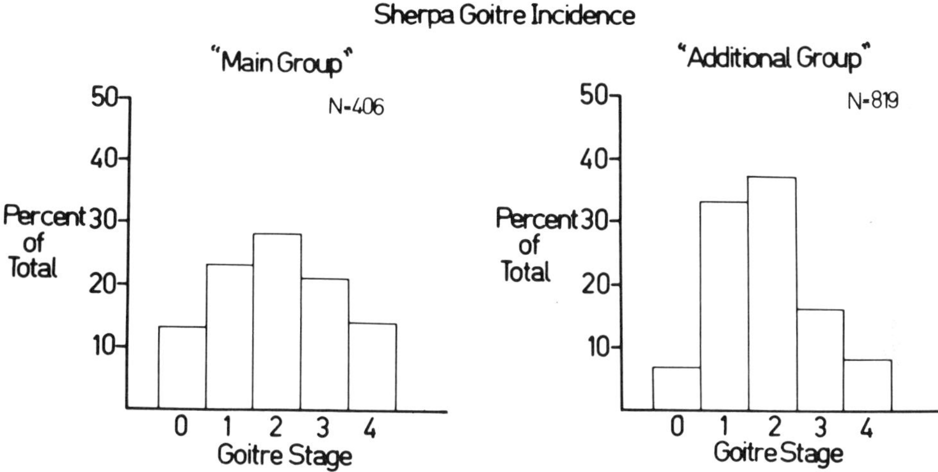

Fig. 2. The incidence and size of goiter amongst 1,225 Sherpas. The "main group" was examined by a single observer.

RESULTS

THYROID ABNORMALITY

The overall incidence of stage 1 - 4 goiters was 92 percent and in 63 percent there was a visible swelling (Fig. 2). Nodules were palpable in half and also in 18 percent of goiters in children younger than 16 years. Thirty percent of 475 Sherpas were judged clinically to be hypothyroid and the serum PBI was less than 4.0μg per 100 ml in 75.6 percent and less than 2.0μg per 100 ml in 43 percent (n=196). In many Sherpas with a very low serum PBI there was no clinical evidence of hypothyroidism. The mean ($\pm$s.d.) urine ^{127}I content was 16.67 $\pm$ 13.2μg per gm creatinine ($\bar{n}$=150). This figure is probably influenced by a small uncontrolled distribution of iodine in the area before the survey began.

NEUROLOGICAL ABNORMALITY

In addition to the widespread goiter and hypothyroidism in this community there was an obvious incidence of physical and mental abnormality. Deafness, speech and intellectual defect,

Table 1: Physical Characteristics

	No.	HEARING Deaf	D/Mute	CLINICAL HYPO.	GROWTH Mean 1S.D.	2S.D.	OBVIOUS MENTAL DEFECT	NEUROMUSC. DEFECT
DEAF	15	15	0	7	12	0	0	0
D/MUTE	22	0	22	12	7	1	±	0
CRETIN	28	4	19	28	21	12	28	6

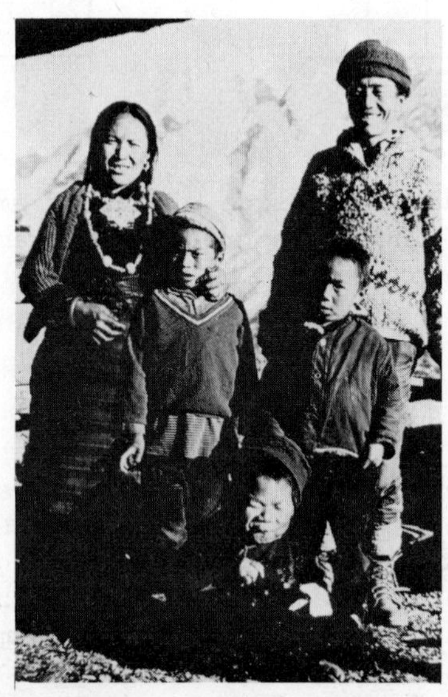

Fig. 3. A typical Sherpa family. The 8 year old boy on the right is euthyroid, with normal hearing and mental function. The 10 year old on the left is euthyroid and deaf-mute without obvious mental defect. The oldest child (16 years) is a classical cretin with hypothyroidism, growth failure, deaf-mutism and severe intellectual defect.

growth failure and neuromuscular disorder were variably associated. Despite the continuous spectrum from slight hearing loss to severe neurological abnormality, two fairly distinct groups could be distinguished (Table 1).

Deaf-mutes. There were 22 Sherpas (13 males) with deaf-mutism alone. The incidence of hypothyroidism was about the same as that in the general population, although in eight the goiter was small or impalpable (Table 2).

Table 2: The Thyroid

	No.	AGE (Mean)	SEX M	SEX F	GOITER STAGE 0	1	2	3	4	GOITER TYPE Diff.	Nod.
DEAF	15	21.7	6	9	2	2	3	4	4	3	9
DEAF-MUTE	22	13.3	13	9	5	3	11	3	0	10	7
CRETIN	28	21.8	11	17	7	6	8	4	3	4	15

Most were of normal height and body proportions were normal. There was no neuromuscular defect nor obvious intellectual defect, but formal testing was not attempted. An additional 15 Sherpas were deaf (Tables 1 and 2) without other distinguishing features and these are not considered further.

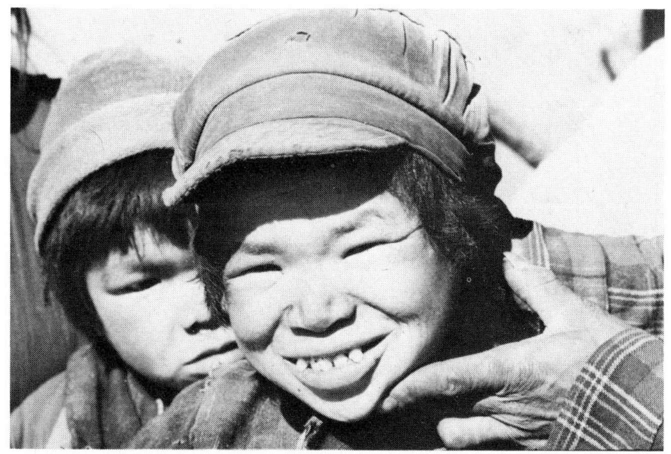

Fig. 4. A 14 yr old female cretin with her similarly affected sister behind.

Classical Cretins. The second group of 28 Sherpas (17 females) all showed immaturity of facial features and were clinically hypothyroid in varying degree. The thyroid gland was small or impalpable in 13, though seven had stage 3-4 goiters. Most in this group had severe intellectual defect and six had pyramidal signs in the legs with extensor plantar reflexes. The majority were short (particularly females) and the height of 12 cretins was less than two standard deviations below the normal mean for this population (Fig. 5).

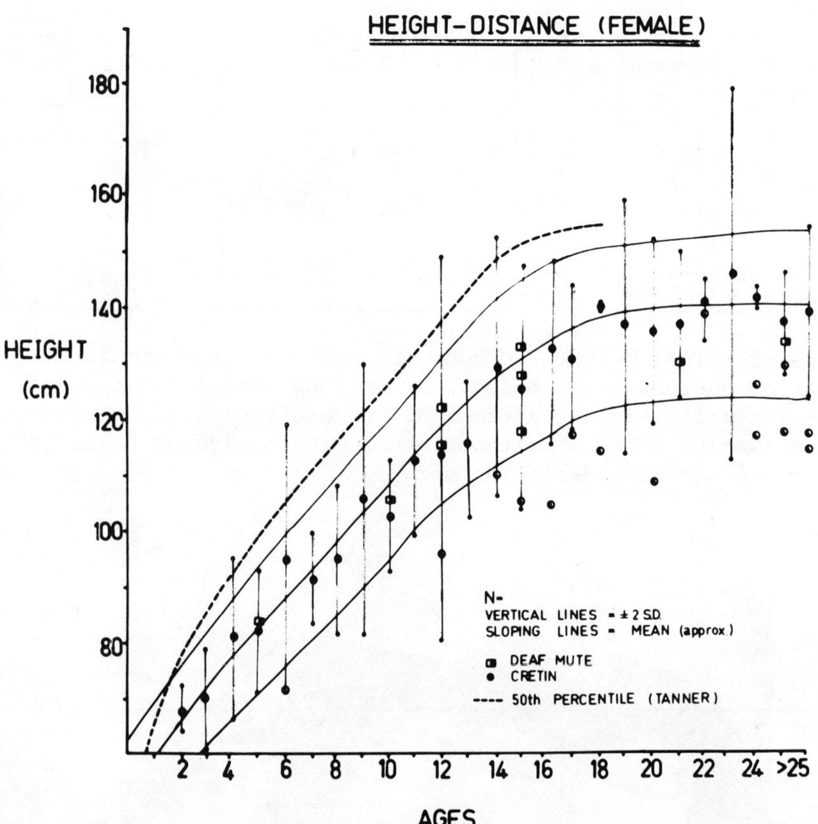

Fig. 5. Approximate height measurements in 161 female Sherpas (Sherpanis). The short stature of the cretins is evident (3).

Ten cretins and nine deaf-mutes had upper/lower body segment ratios above the mean but this was only significantly greater than normal in three cretins. Both height age and skeletal age were significantly retarded in this population as judged by Western standards. There was, however, no disproportionate retardation of skeletal age. In fact, most cretins over the age of 18 years had a greater retardation of height, but the difference was eliminated when correction was made for epiphyseal closure. The absence of disproportionate growth and dissociation between height and skeletal age retardation were unexpected but could relate to the high incidence of hypothyroidism in the so-called "normal" population or possibly to the ethnic differences in skeletal development (4).

Incidence of Deaf-mutism and Cretinism. The total incidence of isolated deafness, deaf-mutism and cretinism amongst 475 Sherpas was 3.1 percent, 4.7 percent and 5.9 percent respectively. The relative absence of cretins in younger age groups may reflect the tendency to keep these children hidden. The incidence was much higher in the village of Porche. Here there were 22 cretins (10.2 percent) and seven deaf-mutes (3.1 percent) amongst 215 inhabitants. All but one of the 15 Sherpas with deafness alone came from this village.

IODINE KINETICS (TABLE 3)

In both deaf-mutes and cretins radioiodine uptake was high and often approached 100 percent at four hours. There was, however, no significant difference from normal persons. In contrast to the "normal" population, uptakes were lowest in Sherpas with small or absent goiters. Failure of uptake and early thyroid ^{131}I clearance to rise following TSH injection suggested that this reflected a reduction in thyroid functional capacity.

Both serum and urine inorganic iodide were low, and serum levels were significantly lower in cretins than in the normal population. The same was true of the serum PBI, which was significantly lower than normal in both deaf-mutes and cretins.

Comparison of neck uptake and serum PBI in individual patients showed a disproportionate reduction in uptake in almost half the cretins. This confirmed a reduced functional capacity. In the remainder, uptakes were above 65 percent in spite of very low PBI's, indicating severe iodine deficiency.

Table 3: Iodine Kinetics

	NORMALS			DEAF-MUTES			CRETINS		
	Mean ±	S.D.	No.	Mean ±	S.D.	No.	Mean ±	S.D.	No.
4 hr ^{131}I Neck uptake (%)	56.70±	23.50	161	70.30±	31.59	13	55.88±	19.4	18
S.P.B. ^{127}I (μg/100ml)	2.86±	1.58*	159	1.71±	1.41	15	1.8 ±	1.85*	18
Serum ^{127}I (μg/100ml)	0.06±	0.07*	113	0.08±	0.10	7	0.04±	0.01*	6
Urine ^{127}I (μg/day)	20.43±	17.72	112	14.77±	12.83	9	17.95±	26.78	12

* P = .05 - .005

Measurement of serum iodinated amino acids following an oral dose of ^{125}I showed an increase in ^{125}I-T_3 percentages in 27 of 39 sera (Fig. 6). The increase was apparent in both "euthyroid" and "hypothyroid" (six cretins) Sherpas. Measurement of absolute T_3 levels was not possible for technical reasons, but, if confirmed,

SERUM TRIIODOTHYRONINE - I 125

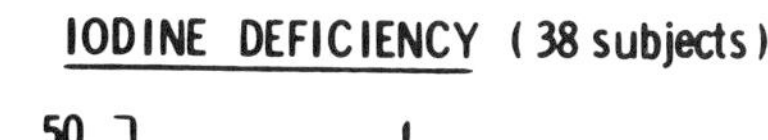

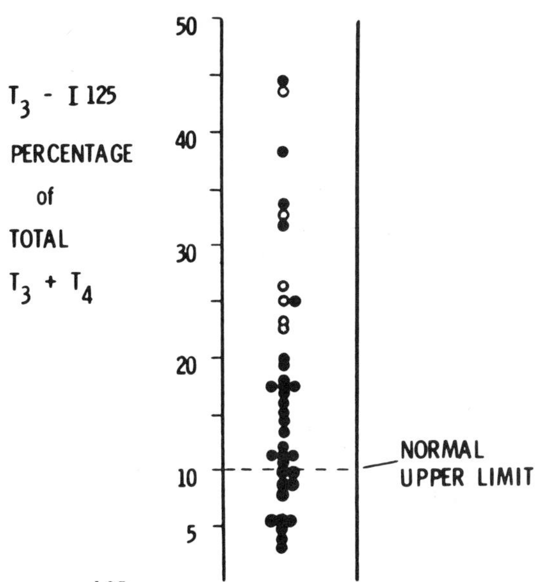

Fig. 6. Serum ^{125}I-triiodothyronine percentage in 32 normal Sherpas and six cretins.

these findings suggest an adaptive mechanism, though limitation of <u>total</u> iodothyronine production by severe iodine deficiency may prevent a significant contribution to the overall metabolic status of the individual.

It is apparent from these studies that although there is an indication of a reduction in functional thyroid capacity in some cretins, neither they nor the deaf-mutes can be clearly distinguished from normal on the basis of iodine kinetic data.

PERIPHERAL INDICES (Table 4)

There was poor correlation between the clinical diagnosis of hypothyroidism and abnormality of serum cholesterol, ECG voltage and ankle reflex time. The mean ECG voltage was lower in cretins than in either normal persons or deaf-mutes (P=0.01), although

Table 4: Peripheral Indices

	NORMAL		DEAF-MUTES		CRETINS	
	Mean ± S.D.	No.	Mean ± S.D.	No.	Mean ± S.D.	No.
S. Cholesterol (mg/100ml)	151.22 ± 25.71	165	152.21 ± 19.16	14	141.50 ± 25.56	20
ECG Voltage (mm) R.	*20.06 ± 7.32	204	22.56 ± 11.18**	19	*16.28 ± 6.33**	24
T.	6.86 ± 2.44		6.07 ± 2.68		4.77 ± 1.80	
Ankle Reflex (msec)	270.46 ± 49.32	148	281.76 ± 55.0	17	287.50 ± 62.60	22

* P = 0.01
** P = 0.025

the range was wide. The serum creatinine phosphokinase was abnormal in only two of 17 cretins and normal in nine deaf-mutes. These results are no doubt influenced by the inclusion in the "normal" population of subjects with subclinical hypothyroidism, by the effects of diet and exercise on the serum cholesterol and ankle reflex, and by the variable metabolic contribution of triiodothyronine.

DISCUSSION

The clinical abnormalities described here provide clear evidence of a continuing endemic of some severity in the Khumbu region of the Nepalese Himalayas. The combined incidence of cretinism and deaf-mutism is high and exceeds that reported in most other areas. Previous reports (1,5) from the Himalayas gave little indications of incidence, although in a recent limited survey in the Gilgit region (6) 2.4 percent of the population were found to be cretins and 1.4 percent deaf-mutes - substantially lower than in the Khumbu.

At first sight the two clinical types are similar to the "nervous" and "myxedematous" cretin described by Robert McCarrison in 1909 (1). There are, however, important differences. Although deaf-mutism is a feature of both groups, severe intellectual defect and neuromuscular disorder is confined to the classical (myxedematous) cretin. Formal testing was not performed but it was clear that gross mental abnormality was not a feature of deaf-mutism alone and that when it did occur other features of the myxedematous cretin were usually present. There is still debate as to whether intellectual potential can be normal in the deaf-mute (3). The continuous clinical spectrum seen here, ranging from mild deafness and speech defect to deaf-mutism, intellectual impairment and motor disorder suggests that selective impairment of neurological tissue does occur.

The cause of the neurological defect in endemic cretinism is still unknown. Fetal iodothyronine deficiency has been incriminated, and although the maternal thyroid hormone contribution to the fetus is usually small (7), severe iodine deficiency will result in a reduction in both the fetal and maternal thyroid hormone level. Variable intellectual impairment is a feature of the sporadic athyreotic cretin and the endemic athyreotic cretin of the Congo (8), but deaf-mutism or neuromotor defect does not occur in either condition. This observation and the reported reduction in nervous cretinism in New Guinea following iodized oil injection (9) suggest that a deficiency of elemental iodine itself may be the etiological agent. A deficiency of this element operating at different critical periods of nervous tissue development could thus be responsible for the spectrum of neurological abnormality. After birth its effects continue to be manifest through severe iodothyronine deficiency which results in a striking immaturity of facial structure, a myxedematous appearance and growth failure.

The presence of neurological abnormality may predispose the individual to a more severe deficiency of thyroid hormone by two mechanisms.

Thyroid functional capacity as judged by the ratio of neck uptake/serum PBI was reduced in almost half the cretins and these subjects had the most severe neurological deficit. Furthermore the intellectual and motor impairment might aggravate an existing iodothyronine deficiency by restricting the individual's capacity to diversify his food (and iodine) intake during the growth period. Thus, despite an intact though limited adaptive mechanism, clinical hypothyroidism, growth defect and the clinical picture of myxedematous cretinism would then become superimposed on an individual who would otherwise be regarded as a "deaf-mute" or "nervous" cretin. Such a sequence would account for the absence of additional neurological abnormality in the deaf-mute population.

There are two obvious discrepancies in the data reported here. The first relates to the absence of clinical hypothyroidism in many subjects (both "normal" and deaf-mute) with serum protein bound iodine levels below 2.0 μg per 100 ml. The demonstration of an increased circulating ^{125}I-triidothyronine percentage may be significant here and could represent an important compensatory mechanism. The serum T_3/T_4 ratio is known to increase with TSH stimulation and serum TSH levels in this population. It is possible, however, that the phenomenon merely represents preferential labelling of a small intrathyroidal pool, and measurement of absolute T_3 serum levels will be necessary to confirm this data. A second difficulty is the absence of confirmation of the clinical diagnosis of hypothyroidism by measurement of indices of peripheral hormone action such as ECG voltage, ankle reflex, serum cholesterol and creatinine phosphokinase. It is tempting to speculate that increased T_3 secretion might also explain this phenomenon and that the clinical assessment of hypothyroidism is incorrect. These subjects were short and myxedema was sometimes florid. It seems much more likely that these conventional though inadequate tests of hormone action are rendered even less reliable by differences in diet and muscular activity which were so apparent in this environment. It is possible also, that <u>partial</u> compensation by circulating T_3 may so modify these indices to allow results to fall within the normal range despite clinical evidence of hypothyroidism, a borderline situation not infrequently seen in normal clinical practice. The striking change in physical appearance in some subjects following iodized oil administration leaves little doubt that tissue levels of thyroid hormone were previously inadequate to sustain normal cellular function.

The postulated sequence of events in the development of cretinism in the Himalayas is shown in Fig. 7. Moderate intrauterine iodine deficiency causes in the fetus variable neurological damage which may include deafness and speech defect. After

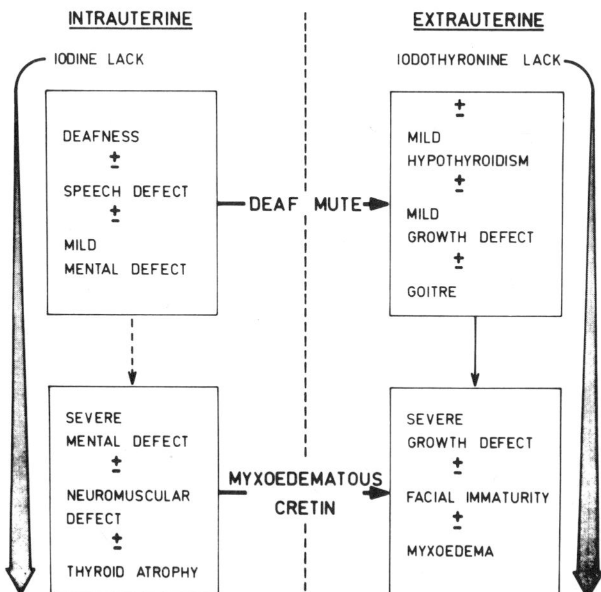

Fig. 7. A tentative scheme to explain the clinical spectrum. The severity of neurological impairment is dependent on the degree of intrauterine elemental iodine deficiency. Postnatal iodothyronine deficiency is responsible for the facial appearance and growth defect of the classical cretin and may also contribute to the intellectual defect.

birth, when iodine deficiency is severe, approximately 30 percent of Sherpas manifest clinical evidence of mild to moderate hypothyroidism, usually without severe growth defect. Occasionally iodothyronine lack is sufficiently marked to produce the clinical picture of myxedematous cretinism. With more severe iodine deficiency during intrauterine development, intellectual impairment and neuromuscular disorder occur. There is often an "atrophy" of thyroid tissue, but it remains to be shown whether this is in any way related to the iodine deficit. Both of these factors predispose the individual to severe iodothyronine deficiency after birth even when the degree of iodine deficiency is less than critical. Such subjects present the clinical picture of the myxedematous cretin with additional severe neurological involvement (Fig. 3). This sequence does not exclude the possibility that iodothyronine deficiency contributes to the intellectual defect, particularly after birth when development of nervous tissue is proceeding. The correlation between the time of beginning treatment and the subsequent mental attainment in sporadic cretinism suggests that this is so (10).

To explain the difference in the clinical spectrum in this study from that recorded by McCarrison it is necessary to postulate a more severe degree of iodine deficiency than was extant in the Gilgit area in 1909. It may be significant that the present incidence of cretinism in that area is much less than in the Khumbu (6).

It seems likely that variations in the clinical features of cretinism seen in this and other endemic areas may be a function of the timing and degree of iodine deficiency. In Zaire the clinical picture is dominated by intrauterine thyroid failure and intellectual impairment is the main expression of the neurological deficit. In New Guinea the development of nervous tissue is severely compromised by a severe iodine deficiency during intrauterine development. After birth relative iodothyronine lack is manifest by growth defect alone. In the Khumbu where the neurological defect is common though less severe, gross iodothyronine lack during childhood results in the clinical picture of the myxedematous cretin whose additional physical features are determined by the presence of severe hypothyroidism. It is possible that these different patterns of development may be determined by variation in social customs and food taboos during pregnancy.

SUMMARY

In a study of 475 Sherpas in the Khumbu region of the Nepalese Himalayas the incidence of isolated deafness, deafmutism and classical (myxedematous) cretinism was 3.1 percent, 4.7 percent and 5.9 percent respectively.

Neither iodine kinetic studies nor measurement of indices of peripheral hormone action allowed distinction from the "normal" population. A variable increase in T3 production may in part be responsible. It is proposed that the neurological defect results from a severe intrauterine deficiency of elemental iodine and that the additional features of the myxedematous cretin are dependent on the degree of postnatal iodothyronine deficiency.

The varying clinical spectrum of endemic cretinism observed in different geographical areas may reflect the timing and degree of iodine deficiency and relate to different behavioral patterns in the community.

ACKNOWLEDGEMENTS

The authors are indebted to Sir Edmund Hillary who led both expeditions. They are grateful to the Staff of the Radioisotope Unit for technical assistance and to Miss P. Brown who typed the manuscript.

Dr. B. Leeming kindly assessed skeletal ages.

Figure 5 is reprinted from (3) by permission of the Institute of Human Biology, Papua, New Guinea.

DISCUSSION BY PARTICIPANTS

DELANGE: Did I understand correctly that you think that hypothyroidism results from something that happens after birth? Do you have some method of estimating when hypothyroidism began in a patient?

IBBERTSON: That wasn't quite the point. We believe that hypothyroidism is caused by two things. One is the amount of functioning thyroid tissue available, which in turn is determined by some intrauterine influence whose nature is not known. The second is the degree of iodine deficiency in the community. The point was that the manifestations we described as clinical myxedematous cretinism are due to iodothyronine deficiency. This deficiency manifests itself after birth in these children who are born apparently normal. Growth defect is a phenomenon of extrauterine development. We are trying to divide the manifestations of cretinism into prenatal - the nervous system abnormalities, and postnatal - the somatic abnormalities which are predetermined only in so far as the thyroid development may be compromised before birth.

DEGROOT: Is that not contrary to the experience that if athyreotic cretins are treated at various ages after birth there is a very clear correlation between time of treatment and later IQ? This suggests that some neurologic development, at least as measured by IQ, occurs after birth.

IBBERTSON: We think that at the level of IQ with which we are concerned, most of the damage occurs early. It is the top 30-40 percent of the IQ, the part you are talking about, that is determined after birth.

DEGROOT: Do the cretins that do not have goiter have high TSH?

DELANGE: In our cretins without goiter, TSH is extremely high, sometimes 100 times higher than in the so-called euthyroid people in the same population.

FIERRO: In Ecuador we have found that in mental defectives with and without goiter the difference in TSH was relative to hormone production (11).

HERSHMAN: In the patients who were assessed as clinically euthyroid, were the TSH levels higher than in a control New Zealand population where there is adequate iodine in the diet?

IBBERTSON: They were higher. Dr. Robert Utiger made about 30 determinations for us. The levels were around 20 in some apparently euthyroid individuals, compared with one to five in normal subjects.

KOENIG: A puzzling fact in McCarrison's paper (1) was the difference between the rich and the poor. If I remember correctly, the rich were myxedematous cretins and the poor tended to be nervous cretins. Did you note any difference in social levels?

IBBERTSON: No, I think it is a very homogenous population.

DELANGE: As further support to the observations of Dr. Ibbertson concerning the increase in the level of the plasma labelled T_3, I would like to point out that we have observed a sharp increase in the level of plasma stable T_3 in euthyroid Idjwi patients. This level becomes higher as that of T_4 is reduced. These findings confirm a preferential secretion of T_3 by the thyroid in endemic goiter (12).

FIERRO: We have the impression that there is no relationship between observed thyroid function and mental capacity. This means that your division between those with very low mental capacity, the myxedematous type, and not-so-low, the nervous type, is not true for Ecuador.

HETZEL: Is there any suggestion that hypothyroidism, as you described it, is correlated with increasing altitude?

IBBERTSON: There is a trek of around 200 miles to get into this area, and as we went up so did the evidence of clinical hypothyroidism. We believe that iodine deficiency also increased, making it very difficult to dissociate these two phenomena.

STANBURY: This is a muddy business. There are statements in the literature that when one gets above a certain altitude, around 11,000 feet, cretinism and goiter no longer are found. This is manifestly not true.

FIERRO: It is our impression that above 3,200 meters [10,500 feet] goiter prevalence decreases. In Guangage village (13,100 ft) we have found no endemic cretinism in spite of severe iodine deficiency (13).

DEGROOT: One can think of an interesting relationship to hypothyroidism at high altitude. Thyroid hormone alters the level of red-cell 2,3 diphosphoglycerate. In hypothyroidism there is low 2,3 diphosphoglycerate, and increased affinity of hemoglobin for oxygen. Hypothyroidism would therefore theoretically accentuate any deficiency of oxygen. Do you think that phenomena occurs?

IBBERTSON: I think it is possible. It is interesting to speculate what iodine will do to this effect, in terms of metabolic efficiency at high altitude.

PRETELL: We have been carrying out a study on acute exposure of natives at sea level by taking them to 14,000 feet in five hours, keeping them at that altitude for 24 hours and then studying them. We have found that there is an impairment in the synthesis of thyroid hormones - a decrease in the synthesis of T_4 and T_3 and an increase in time of $\frac{MIT + DIT}{T_3 + T_4}$, and also an increase of $\frac{MIT}{DIT}$, which probably is an impairment due to the lack of oxygen. In regard to the correlation of goiter with high altitude, I do not think one can make a rule that over a certain altitude goiter disappears. In a study carried out in Peru on 505 villages, we have found a rather close correlation between the prevalence of goiter and altitude. However, there were many villages as high as 14,000 feet without goiter. I think it is related to the geographic distribution of iodine deficiency.

STANBURY: Will you concede, Dr. Fierro, that the lack of cretinism in your village of Guangage might be due to their not surviving there?

FIERRO: It is possible. But in Guangage there is seven μg of iodine intake and we have not found endemic cretins. Perhaps hypoxia kills them.

PRETELL: The death rate at high altitude is very high. The birth weight is also significantly lower than at sea level, correlating well with the placental weight. This means that altitude itself is a negative factor in the survival of babies.

REFERENCES

1. McCarrison, R.: Observations of endemic cretinism in the Chitral and Gilgit Valleys. Lancet 2:1275-1280, 1908.

2. Lang, S.D.R., Lang, A.: The Kunde hospital and a demographic survey of the Upper Khumbu, Nepal. N.Z. Med. J. 74:470, 1971.

3. Ibbertson, H.K., Tait, J.M., Pearl, M., Lim, T., McKinnon, J. and Gill, M.B.: Endemic cretinism in Nepal. In: Endemic Cretinism. Monogr. Series No. 2 (B.S. Hetzel and P.O.D. Pharoah, eds.). Inst. Human Biology, Papua, New Guinea, 1971. pp. 71-88.

4. Garn, S.M.: The applicability of North American growth standards in developing countries. Can. Med. Assoc. J. 93:914-919, 1965.

5. Stott, H., Bhatia, B.B., Lal, R.S. and Rai, K.C.: The distribution and cause of endemic goitre in the United Provinces. Indian J. Med. Res. 18:1059-1086, 1931.

6. Grant, I.S., Chapman, J.A., Mahmud, K., Sardar-ul-Mulk, Shahid, M.A. and Taylor, G.: Endemic goitre in the Gilgit Agency West Pakistan. Report UK/HA/10 International Biological Programme on Wellcome Trust Anglo-Pakistan Goitre Survey, 1968.

7. Ibbertson, H.K.: Reproductive physiology. In: The Thyroid. (R. Shearman, ed.). Blackwell, London, 1972.

8. Delange, F., Ermans, A.M., Vis, H.L. and Stanbury, J.B.: Endemic cretinism in Idjwi Island. In: Endemic Cretinism. Monogr. Series No. 2 (B.S. Hetzel and P.O.D. Pharoah, eds.). Inst. Human Biology, Papua, New Guinea, 1971. pp. 33-49.

9. Pharoah, P.O.D., Buttfield, I.H. and Hetzel, B.S.: Neurological damage to the fetus resulting from severe iodine deficiency during pregnancy. Lancet 1:308-310, 1971.

10. Smith, D.W., Blizzard, R.M. and Wilkins, L.: The mental prognosis in hypothyroidism of infancy and childhood: a review of 128 cases. Pediatrics 19:1011-1022, 1957.

11. Stanbury, J.B., Fierro-Benítez, R., Estrella, E., Milutinovic, P.S., Tellez, M.U. and Refetoff, S.: Endemic goiter with hypothyroidism in three generations. J. Clin. Endocrinol. Metab. 29:1596-1600, 1969.

12. Delange, F., Camus, M. and Ermans, A.M.: J. Clin. Endocrinol. Metab., in press.

13. Fierro-Benítez, R., Paredes, M. and Peñafiel, W.: Aspects of thyroid physiopathology at 4,000 m. above sea-level. VIth Pan American Congress of Endocrinology, Mexico, Excerpta Med. Int. Congr. Ser. No. 99, 1965.

THE CLINICAL PATTERN OF ENDEMIC CRETINISM IN PAPUA, NEW GUINEA

P.O.D. Pharoah

Institute of Human Biology

Goroka, Papua, New Guinea

There remains today considerable diversity of opinion as to the proper definition of endemic cretinism. Two factors have largely contributed to this confusion. The term cretinism has been used to include both the endemic type of the syndrome which is geographically associated with endemic goiter and sporadic cretinism in which the defect is solely related to hypothyroidism. Secondly, endemic cretinism shows regional variations in signs and symptoms. Clinical hypothyroidism is the major feature in some endemias (1), while hypothyroidism is absent or uncommon in other endemic foci of the disease where the syndrome presents usually with mental retardation, abnormalities of hearing and speech and congenital diplegia (2,3,4,5,6).

The usual teaching in English and American medical schools that cretinism is synomymous with hypothyroidism is epitomized by the statement of Osler (7), "that the changes characteristic of cretinism, endemic as well as sporadic, result from the loss of function of the thyroid gland". Gordon (8,9), reviewing the cases of childhood myxedema in the United States literature was most precise in his distinction between endemic and sporadic cretinism. He suggested that the term "sporadic cretinism" be dispensed with in favor of the term "childhood myxedema", because cretinism as described in Europe is a clinically distinct entity from sporadic hypothyroid cretinism. However, the writings of Gordon have gone unheeded and some confusion between sporadic and endemic cretinism has persisted.

Endemic cretinism has been described from both parts of New Guinea. In the Mulia Valley of Western New Guinea (now West

Irian); Choufoer *et al.* (5), described mental deficiency, deaf-mutism and motor abnormalities as the most frequent defects. The motor abnormalities in young children were manifest by an inability to sit or stand, a sagging of the head and a characteristic extension and internal rotation of the legs suggestive of a spastic diplegia. The adults had a characteristic gait and stance, with flexed knees and flexion, adduction and internal rotation of the hips. Radiographic assessment of bone maturation and measurements of height were not significantly different between the defectives and non-defectives, and the authors concluded that hypothyroidism is not a feature of the syndrome of endemic cretinism as seen in the Mulia Valley.

In East New Guinea, McCullagh (2,3) described the syndrome as seen in adults in the Huon Peninsula. Amentia (or hypomentia) partial or complete deaf-mutism and motor incoordination were the main defects. McCullagh saw no case of classical cretinism in the area, i.e., no "hypothyroid" cretin. It is patently evident that an identical syndrome has been described quite independently from widely separated areas in New Guinea, and this syndrome is very similar to McCarrison's (11) "nervous" cretinism in the Himalayas.

The following account of the syndrome is derived largely from patients seen in the Jimi Valley in the Western Highlands of New Guinea; all statistical figures are from this area. Studies have also been carried out in the Waria and Ono Valleys in Papua, and in the Nomane and Dom subdistricts in the Highlands.

As part of an experiment on the use of iodized oil as a prophylactic for endemic cretinism (11), approximately half the cretins received an intramuscular depot injection of iodized oil in 1966; the remainder received as a placebo a saline injection or had no treatment at all.

PATIENTS AND METHODS

The examination and investigation of the endemic cretins in the Jimi Valley was carried out during a series of patrols to this area commencing in May, 1967. Patrolling has been limited to the middle valley and 13 villages with a population of 8,000 have been visited, each on a number of occasions.

The total population of each village with the names of every person in it were available from the records of the census that was conducted in 1966. These records were used throughout the survey.

At each village inquiries were made for abnormalities of hearing or speech in members of the population and those with any such abnormality were requested to present themselves for clinical examination. People in whom deafness was of late onset or in whom there was evidence of middle ear disease such as otitis media were excluded from the study.

The ages of the majority of cretins born prior to 1966 are not accurately known. In the census of 1966 an estimate was made of the age of each person using as a guideline estimates made in previous census patrols which have been conducted since about 1956. Since the great majority of cretins seen were under the age of 16 years, inaccuracies of more than three years in the age estimation were unlikely.

The presence of deafness or speech abnormalities or both was elicited mainly from the history taken in Pidgin English with an interpreter translating into the local dialect. In most cases a history of deafness was substantiated by observing how communication between the patient and other people was maintained, e.g. whether mime or a raised voice was used.

Clinical examination was aimed primarily at detecting abnormalities of the central nervous system and evidence of hypothyroidism. Particular attention was paid to gait, sitting and standing postures, the external ocular movements, tendon reflexes, plantar responses, muscle tone and the presence of clonus.

Standing height was determined using a Harpenden anthropometer. Electrocardiographic records were obtained using a portable battery operated Phillips Cardiopan 531A electrocardiograph running at a paper speed of 25 cm per second. Standard limb leads I, II, III, aVl, aVf and precordial leads V1 to V6 were recorded in each case.

A formal evaluation of mental ability was not attempted.

RESULTS

A total of 107 endemic cretins have been examined clinically on at least one occasion. This total is comprised of 63 males and 44 females, giving a Male to Female ratio of 1.4.

In no case were the clinical features of hypthyroidism evident, such as large protruding tongue, dry puffy skin, umbilical hernia, low-set hairline or delayed relaxation of the ankle jerk.

An electrocardiogram was performed in 33 subjects and in none was there evidence of reduced voltage of the P wave or QRS complex, or flattening or inversion of the T wave.

Speech was invariably affected in all those who had severe partial or complete deafness; these were designated deaf-mutes. There were 93 patients (87.0 percent) in this group.

A second group constituted those who had partial hearing and in whom speech was not normal, being limited to a few words such as the names of sibs or close associates. There were nine in this category or 8.4 percent.

A third group consisted of those in whom speech was severely affected, amounting at times to mutism, but in whom hearing appeared to be normal. If a degree of deafness did exist it was disproportionate to the severity of the speech abnormality. There were five such patients (4.7 percent).

The neuromuscular abnormalities were those of a congenital diplegia. In young infants this was manifest as hypotonia and delay in attaining the motor milestones. Head control was poor and often drew attention to the child who was being carried because the head hung limply to one side. This feature was also evident when the child was pulled to sitting from lying supine. Normally there is no head lag after the age of about 24 weeks, but in the endemic cretin this may persist until well over 12 months of age (Fig. 1). Sitting unsupported is usually possible in the normal infant by eight or nine months and the spine is straight, (Fig. 2) but in the cretin sitting can be delayed for years, and often the child sits forward supporting the head and trunk with the hands. Even when able to sit unsupported there is usually a marked kyphosis of the thoraco-lumbar spine. (Fig. 3). Crawling is also abnormal in the cretin. Characteristically the infant is unable to properly raise its pelvis from the floor, so that a frog-like attitude is maintained and the movements of crawling are ineffective.

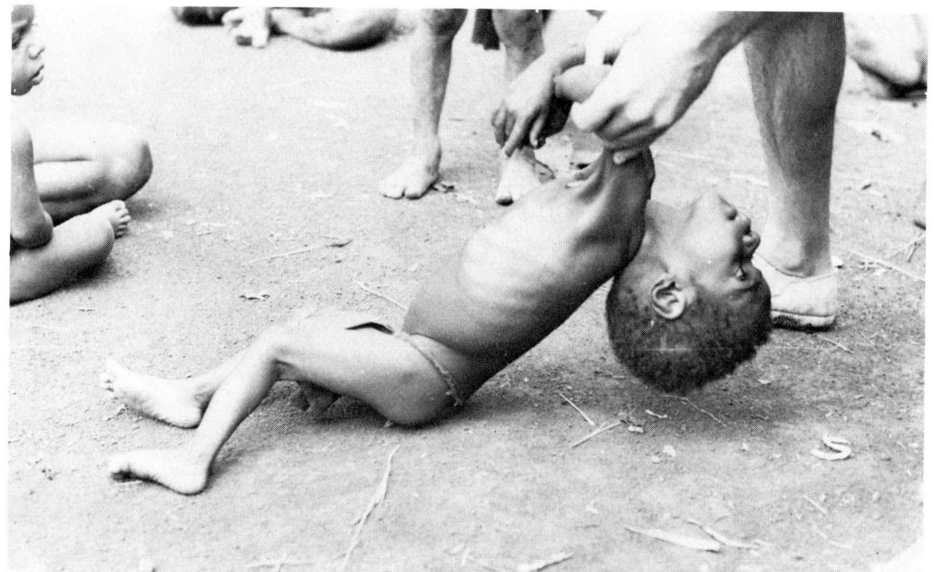

Fig. 1. Extreme lack of head control in a three year old endemic cretin when raised from the lying to the sitting position.

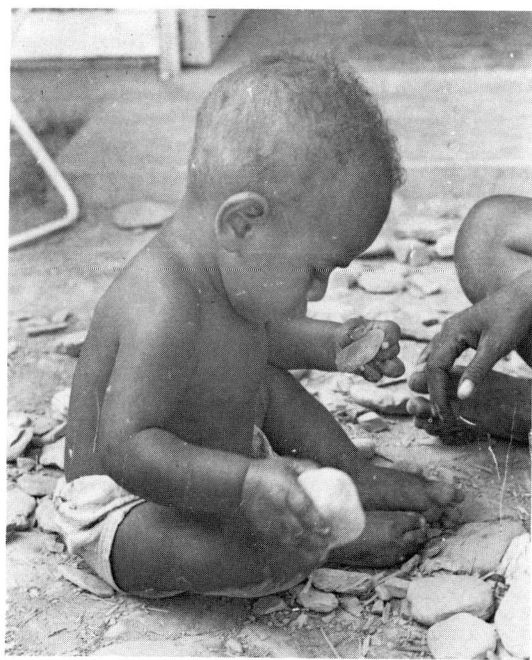

Fig. 2. Normal 10 month old child showing relatively straight spine when sitting upright. Cf. Fig. 3.

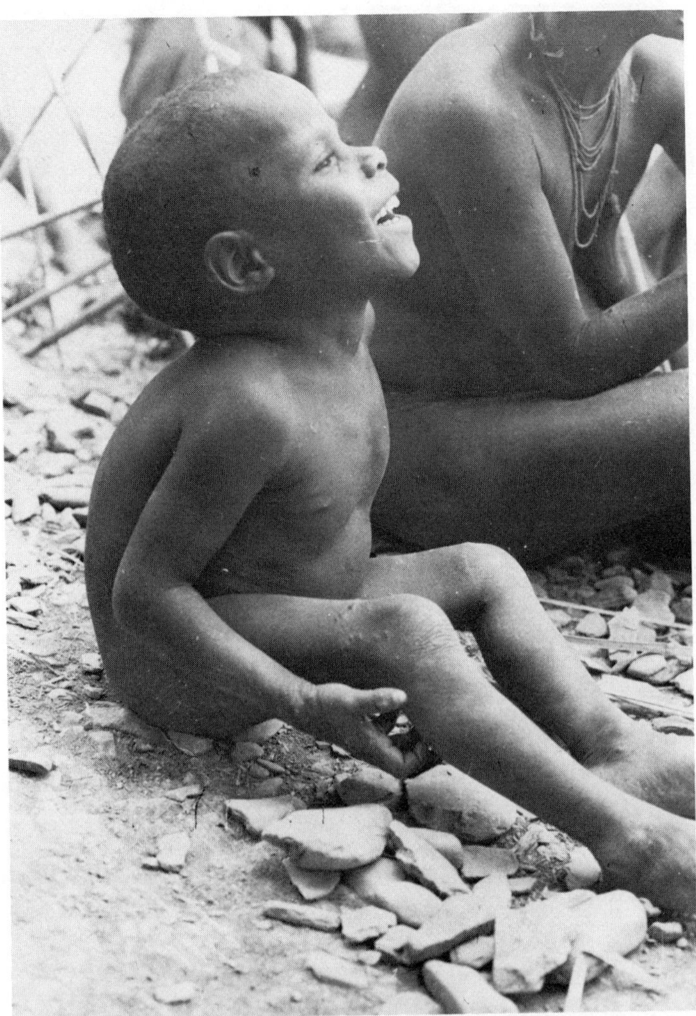

Fig. 3. Five year old endemic cretin demonstrating marked curvature of thoraco-lumbar spine. The characteristic posture of the head with the neck in extension.

When standing, the posture adopted is with the legs apart and the knees and hips partially flexed (Fig. 4). There is usually some internal rotation at the hips also. The gait is wide-based, stiff-legged, shuffling and sometimes with a stamping quality to it. A partial flexion of hips and knees gives a stooping appearance and is maintained while walking. The effect of stooping may be accentuated by the presence of a kyphosis.

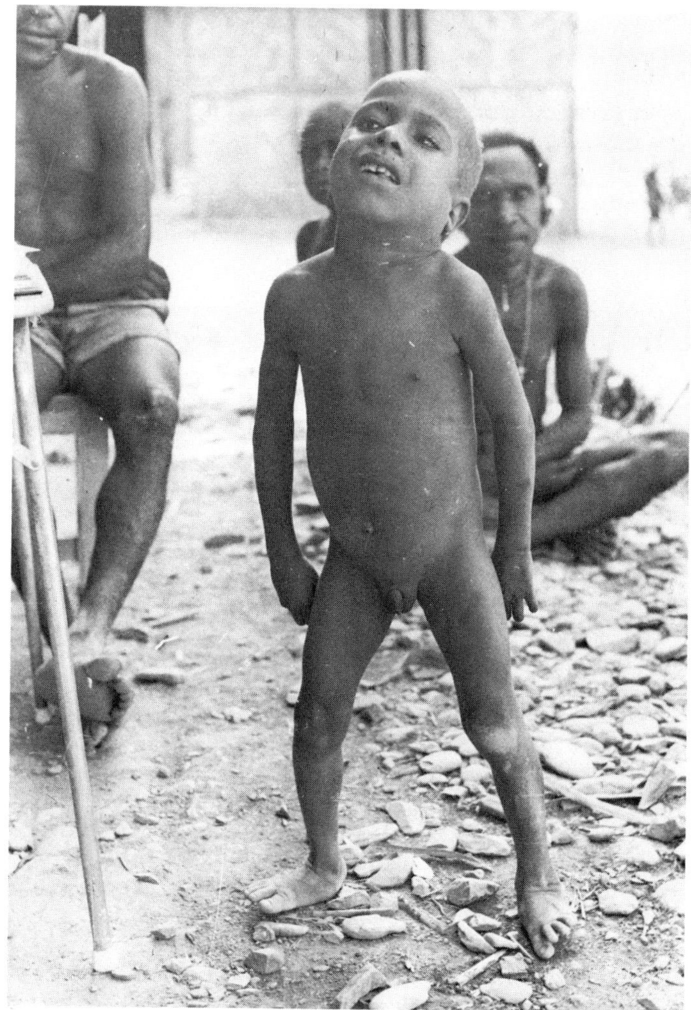

Fig. 4. Seven year old endemic cretin showing characteristic standing posture with wide base and partial flexion of hips and knees. Head is held with neck in extension.

The upper limbs are not as frequently affectd as the lower, but when affected, show a clumsiness of movement. An example of this is inability to pick up an object with the thumb and forefinger, the hand adopting a main en griffe posture.

Tone is variably increased in different muscle groups; predominantly affected are quadriceps, hamstring and adductors of the thighs. This was often accompanied by pathologically brisk tendon reflexes.

A prolonged ankle or patellar clonus was only rarely elicited but a clonus of three or four beats was a common finding. In many cases a satisfactory plantar response could not be obtained owing to the callus formation on the soles of the feet. The reflex was found to be extensor in approximately 40 percent of cases in which it was elicited.

In summary 87 of 107 cretins (81.4 percent) had abnormalities of motor function.

Strabismus occurs with sufficient frequency to be considered as a feature of endemic cretinism. It was usually found in the more severely affected patients. Usually it is an internal strabismus; and often is present transiently and may alternate between one eye and the other. In one extremely severe instance a coarse nystagmus was also present. Twenty-seven (25.2 percent) of the cretins had strabismus. Table 1 provides a summary of the incidence of these various abnormalities.

The mean height for 127 normal adult males was 154.6 cm (range 145.0 - 165.1) and for 227 normal adult females was 145.3 cm (range 131.0 - 158.4 cm). Although height measurements were made on all age groups, adequate numbers were not obtained to permit the construction of a growth curve. As an alternative, the growth curve obtained by Malcolm (13) for Bundi (an adjacent valley to the Jimi) children, was used. He obtained mean adult heights of 156 and 147 cm for males and females respectively. These are not significantly different from the values in the Jimi valley. Since the adult heights for the Bundi and Jimi people are the same, it is assumed that the growth pattern is also comparable. This is shown in Fig. 5 which also shows the height/age distribution of 59 endemic cretins. There are two groups of cretins represented - those who received an iodized oil injection five years earlier and those who were untreated. It is evident that the majority of cretins are within the normal height range and that dwarfism is rare. Furthermore, there is no obvious difference in height between those who had received iodized oil and those who were untreated.

Although no formal mental assessment was made in any patient, the impression was obtained that some, albeit a minority, of those with a disorder of hearing or speech may have had a normal intelligence.

Table 1: Clinical disorders in 107 cretins from the Jimi Valley, Papua, New Guinea

TOTAL 107	ABNORMALITIES OF SPEECH AND HEARING			NEUROMUSCULAR ABNORMALITIES	STRABISMUS
	Deaf-mutism	Partial Speech and Hearing Loss	Predominant Abnormality of Speech		
Number	93	9	5	87	27
Percentage	87.0%	8.2%	4.7%	81.4%	25.2%

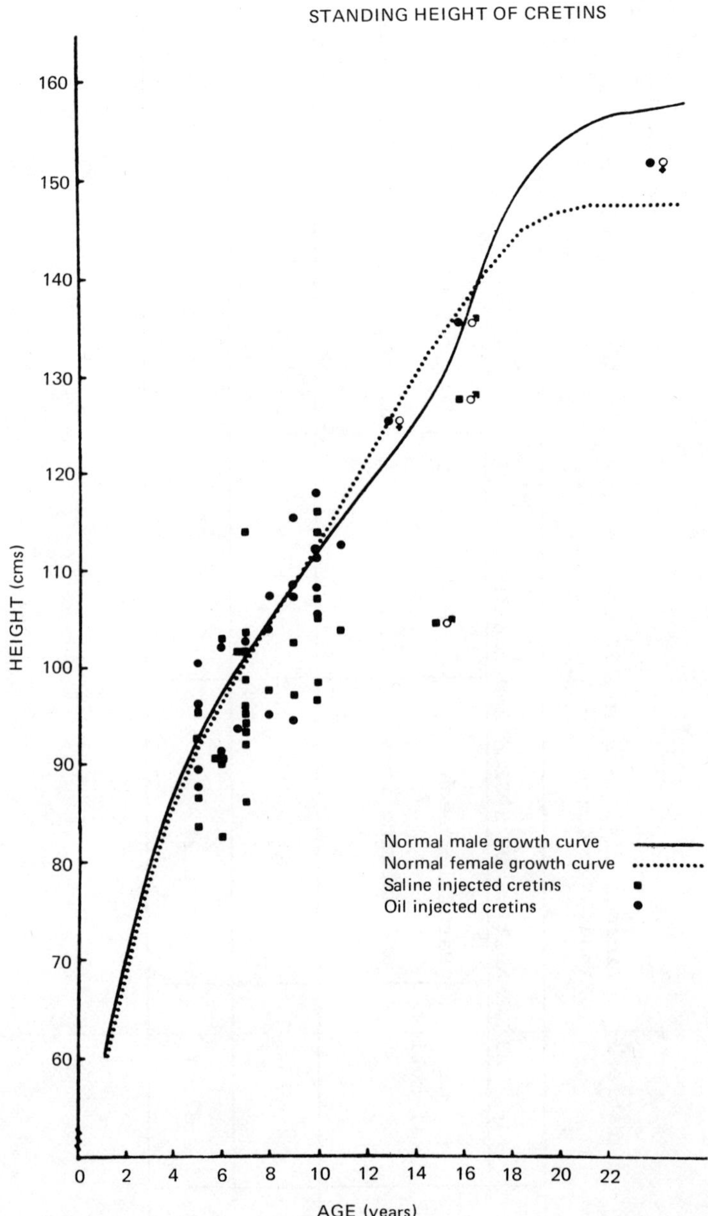

Fig. 5. Relation between height and age in a group of cretins either injected with saline or iodized oil compared to distribution of height by age in an adjoining region where endemic cretinism is not found.

DISCUSSION

The occurrence of deaf-mutism or abnormalities of hearing or speech as part of the syndrome of endemic cretinism is accepted. However, in a goiter area, patients who have as their sole defect an abnormality of hearing or speech, are not considered by some observers to be endemic cretins. Costa et al. (6) did not study endemic deaf-mutes because "in the large majority of cases, the endemic deaf-mute is not a cretin". Fierro-Benitez et al. (10) classified endemic cretinism as Types I and II and considered those with deaf-mutism, deafness and mutism as separate entities. The author postulates that patients with abnormalities of hearing and speech, even if the sole abnormality, should be considered as part of the spectrum of endemic cretinism.

The mutism that occurs is usually presumed to be secondary to the congenital deafness, but in a small minority the mutism appears to be out of proportion to the degree of deafness. It may be inferred from the report on the cretins in the Andes (14) that a similar situation exists there. What is the cause of the mutism? It may be due to a hearing deficit which is not immediately apparent, but which may become evident with more sophisticated tests. As a second possibility, mental deficiency is a prominent cause of speech retardation although it does not usually produce mutism unless severe. The third possibility is that mutism is due primarily to damage to the speech centers of the cerebral cortex.

The height of cretins has been another contended point, i.e. whether dwarfism is or is not a feature of the syndrome. Dwarfism is unequivocal (1) in an endemic where overt hypothyroidism is evident. However, in those areas where the neurological form of the syndrome predominates, dwarfism is uncommon. Costa et al. (6) referring to cretins in the Piedmont of Italy, stated that their stature was on average smaller than normal, ranging from 150 to 160 cm. True dwarfism was uncommon and a normal or greater than normal stature was not exceptional. Choufoer et al. (5) in West New Guinea found that the mean adult height of defectives was slightly below the mean of the normal population, but the majority fell within the normal range. In the Andean study, two types of cretins were defined. The most prevalent, which was 10 times more prevalent than the second, was of normal stature (14).

If cretins are of normal or near normal stature, then hypothyroidism of any severity during the growth period can be excluded. The minor growth retardation that occurs in some cretins could be related largely to malnutrition. The mental deficiency and the reduced mobility secondary to the diplegia must make the infant much less able to forage successfully. Certainly a degree of malnutrition is common among the New Guinea cretins.

In the Pan American Health Organization defintion of endemic cretinism, mental deficiency is a _sine qua non_ of the syndrome (15). Is this really true? No formal mental testing was attempted in the present study. Nevertheless the impression was obtained that some, albeit a minority, did perhaps have normal intelligence. In many studies of endemic cretinism mental deficiency has been taken as essential to the diagnosis. This was so in the report on the Andes (14) yet there was a group of patients with abnormalities who were not classified as cretins, presumably because they were not mentally deficient. Furthermore, it was stated that some deaf-mutes presented "normal" intelligence.

Similarly in the reports on Piedmont and Mendoza (6,16) the inmates of certain mental institutions were studied after excluding deaf-mutes, who were numbered among the normal population. On the other hand, Choufoer _et al_. (5) state that in at least two complete deaf-mutes there was sufficient proof of a good intelligence. In the focus of cretinism in 19th-century England, two deaf-mutes were described "who have been educated and are said to be possessed of remarkably quick parts" (17). Unfortunately none of these studies are backed by adequate quantitative mental evaluation of the patients. This has often been due to wide cultural and language differences between investigator and patient, added to which is the inherent difficulty of assessing mental ability in a deaf-mute. Thus, while the majority of endemic cretins are mentally retarded, proof is lacking that they are all retarded. Equally, proof is lacking that some are of normal intelligence.

SUMMARY

The syndrome of endemic cretinism in Papua, New Guinea, is described. The disorder encompasses a wide spectrum, with severe mental retardation, deaf-mutism, congenital diplegia and strabismus representing one extreme. The other end of the spectrum is perhaps a sole defect of hearing or speech; the case for mental retardation as a _sine qua non_ of the syndrome is unproven. Clinical hypothyroidism is not a feature of the syndrome as seen in Papua, New Guinea.

ACKNOWLEDGEMENTS

Supported by Department of Public Health, Papua, New Guinea.

DISCUSSION BY PARTICIPANTS

PITTMAN: Is there any evidence of progression in the disease with these people? Could it not be confused with kuru or any other disease?

PHAROAH: I have found no evidence of progression in examining them since 1967.

HERSHMAN: Is there any change in the dietary habits of pregnant women so that iodine deficiency might be more severe during pregnancy?

PHAROAH: There are some taboos on a woman when she becomes pregnant. They do not eat much pumpkin anyway, but it is taboo during pregnancy. There are other taboos with which I am not familiar.

IBBERTSON: There is a difference between our Sherpas who don't have taboos during pregnancy and your people who do. This could possibly explain the difference in neurological involvement between these two populations.

ROSMAN: With regard to the basis of the mutism, there is no clinical evidence that an injury to the speech area either before or after birth causes a child to become mute. Even a child who becomes aphasic from a severe injury to the speech area only very exceptionally will remain mute. I think your other two suggestions are more likely to be the basis of the mutism - either it is a manifestation of severe mental retardation or a manifestation of hearing impairment.

COSTA: I wonder if we are allowed to use the term "endemic cretin" for a person who is not mentally deficient. The meaning of this term has been fixed for some centuries: it is related to the concept of a Christian docility and innocence. When and where this disease has been described, mental deficiency has been a *conditio sine qua non* for the use of this term. If there are people who repeat the somatic features of the endemic cretin, but are not idiots, we can say that they are like cretins, but not "endemic cretins".

HETZEL: I think it is true that as knowledge increases, definitions of disease do change. Usually it is the pathologist that first describes the disease and as further studies are made the picture becomes blurred. Less flagrant pictures are identified as related to a syndrome rather than disease entities in themselves.

IBBERTSON: Let us get the term cretinism out of the way, and accept that they are stupid individuals. We must coin a new term to define those individuals with significant physical or thyroid abnormality or both but without obvious intellectual defect.

QUERIDO: The point is that when we examine carefully we may find the initial assessment to be in error. Dr. Dodge examined a deaf-mute in Tocachi, whom we all thought, Dr. Fierro, Dr. Stanbury, and myself - and the community as well - to be normal. Then we discovered that in an acultural assessment of performance this cretin did not achieve above three or four years of age.

IBBERTSON: But Dr. Fierro's studies show that some of his cretins come up into the low or borderline normal range for his population.

FIERRO: Borderline, low normal range.

IBBERTSON: But a large part of your normals were in the borderline range, suggesting that the method of testing was not adequate for your normal population.

QUERIDO: I think that what Dr. Fierro has shown is that mental development of the whole population is not bimodal, but is a universe. If one accepts that there are not two Gaussian curves for the whole population, the interpretation of the data as to incidence becomes different. The prevalence may be higher than suspected. You quoted me as saying that we have seen two deaf-mutes who were mentally normal. That I withdraw. I made this error in Ecuador and Dr. Dodge showed me that I was wrong. For deaf-mutism the situation is even more complicated, because I am told that if it is not detected before a child is three, and then special training is started, normal performance at a later age cannot be achieved.

COSTA: With an endemic deaf-mute it is possible to achieve a mental age comparable to that of a normal person. On the other hand the endemic cretin has such a deficiency and alteration of the mental faculties that it is not possible to compare him with the intellectual capacity and the psychological pattern of a normal person of any age.

ROSMAN: Certainly the patients can catch up a lot. The question is can they catch up completely. I don't think that is known in terms of auditory stimuli. There is some experimental evidence concerning visual stimuli. Hubel and Wiesel (18) showed that if kittens were visually deprived early in life, there was a disruption of cortical connections. If a parallel situation exists in human audition, a young child who has been auditorally deprived for a finite period, and then has hearing restored, may lack the potential for complete recovery. If a child is not exposed to speech, he will never speak; once exposed, he will begin to learn to speak. I do not believe anyone knows for certain if he has the potential for the eventual development of normal speech if the exposure to speech is delayed beyond a certain time. Another important point is the nature of psychological testing. Dr. Fierro used three types of testing. One of them, the Leiter Test, is an excellent test for deaf children. The Stanford-Binet test, which he used, is rather inappropriate for patients who hear and speak poorly because it is highly verbal.

FIERRO: The verbal tests were used only when the patients were able to answer the questions.

REFERENCES

1. Dumont, J.E.; Ermans, A.M. and Bastenie, P.A.: Thyroidal function in a goiter endemic. IV. Hypothyroidism and endemic cretinism. *J. Clin. Endocrinol. Metab.* 23:325-335, 1963.

2. McCullagh, S.F.: The Huon Peninsula Endemic: IV. Endemic goiter and congenital defect. *Med. J. Aust.* 1:884-890, 1963.

3. Buttfield, I.H. and Hetzel, B.S.: Endemic cretinism in eastern New Guinea. *Aust. Ann. Med.* 18:217-221, 1969.

4. Lobo, L.C.G.; Pompeu, F.; Rosenthal, D.: Endemic Cretinism in Goiaz, Brazil. *J. Clin. Endocrinol. Metab.* 23:407-412, 1963.

5. Choufoer, J.C.; Van Rhijn, M. and Querido, A: Endemic goiter in western New Guinea. II. Clinical picture, incidence and pathogenesis of endemic cretinism. *J. Clin. Endocrinol. Metab.* 25:385-402, 1965.

6. Costa, A.; Cottino, F.; Mortara, M. and Vogliazzo, U.: Endemic cretinism in Piedmont. *Panminerva Med.* 6:250-259, 1964.

7. Osler, W.: Sporadic cretinism in America. Trans. Am. Congr. Physicians Surgeons 4:169, 1897.

8. Gordon, M.B.: Childhood myxoedema or so-called sporadic cretinism in North America. Endocrinology 6:235-254, 1922.

9. Gordon, M.B.: Childhood myxoedema (sporadic cretinism) in the United States. Transactions of the Third International Goiter Conference, 1938. pp. 114-129.

10. Gajdusek, D.C.: Congenital defects of the central nervous system associated with hyperendemic goiter in a neolithic highland society of Netherlands New Guinea. Pediatrics 29:345-363, 1962.

11. McCarrison, R.: Observations on endemic cretinism in the Chitral and Gilgit Valleys. Lancet 2:1275-1280, 1908.

12. Pharoah, P.O.D.; Buttfield, I.H. and Hetzel, B.S.: Neurological damage to the foetus resulting from severe iodine deficiency during pregnancy. Lancet 1: 308-310, 1971.

13. Malcolm, L.A.: Growth and development in New Guinea. A study of the Bundi people in the Madang district. Institute of Human Biology, Monogr. Ser.1, Papua,New Guinea 1970.

14. Fierro-Benítez, R.; Penafiel, W.; De Groot, L.J. and Ramirez, I.: Endemic goiter and endemic cretinism in the Andean Region. New Engl. J. Med. 6:296-302, 1969.

15. Report of the Pan American Health Organization Scientific Group on Research in Endemic Goiter. Pan American Health Organization Advisory Committee of Medical Research, Washington, 1963.

16. Stanbury, J.B.; Brownell, G.L.; Riggs, D.S.; Perinetti, H.; Itoiz, J. and Del Castillo, E.B.: Endemic Goiter; The Adaptation of Man to Iodine Deficiency. Harvard University Press, Cambridge, 1954.

17. Norris, H.: Notice of a remarkable disease analagous to cretinism existing in a small village in the west of England. The Med. Times 17:257-258, 1847-48.

18. Hubel, H. and Weisel, T.N.: The period of susceptibility to the physiological effects of unilateral eye closure in kittens. J. Physiol. 206:419-436, 1970.

ENDEMIC CRETINISM IN IDJWI ISLAND (KIVU LAKE, ZAIRE REPUBLIC)

F. Delange, A.M. Ermans, J.B. Stanbury

CEMUBAC Medical Team, Department of Pediatrics and Radioisotopes, School of Medicine, St. Peter Hospital, University of Brussels, Belgium. IRSAC, Lwiro, Zaire Republic. Massachusetts Institute of Technology, Cambridge, Mass.

The term "endemic cretin", as defined by the Pan American Health Organization (1), describes mentally deficient subjects born in an endemic goiter area who exhibit some of the following characteristics which are not readily explained by other causes:

1) Irreversible neuromuscular disorders;
2) Irreversible abnormalities in hearing and speech which sometimes lead to deaf-mutism;
3) Impairment of somatic development;
4) Hypothyroidism (2)

This definition covers two very different but overlapping syndromes (3,4). One is characterized primarily by abnormalities of hearing and speech associated with neuromuscular disorders, but with little or no impairment of thyroid function. Patients of the second syndrome are severely hypothyroid. These syndromes have been called "nervous" and "myxedematous" cretinism respectively (2). We use the general term "endemic cretinism" for both syndromes because the geographic distributions of endemic goiter and cretinism are superimposed (5), and because both disorders disappear progressively from the population with the introduction of iodine prophylaxis (4,6-8).

The relative frequency of the two types of cretinism varies considerably from one endemia to another. In many endemias, most cretins (3,4,9-11), if not all (6,12-15) are of the first type. In others, the large majority are clearly hypothyroid, as in the Uele endemia in the northeastern part of the Zaire Republic (16,17).

Dumont et al. showed that the degree of mental retardation in the Uele cretins is related to the degree of thyroid deficiency (17), which results from an extreme reduction of the hormonal content of the gland (18). Their studies appear to exclude inborn errors of the thyroid as the cause of this cretinism in the Uele.

Cretins similar to those of the Uele live in another area of central Africa, Idjwi Island, situated in the Kivu Lake in the eastern part of the Zaire Republic (19). Clinically identical patients are also found in the Ubangi region in northwestern Zaire. We present a report on the epidemiologic, clinical and biologic characteristics of endemic cretinism on Idjwi island.

SUBJECTS AND METHODS

A medical survey was performed on 12,557 inhabitants of the Island, 9,000 living in the North, and 3,557 in the South-west. The survey included almost the total population of the two regions. Prevalence of goiter was determined according to Perez et al. (20.) Measurements of the heights of all subjects established the normal growth curve for the Idjwi population. Endemic cretins were catalogued from a clinical examination according to the recommendations of PAHO (1) and identified either as the nervous or the myxedematous type.

The study was performed in 21 random myxedematous cretins who were clinicall hypothyroid. All lived in the northern part of the island; their ages ranged from 6 to 26 and their mean age was 16.9 years.

METABOLIC, RADIOLOGIC, AND ELECTROCARDIOGRAPHIC STUDIES IN CRETINS

Iodine Metabolism. The 24 hour ^{131}I thyroidal uptake, the level of the plasma $PB^{127}I$ and of the $PB^{125}I$ at the 24th hour were determined by standard methods (19). The results were compared with those reported previously for euthyroid adults in the same area (19).

The following measurements were made in a smaller number of cretins:

1) $NBE^{125}I$ expressed in percent of the $PB^{125}I$.
2) T_3 resin uptake test [Triosorb (Abbott)]. The results were expressed in percentage of the value found for a

pool of normal serum in Brussels. Results found in euthyroid Belgian adults range from 85 to 110 percent.

3) Thyroglobulin antibodies in the serum were determined by the tanned red-cell agglutination method of Boyden (21) slightly modified (22).
4) Serum TSH level*.
5) Thyroid scanning. The scannings were made with a Nuclear scanner 1,700 A. The surfaces of the thyroid scannings were measured by planimetry and compared with those from five euthyroid non-goitrous control patients from a non-goitrous area on the shores of Kivu Lake, whose heights were identical to those of the cretins. The results were compared by the test for paired samples (25).

X-ray Studies. X-rays of the skull, the hand and wrist, the knee and the pelvis were performed on eight hypothyroid cretins. A 24-year-old clinically euthyroid man with a stage II goiter was used as control. The bone maturation of the hand and wrist was estimated according to Greulich and Pyle (26) and that of the knee after Pyle and Hoerr (27).

Electrocardiograms. Standard ECG's were recorded for the same subjects as had x-ray studies. The sum of the absolute values of QRS complexes and T waves in standard limb leads (I + II + III) and in unipolar chest leads ($V_1 + V_5$) were computed. The results were compared to those reported by Lepeschkin (28) for normal adults.

EFFECTS OF TRIIODOTHYRONINE (T_3) ON UPTAKE AND ECG IN CRETINS

A thyroid suppression test with T_3 was performed on eight cretins. Because of their small weight, the mean being 24.8 kg, and the severe thyroidal deficiency, the dose of T_3 was only 25μg per day on five consecutive days. In spite of this small dose, the treatment had to be interrupted in two subjects because of a pulse rate of more than 100 per minute. ECG and 24 hour ^{131}I thyroidal uptake were recorded before and on the sixth day after treatment was begun. The results were compared by the t test for paired samples (25).

FIVE-YEAR FOLLOW-UP OF MYXEDEMATOUS CRETINS

Five myxedematous cretins were reexamined two or three times during a five-year period. The follow-up included height measurements, estimation of the thyroid volume, and determination of the 24 hour ^{131}I thyroidal uptake and of the $PB^{127}I$.

*Kindly determined by Dr. J.M. Hershman using the method of Odell et al. (23) slightly modified (24).

RESULTS

EPIDEMIOLOGIC SURVEY AND CLINICAL ASPECT OF CRETINISM IN IDJWI ISLAND

Detailed results of the medical survey have appeared elsewhere (19). The prevalence of goiter is 5.3 percent in the southwest of the island and reaches 54.4 percent in the north. No cretin has been observed in the southwest area. In contrast, 99 cases of cretinism were recorded in the north area. Only 11 of the 99 cretins are clinically euthyroid. All these 11 cretins are deaf-mutes and seven have a spastic diplegia of the lower limbs. The remaining 88 are clinically hypothyroid as follows:

1) Growth retardation, as shown in Fig. 1. Height expressed in percent of the normal height for this population varies from 56 to 95. The mean value observed was 77 percent.

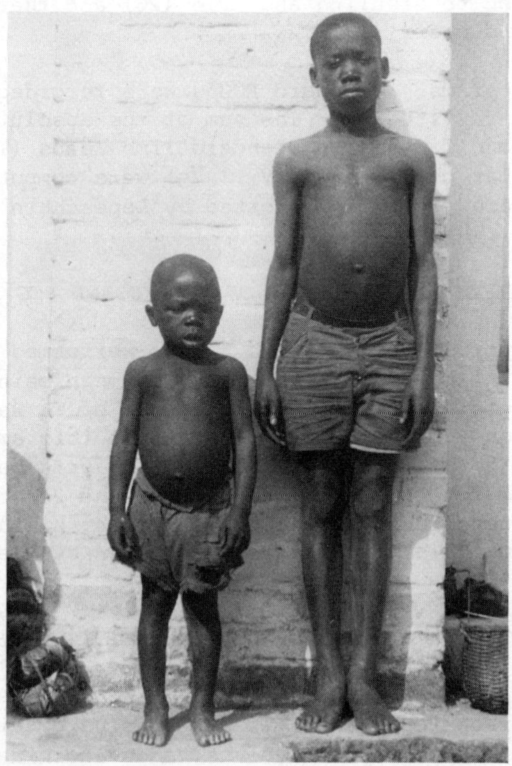

Fig. 1: Growth retardation in Idjwi myxedematous cretins: on the left, a 12 year-old cretin with a height of 96 cm; on the right, a normal 12 year-old boy with a height of 136 cm.

2) Marked mental retardation, which could not be measured because of the absence of standardized psychomotor tests for this population. The degree of mental retardation varied considerably from one patient to another, but most understood simple orders and participated in some way in the more rudimentary activities of the family.

3) Characteristic posture with marked lumbar lordosis, prominent abdomen and frequent umbilical hernia. A typical myxedematous cretin is shown in Fig. 2.

4) Myxedematous thickening of the skin with puffy features, as in Fig. 3.

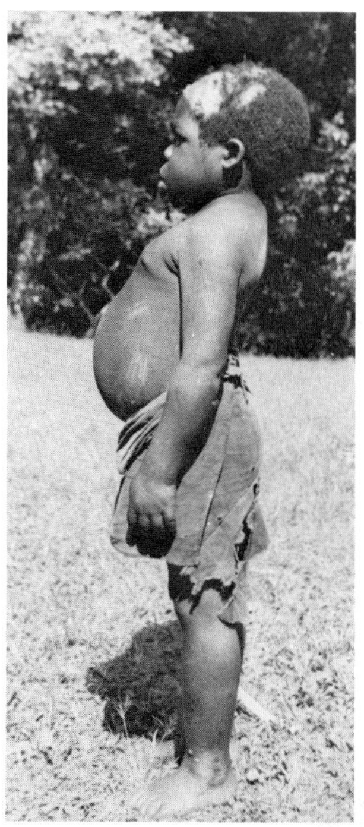

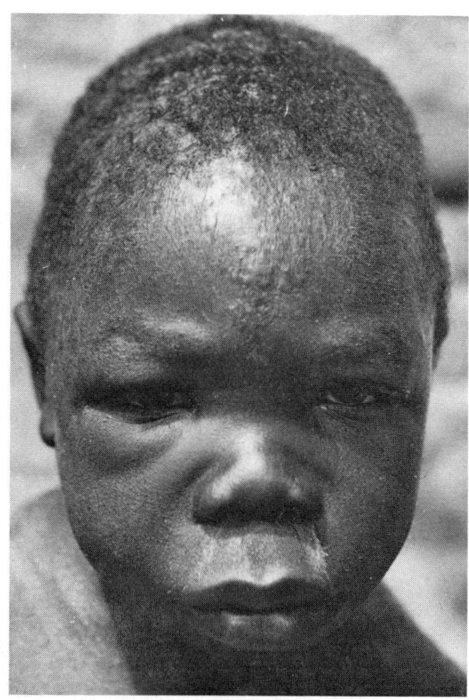

Fig. 2: Characteristic posture of cretins: marked lumbar lordosis and prominent abdomen. Subject aged 21 years, height 105 cm (64 percent of normal), $PB^{127}I$: 0.4 μg/100 ml.

Fig. 3: Myxedematous thickening of the skin causing puffy features. The failure of feature maturation and naso-orbital configuration is obvious; the bridge of the nose remains flat and broad. Subject aged 15 years, height 82.5 cm (58 percent of normal), $PB^{127}I$:0.3 μg/100 ml. Reprinted from (29)

5) Skin dry and scaly, as in Fig. 4.
6) Marked delay in sexual development.
7) Prolonged relaxation time of tendon reflexes. Babinski sign was carefully looked for in 12 cretins; a bilateral sign was found in four and a unilateral sign in one. Motor behavior was extremely slow but neurological examination was otherwise normal except for one case of spastic diplegia. None was deaf-mute.

This group of 88 myxedematous cretins includes 29 females and 59 males; 22 are goitrous but the enlargement of the gland is minimal. Their ages range from less than one to 31 years, their mean age being 12.2 years.

A clear familial aggregation of endemic cretinism is evidenced by the fact that 28 patients, or 32 percent, have one, two, three or more cretin relatives.

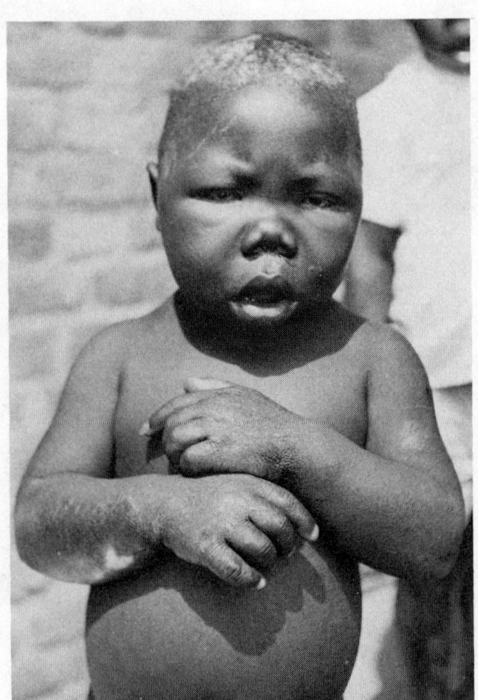

Fig. 4: Skin dry and scaly. Subject aged 15 years, height 82.5 cm (58 percent of normal), $PB^{127}I$:0.4 μg/100 ml.

METABOLIC, RADIOLOGIC AND ELECTROCARDIOGRAPHIC STUDIES

Iodine Metabolism. The 24 hour ^{131}I thyroidal uptake, the levels of the plasma $PB^{127}I$ and $PB^{125}I$, the $NBE^{125}I$ in myxedematous

Table I. Comparison of the main parameters of iodine metabolism in myxedematous cretins and in clinically euthyroid adults living in North Idjwi.

	Euthyroid controls (adults)	Myxedematous cretins	t test Value of P
24 hr thyroid uptake (% dose)	79.5 ± 0.7* (376)**	40.0 ± 4.7 (18)	< 0.001
Plasma $PB^{127}I$ (µg/100ml)	3.7 ± 0.1 (301)	1.3 ± 0.2 (21)	< 0.001
Plasma $PB^{125}I$ 24 hr (% dose/liter)	0.17 ± 0.02 (105)	1.09 ± 0.18 (19)	< 0.001
Plasma $NBE^{125}I$ (%$PB^{125}I$)	10.5 ± 1.2 (33)	8.5 ± 2.0 (7)	> 0.4

* Mean ± SEM
** Number of subjects

cretins and in euthyroid controls from the same area are compared in Table I. Uptake and $PB^{127}I$ were lower and $PB^{125}I$ were higher in cretins than in normal adults respectively ($P < 0.001$). However, the $NBE^{125}I$ was approximately the same in both groups ($P > 0.4$).

As shown in Figs. 5 and 6, a significant correlation was found between height retardation and uptake and between height retardation and PBI ($P < 0.001$). Uptake and PBI also correlated significantly ($P < 0.001$).

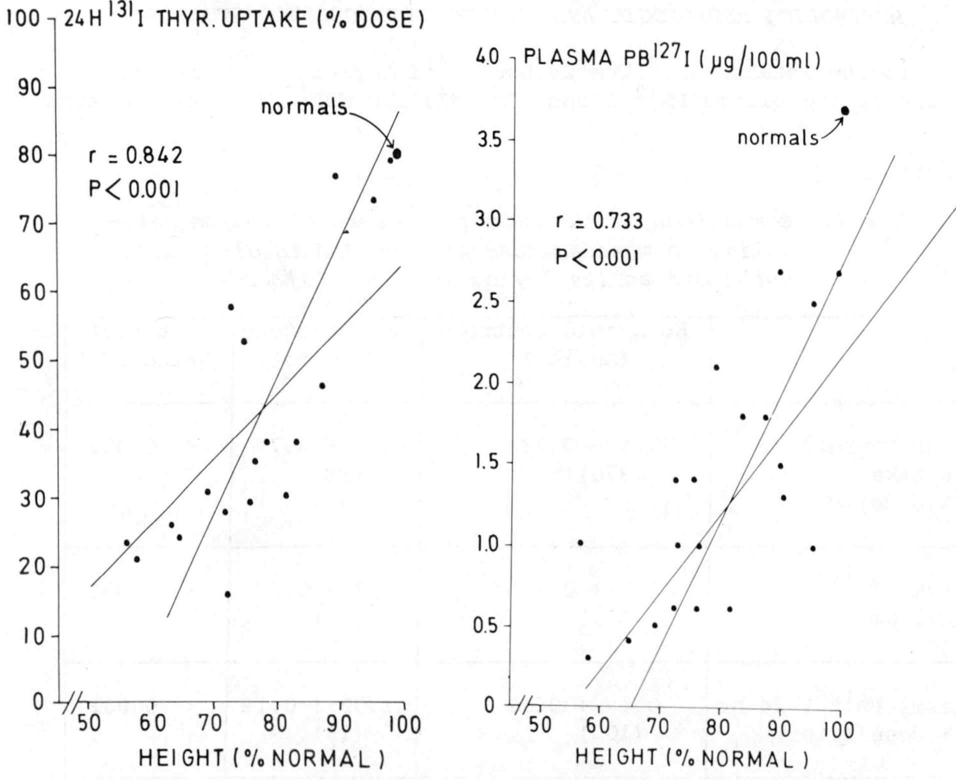

Fig. 5. Correlation between height retardation and uptake in cretins. From Delange, et al. (42)
Fig. 6. Correlation between height retardation and $PB^{127}I$ in cretins. From Delange, et al. (42)

The T_3 resin uptake test and the plasma TSH levels were measured in 11 and 10 cretins respectively. The results for the T_3 resin uptake test ranged from 64 to 92 percent, the mean value being 74 ± 3 percent*. All were lower than 85 percent except for one cretin with a T_3 uptake of 92 percent. The TSH levels varied from 220 to 1,140 microunits per ml, with a mean value of 580 ± 125* microunits per ml. These levels are 10 to 100 times higher than those from the same laboratory for 55 euthyroid patients living in the same area as the cretins (30).

*Standard error of the mean.

Thyroid scanning showed that in all patients the thyroid gland was in normal position. The surface areas of the scans are compared with those of normal subjects in Table II. The thyroid surfaces of the control were always greater than these of the cretin member of each pair. However, the difference in the results for both groups is not significant (P >0.2). In five patients the scan appeared normal. Scans of the remaining three had a pitted and heterogeneous aspect, as shown in Fig. 7. Thyroglobulin antibodies were absent from the serum of 11 cretins tested.

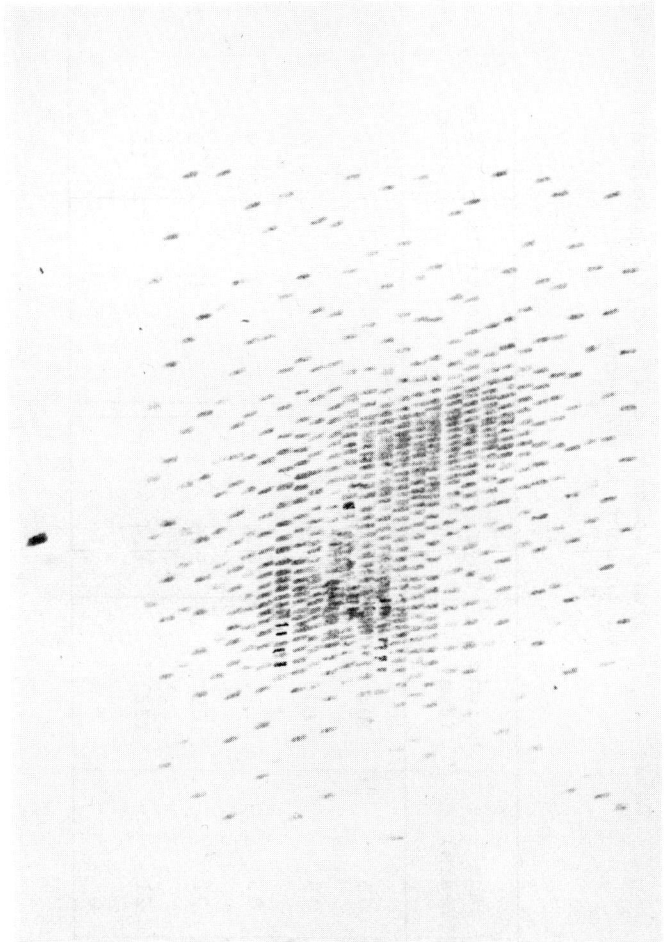

Fig. 7. Thyroid scanning in cretins: split and heterogeneous aspect of the gland. Subject aged 25 years, height 112.5 cm (69% of normal), $PB^{127}I$: 0.5 µg/100ml, 24th hour $PB^{125}I$: 1.45 % dose/liter (cretin n° 7 in Table II).

Table II. Thyroid scanning surfaces in myxedematous cretins and in control subjects

Cretins	Age (Years)	Height (cms)	Thyr. surf. (cm^2)	Controls	Age (years)	Height (cms)	Thyr. surf. (cm^2)
4	15	104	8.2	4	7.5	104	13.1
5	15	82.5	5.0	5	4	83	5.2
7	25	112.5	10.4	7	9	113	10.8
8	21	105	9.6	8	8	105	10.4
9	21	132	8.4	9	12	132	18.4

Electrocardiograms. Regular sinus rhythm or sinus arrhythmia was observed in all patients. The P-R and the corrected Q-T intervals were normal. The voltages of QRS complexes and of T waves in the cretins are compared with normal values in Table III. The voltages found in the cretins were much lower than normal, particularly in the unipolar chest leads ($P < 0.01$). A typical ECG appears in Fig. 8. The results for the control subject were in the normal range.

Table III. Comparison of voltages of QRS complexes and T waves in cretins and in normal adults (28)

ECG waves and complexes (mv) Absolute values	Normals	Myxedematous cretins (8)**	t test Value of P
QRS (I + II + III)	3.09 ± 1.64* (104)**	1.64 ± 0.53	< 0.025
QRS (V1 + V5)	2.48 ± 1.23 (150)	0.90 ± 0.58	< 0.010
T (I + II + III)	0.63 ± 0.37 (104)	0.26 ± 0.22	< 0.010
T (V_1 + V_5)	0.37 ± 0.32 (150)	0.11 ± 0.08	< 0.025

* Mean ± SD

** Number of subjects

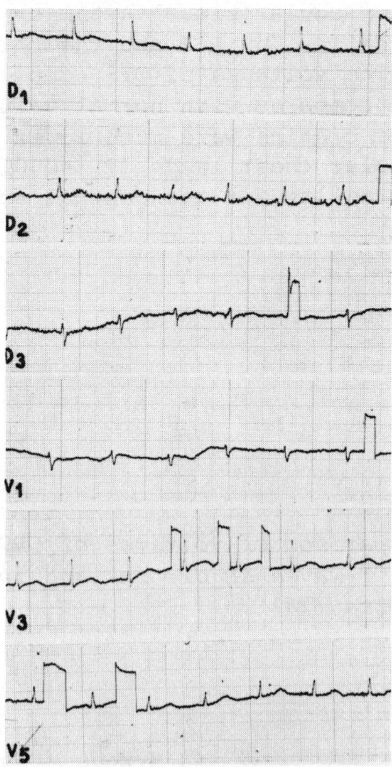

Fig. 8. ECG: low voltages of QRS and T (cretin n° 7)

X-ray Studies. X-rays of the control subject showed normal skeletal development for age according to the criteria used. X-rays of the cretins revealed for each instance obvious abnormalities, including marked retardation in bone maturation, epiphyseal and metaphyseal dysgenesis (31,32) and failure of modeling (33). The pelvis x-ray of a 20-year-old cretin appear in Fig. 9. The ilia are hypoplastic and there is bilateral dysgenesis of the femoral heads. Fig. 10 shows the knee x-ray of a 15-year-old cretin. There is marked epiphyseal dysgenesis in both femur and tibia, and failure of modeling.

The x-ray studies permit an estimate of the ages at which hypothyroidism appeared in six of eight cretins. In three, 15, 17 and 21 years old respectively at the time of study, the existence of epiphyseal dysgenesis in the knees proves that hypothyroidism developed before or around birth (33,34). In three others, 20, 21 and 25 years old respectively, normal knees but dysgenesis in the femoral heads indicate hypothyroidism before

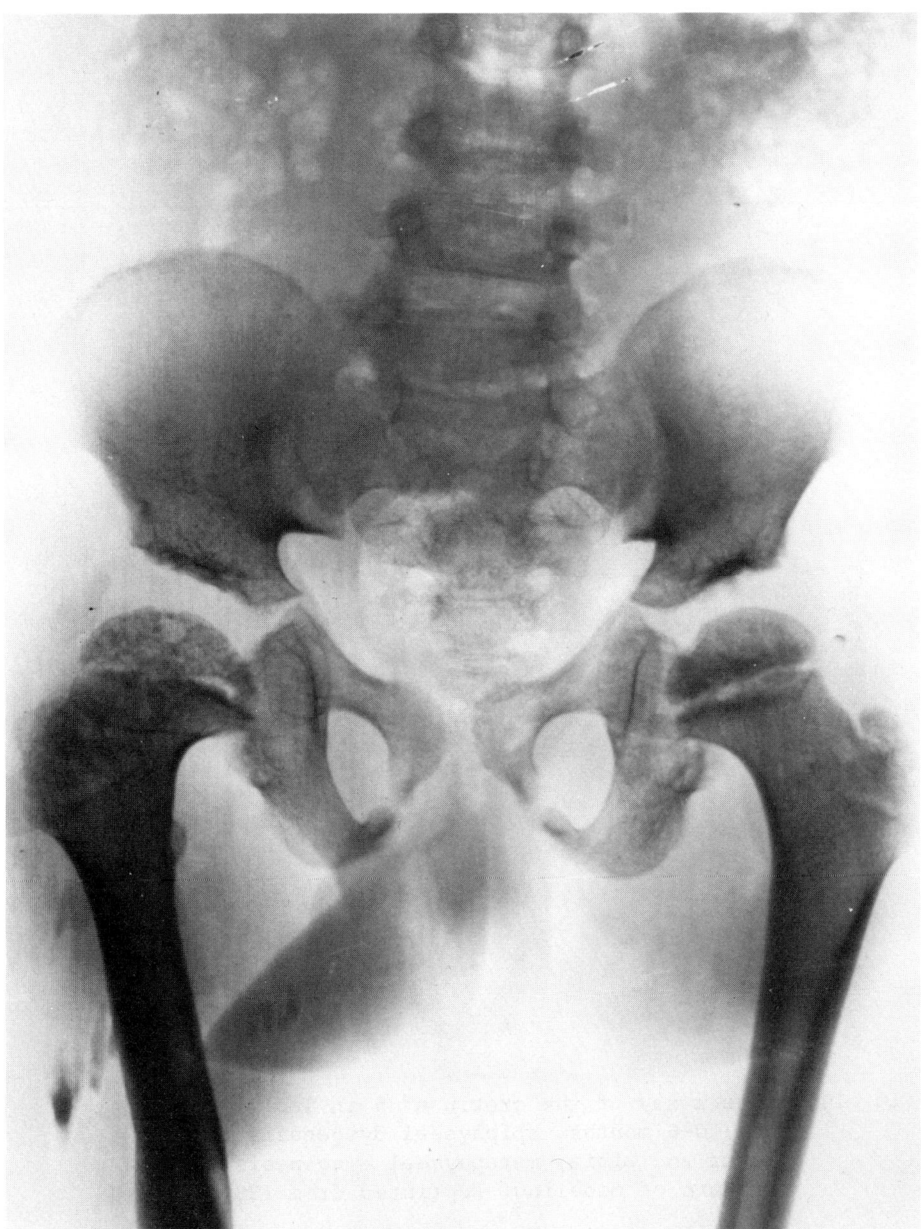

Fig. 9. Pelvis x-ray of the cretin n° 2 in Table IV. Subject aged 20 years, height 123 cm (75% of normal). PB^{127}I: 0.6 μg/100 ml. Hypoplastic ilia and marked retardation in bone maturation. Bilateral dysgenesis of the femoral heads.

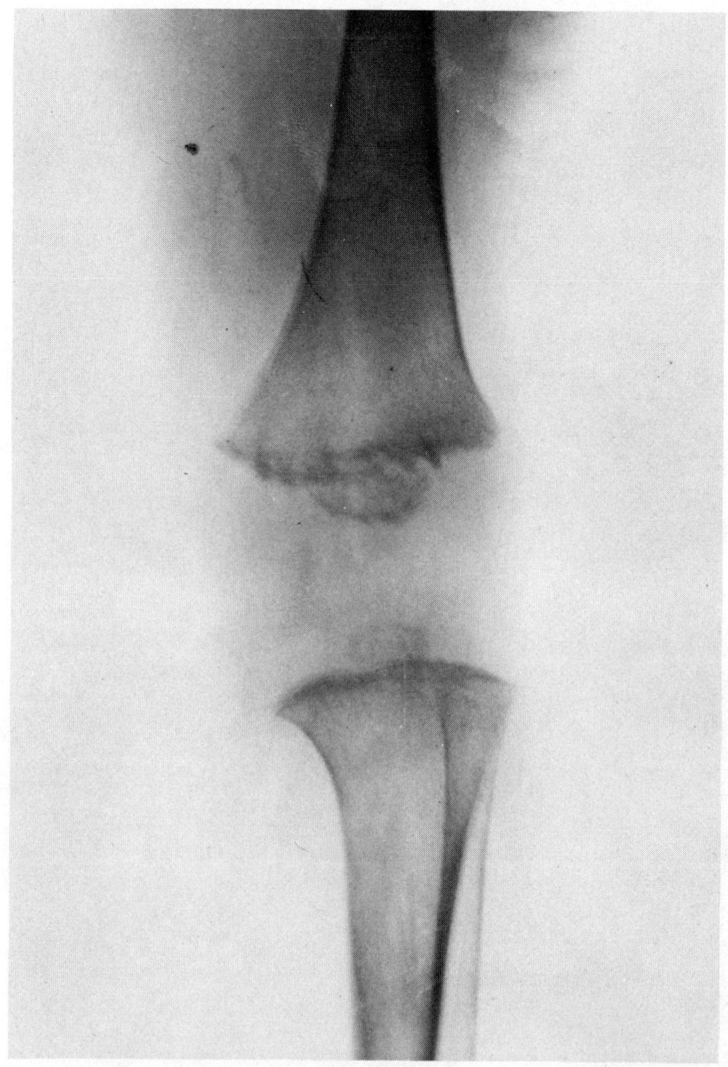

Fig. 10. Knee x-ray of the cretin n° 5 in Table II. Bone age: 0-6 months, epiphyseal dysgenesis in both femur and tibia, metaphyseal dysgenesis and failure of modeling. Reprinted from (29).

the age of one year (33,34). In the two remaining cretins, long-standing hypothyroidism is strongly implied by marked retardation of bone maturation, but the absence of dysgenesis on the available x-rays does not permit accurate establishment of the date of origin of the disease. The present x-ray data do not necessarily indicate that bone maturation was normal up to a particular age.

EFFECTS OF T_3 ON UPTAKE AND ECG IN CRETINS

The 24 hour ^{131}I thyroidal uptake recorded in six cretins before daily administration of 25 µg of T_3 and six days later are compared in Table IV. None of the subjects showed decreased uptake; on the contrary, it was slightly increased in three patients.

Treatment with T3 induced a significantly increased heart rate and voltages of QRS complexes and T waves in the unipolar chest leads in all the patients ($P < 0.05$). In the standard limb leads, the voltages of the T waves were significantly increased ($P < 0.005$), but the QRS complexes were not significantly modified ($P > 0.05$).

Table IV. Comparison of 24th hour ^{131}I thyroidal uptake in six cretins before the daily administration of 25 µg of T_3 and six days later

Cretins	24 hr thyroid uptake (% dose)	
	Before Treatment	After treatment
2	28.9	35.7
4	57.4	57.7
5	20.3	24.1
6	27.2	31.0
7	30.5	38.3
8	24.0	30.2

FIVE-YEAR FOLLOW-UP OF MYXEDEMATOUS CRETINS

The results for these five patients appear in Table V. Height retardation became more marked in two patients, and the uptake and PBI were stable or decreased with time. The differences observed between the first and the last results are not significant for the uptake ($P > 0.2$), but are significant for the PBI ($P < 0.05$).

Table V. Five-year follow-up of five myxedematous cretins

Subject	Age (yr)	Goiter	Height cm	Height %normal	24 hr. thyr uptake (% dose)	$PB^{127}I$ (μg/100ml)
2	15	0	105	73	---	---
	17	-	---	--	44.7	0.9
	20	0	123	75	28.9	0.6
3	12	0	82	65	36.4	2.0
	14	-	--	--	34.6	0.9
	17	0	87.5	56	23.2	1.0
4	10	0	87	73	----	---
	12	-	--	--	60.3	1.2
	15	0	104	73	57.4	1.0
7	20	0	109	69	27.5	1.4
	25	0	112.5	69	30.5	0.5
9	16	0	128	86	33.1	1.0
	21	0	132	81	29.8	0.6

DISCUSSION

This study has demonstrated the high prevalence of endemic cretinism in the north of Idjwi Island. The figure obtained was 1.1 percent of the population, but considering the probable high mortality of defective persons in the first years of life, the true incidence is probably underestimated.

Only 10 percent of the cretins were clinically of the type prevalent in other endemic areas in Oceania (6,12), South America (10,13,15), Asia (14) and Europe (3,4,9,11). In those cretins the predominant characteristics are idiocy and neurologic defects including spasticity and deaf-mutism. They are euthyroid, whereas 90 percent of the Idjwi cretins are clinically strikingly hypothyroid. Hypothyroidism is confirmed by a decrease of PBI and uptake in comparison with euthyroid inhabitants of the same area, and by the radiologic and electrocardiographic findings typical of severe hypothyroidism (33,35). It may be noted that extensor plantar responses of some of the Idjwi myxedematous cretins have been recorded as an isolated neurologic finding in myxedema (36), but are not necessarily indicative of generalized spasticity. Clinically and biologically, these patients are comparable to those in the Uele area previously observed by Bastenie _et al._ (16) and Dumont _et al._ (17,18). Although observed sporadically in other goitrous endemias (3,4,7,9-11), myxedematous cretinism seems particulary prevalent in Central Africa. Its association with endemic goiter is confirmed by the fact that no cretin has been encountered in southwest Idjwi where the prevalence of goiter is much lower than in the North (19). The populations in both areas belong to the same race and live in identical nutritional and socio-economic conditions (19).

The high values of $PB^{125}I$ at the 24th hour in cretins agree with those observed by Dumont _et al._ (18) and indicate considerable reduction of the intrathyroidal iodine pool. This indication is confirmed by our scanning studies which revealed small thyroid glands in normal position. The unusually high blood TSH levels indicated primary hypothyroidism. The hyperactivity of the pituitary agrees with the enlargement of the sella turcica previously observed in the Uele cretins by Belgian authors (38). The magnitude of this stimulation by the pituitary probably also explains why thyroidal uptake is not depressed after T_3 administration in small doses during a short period, as was also observed in the Uele cretins (18).

Our x-ray findings support the hypothesis of Dumont _et al._ that this type of cretinism could result from thyroid damage during fetal life or early infancy (18). They show that six out of eight cretins studied developed hypothryoidism by the time of birth or during the first months of life (33,34).

The studies, and particularly the scanning data, from the Uele and Idjwi areas suggest that hypothyroidism of the African myxedematous cretins could result from a degenerative process of the thyroid. This could explain the apparent aggravation of hypothyroidism evidenced in some Idjwi cretins. Such a degenerative process has been suggested by de Quervain and Wegelin in non-goitrous myxedematous cretins of Switzerland (3).

Two essential points must be borne in mind when considering the relation between the iodine deficiency and myxedematous cretinism on Idjwi. The first is that, as in other regions of the world, endemic cretinism exists in a region subjected to an extremely severe iodine deficiency. The role played by this deficiency in cretinism seems undeniable since no fresh cases of cretinism have been observed on the island since the introduction of iodized oil prophylaxis (39). The second point is that no case of cretinism is observed in the southern non-goitrous area of the island although this region suffers an iodine deficiency identical to that of the north.

The difference in goiter prevalence between the north and south of the island led us to the idea that the iodine deficiency on Idjwi constitutes a permissive but not a causal factor in the development of endemic goiter (19).

The question arises as to whether this hypothesis does not also apply in endemic cretinism, and whether an additional goitrogenic factor acting specifically in the north does not constitute the decisive factor in both endemic goiter and endemic cretinism.

Other investigations by Delange _et al_. (40) suggest that the factor in question could be thiocyanate, resulting from detoxification of considerable quantities of cyanide. Cyanide is known to be produced by hydrolysis of linamarin (41), which is contained in large quantities in cassava, a principal Idjwi dietary item (19). The hypothesis that this toxic factor, acting in conjunction with iodine deficiency, could directly influence the thyroid during critical periods of early development remains to be studied.

SUMMARY

Endemic cretins comprise 1.1 percent of the population of the northern part of Idjwi Island (Kivu Lake, Zaire Republic). Goiter is common in this part of the island, while no cretin was found in the southwest of the island where goiter is much less prevalent. Only 10 percent of the Idjwi cretins are clinically euthyroid, and most of those are deaf-mute and spastic. Ninety percent of the Idjwi cretins are severely hypothyroid, possibly as a result of a degenerative process of the thyroid gland occurring by birth or in early infancy. The cause of this phenomenon is unknown.

ACKNOWLEDGEMENTS

Supported in part by International Atomic Energy Agency, Vienna (Contract 216/R1/OB), Fonds de la Recherche Scientifique Medicale, Institut Belge d'Alimentation et de Nutrition, Belgium, and Euratom, Universities of Pisa and Brussels (Contract BIAC 026-63-4).

Our gratitude is primarily due to Dr. H.L. Vis, Director of the CEMUBAC Medical Team, who made this study possible.

The authors wish to acknowledge Professors M. Millet, R. Dubois and P.A. Bastenie, Brussels University and Dr. U. Rahm, Director of the IRSAC for their generous support, Dr. N. Cremer and Dr. O. Polis for their valuable help, Miss G. Willems and Mr. C. Walschaerts for their helpful technical assistance.

The authors wish to express their particular gratitude to Dr. J. M. Hershman, Veterans Administration Hospital, Birmingham, Alabama for having performed the TSH radioimmunoassays.

The chemical assays of iodine were kindly performed by Mrs. M. Camus.

Figures 5 and 6 are published by kind permission of the *Journal of Clinical Endocrinology and Metabolism*; Figures 3 and 10 by kind permission of *Hormone and Metabolic Research*.

DISCUSSION BY PARTICIPANTS

QUERIDO: Were there enzyme defects in this population?

DELANGE: Such studies were not performed in Idjwi. They were in the Uele cretins and they led to the conclusion that there was no enzyme defect (18). Furthermore, when a defect exists, hypothyroidism is usually accompanied by goiter. This is not the case in Idjwi.

STANBURY: I have photographs showing the same disorder extending to the Northwestern part of the Zaire Republic. This myxedematous type of cretinism extends for 1,500 miles across the country!

PHAROAH: You say that the myxedematous cretins are not deaf-mutes while the deaf-mutes are euthyroid. You stated in your paper of 1969 that you thought there were two types of cretins. Do you still maintain this?

DELANGE: We saw 99 patients with endemic cretinism. Eleven closely resemble the picture found in other countries, i.e. the nervous type. The other 88 are myxedematous cretins. However, we do not believe that there are only two types, but a whole spectrum of disease, as nicely pointed out by Dr. Ibbertson.

PITTMAN: Did any of the patients have gynecomastia? I wondered about abnormal prolactin levels.

DELANGE: I personally never saw it in the cretins in North Idjwi.

PITTMAN: And mycotic infections? We have seen hypothyroid people with mycoses which have disappeared when they were made euthyroid.

DELANGE: Mycotic infections are common in this country, whether the patient is hypothyroid or not.

IBBERTSON: In those deaf-mutes who were euthyroid, were PBIs low?

DELANGE: We have just one measurement, which is normal.

DUNN: Have you treated any of these hypothyroid cretins?

DELANGE: Yes, With T_3. We gave very small doses of T_3 - 25 micrograms per day for five days - as we were worried about their being severely hypothyroid. In two of them we had to stop because of the appearance of tachycardia and signs of ischemia in the ECG. There was only a slight improvement in the cretins.

We have organized a system of detection of cretinism in the newborns in the north. Until now we have detected 10 hypothyroid cretins below the age of six months. They were treated with T_3 with much better results.

ERMANS: A few months ago, I saw three young cretins in Idjwi treated with triiodothyronine from one year. Local conditions did not permit accurate control of the administration of the drug. However, the parents were surprised to observe that the children started walking and talking after a few months.

HERTZEL: What are other factors in morbidity in this population?

DELANGE: I do not have precise figures. The population has severe epidemic diseases of all kinds. The mortality in children is 70 percent before 10 years of age. This seems to be the same in goitrous and non-goitrous areas.

PRETELL: I think it is very speculative to say that in cretinism iodine is a permissive factor on the basis of previous fetal impairment of the thyroid gland. Also, it has been demonstrated that, in iodine deficiency, T_4 is low, but T_3 compensates at times.

DELANGE: The permissive role played by iodine deficiency in the etiology of both endemic goiter and cretinism is stressed by the fact that iodine deficiency is the same in the North and in the South of the island, and that both diseases exist only in the North. Concerning the second point, we have some preliminary data showing that the cretins have T_3 in their serum, but that the level is lower than in euthyroid people in the same region.

ERMANS: It seems likely that the primary impairment in this type of cretin corresponds to a degeneration of the thyroid tissue beginning during fetal life.

DELANGE: Our only evidence that the thyroid impairment began in fetal life is the x-rays of the knees. Dysgenesis of the knees is considered to be a sign of hypothyroidism beginning at the time of their formation in fetal life.

STANBURY: Epiphyseal dysgenesis does not mean fetal hypothyroidism, does it? It is the failure of the epiphysis to appear that means fetal hypothyroidism.

DELANGE: Dysgenesis is more specific of hypothyroidism than delayed bone maturation. If these x-rays had been taken in a European or American population, where it is known that the lower epiphysis of the femur is constituted at birth, I think we could have said that hypothyroidism began in fetal life. Dysgenesis in the lower femoral epiphysis, as far as I know, is the best way to make the diagnosis of fetal hypothyroidism. The point is that we have seen x-rays for only cretins at least 15 yr. old. It is possible that the appearance of the femoral epiphysis was delayed through local nutritional or other factors. For that reason, I say there was possibly fetal hypothyroidism.

BECKERS: You say that the thyroid is destroyed by a degenerative process, but you have also shown that there is a high turnover rate in these glands. What data shows that there is impairment in hormonal synthesis? For example, if you give physiological doses of iodine, does T_4 iodine increase? There may be just iodine deficiency. Is there any difference in iodine excretion compared with people in the same region?

DELANGE: The evidence that they cannot synthesize thyroid hormone is that they are hypothyroid using all the criteria one has. We have no data on iodine excretion compared with people in the same region. We also did not try giving them iodine.

ERMANS: All data collected about iodine metabolism in this type of cretins indicate that the thyroidal machinery is normal from a qualitative point of view. This point was clearly evidenced by Dumont *et al.* (18) who were able to discard all types of congenital defects. The failure is only related to a tremendous reduction of the iodine stores of these thyroid glands.

STANBURY: Isn't this what you would find in Hashimoto's thyroiditis or in a fibrosed thyroid? There is a small pool with a rapid turnover, an uptake lower than that in the community at large (where people do have goiter), and a very high TSH concentration.

PHAROAH: The thyroid scans surely do not look like those in degenerative disease. The gland is very small. With degeneration you get a larger gland with patchy degeneration.

DELANGE: We shouldn't say degenerative. All we can say is that there seems to be an extremely small active hormonal pool in the thyroid. Maybe there is degeneration. Maybe, for reasons we do not know, there was not normal growth.

COSTA: If it is an exhaustion atrophy, why is there not goiter in some period of life? As a second point, if this type of cretinism, sustained by thyroid atrophy, also disappears from a country after iodine prophylaxis, there would be two possible actions of iodine prophylaxis: first, correcting an iodine deficiency; secondly, to negate this unknown process causing atrophy of the gland.

DELANGE: Concerning exhaustion atrophy, it is only a working hypothesis (18). We have not followed the cretins every six months for 15 years to determine whether they had goiter and whether this subsequently disappeared. I cannot answer how iodine prophylaxis works.

KOENIG: We got the same results in our population of dwarfed cretins. In two whom we autopsied, we were impressed by the fibrous atrophy with small clumps of hyperactive, parenchymatous thyroid cells. When we worked these patients up with radioiodine, they showed the same results as patients with small ectopic thyroids - low uptake and quick turnover with a relatively high $PB^{131}I$ and relatively how $PB^{127}I$.

ERMANS: If these patients did produce goiter, as Dr. Costa suggested, they would not be cretins.

PRETELL: We have observed the same thing as Dr. Koenig has in some of our patients. We had a chance to study only four adults in our series. Was there a difference between older and younger patients in your series?

DELANGE: They were from six to 26 years old, with a mean age of 17 yr. There was no difference according to age.

IBBERTSON: In the Himalayas, we never found a cretin with hypothyroidism, presenting the same sort of picture you describe, who had responded to TSH by an increase in clearance or uptake. A number of the cretins who had goiters did show such an increase. It underlines that these patients do have an impaired synthetic capacity, because of lack of tissue.

REFERENCES

1. Report of the Pan American Health Organization Scientific Group on Research in Endemic Goiter. Pan American Health Organization Advisory Committee on Medical Research: PAHO, Washington, 1963.

2. Dumont, J.E.; Delange, F. and Ermans, A.M.: Endemic cretinism. In: Endemic Goiter. Report of the meeting of the PAHO Scientific Group on Research in Endemic Goiter held in Mexico, 1968. (J.G. Stanbury, ed.). PAHO Scientific Publication No. 193. Washington, 1969 pp 101-117

3. De Quervain, F. and Wegelin, C.: Der endemische Kretinism, Springer, Berlin, 1968.

4. Koenig, M.P.: Die Kongenitale Hypothyreose und der endemische Kretinismus. Springer, Berlin, 1968.

5. Clements, H.W.: Health significance of endemic goiter and related conditions. Endemic Goitre. Geneva, WHO:235-260, 1960.

6. Buttfield, I.H. and Hetzel, B.S.: Endemic cretinism in Eastern New Guinea. Austral. Ann. Med. 18:217-221, 1969.

7. Pharoah, P.O.D., Buttfield, I.H. and Hetzel, B.S.: Neurological damage to the fetus resulting from severe iodine deficiency during pregnancy. Lancet 1:308-310, 1971.

8. Fierro-Benítez, R.; Ramirez, I.; Estrella, E.; Querido, A. and Stanbury, J.B.: The effect of goiter prophylaxis with iodized oil on the prevention of endemic cretinism. Proceedings of the Sixth International Thyroid Conference, Vienna, 1970. p. 16.

9. Costa, A. and Mortara, M.: A review of recent studies of goiter in Italy. WHO Bull.22:493-502, 1960.

10. Lobo, L.C.G.; Pompeu, F. and Rosenthal, D.: Endemic Cretinism in Goiaz, Brazil. J. Clin. Endocrinol. Metab. 23:407-412, 1963.

11. Mortara, M. and Rubino, R.: Cretinismo Endemico - La Malattia - I suoi aspetti neurologici. Roma, Consiglia Nasionale delle Richerche (Quaderni de la Ricerca Scientifica No. 62), 1970. pp. 1-59.

12. Choufoer, J.C.; Van Rhijn, M. and Querido, A.: Endemic goiter in Western New Guinea. II. Clinical picture, incidence and pathogenesis of endemic cretinism. J. Clin. Endocrinol. Metab.25:385-402, 1965

13. Fierro-Benítez, R.; Stanbury, J.B.; Querido, A.; De Groot, L.J.; Alban, R. and Cordova, J.: Endemic cretinism in the Andean region of Ecuador. J. Clin. Endocrinol. Metab.30:228-236, 1970.

14. Srinivasan, S.; Subramanyan, T.A.V.; Sinha, A.; Deo, G. and Ramalingaswami, V.: Himalayan endemic deaf-mutism. Lancet 2: 176-178, 1964.

15. Stanbury, J.B.; Brownell, G.L.; Riggs, D.S.; Perinetti, H.; Itoiz, J. and Del Castillo, E.B.: Endemic Goiter, the Adaptation of Man to Iodine Deficiency. Harvard University Press, Cambridge, 1954.

16. Bastenie, P.A.; Ermans, A.M.; Thyrs, O.; Beckers, C.; Van Den Schrieck, H.G. and De Visscher, M.: Endemic goiter in the Uele region. III. Endemic cretinism. J. Clin. Endocrinol. Metab. 22:187-194, 1962.

17. Dumont, J.E.; Ermans, A.M. and Bastenie, P.: Thyroidal function in a goiter endemic. IV. Hypothyroidism and endemic cretinism. J. Clin. Endocrinol. Metab. 23:325-335, 1963.

18. Dumont, J.E.; Ermans, A.M. and Bastenie, P.A.: Thyroidal function in a goiter endemic. V. Mechanism of thyroid failure in the Uele endemic cretins. J. Clin. Endocrinol. Metab. 23:847-860, 1963.

19. Ermans, A.M.; Thilly, C.; Vis, H.L. and Delange, F.: Permissive nature of iodine deficiency in the development of endemic goiter. In: Endemic Goiter. Report of the meeting of the PAHO Scientific Group on Endemic Goiter held in Mexico, 1968 (J.B. Stanbury, ed.). PAHO Scientific Publication No. 193. Washington, 1969. pp.101-117.

20. Perez, C.; Schrimshaw, N.S. and Munoz, J.A.: Technique of endemic goitre surveys. In: Endemic Goitre. Geneva, WHO, 1960. pp. 369-384.

21. Boyden, S.V.: The absorption of proteins on erythrocytes treated with tannic acid and subsequent haemagglutination by antiprotein sera. J. Exp. Med. 93:107-120, 1951.

22. Bastenie, P.A.; Neve, P.; Bonnyns, M.; Van Haelst, L. and Chailly, M.: Clinical and pathological significance of asymptomatic atrophic thyroiditis. A condition of latent hypothyroidism. Lancet 1:915-918, 1967.

23. Odell, W.D.; Rayford, P.O. and Ross, G.T.: Simplified partially automated method for radioimmunoassay of human thyroid stimulating, growth, luteinizing and follicle-stimulating hormones. J. Lab. Clin. Med. 70:973-980, 1967.

24. Hershman, J.M.; Read, D.G.; Bailey, A.L.; Norman, V.D. and Gibson, T.B.: Effect of cold exposure on serum thyrotropin. J. Clin. Endocrinol. Metab. 30:430-434, 1970.

25. Snedecor, G.W. and Cochran, W.G.: Statistical Methods. The Iowa State University Press, Ames, 1968. p. 94.

26. Greulich, W.W. and Pyle, S.I.: Radiographic Atlas of Skeletal Development of the Hand and Wrist. Stanford University Press, Stanford, 1959.

27. Pyle, S.I. and Hoerr, N.L.: Radiographic Atlas of Skeletal Development of the Knee. Charles C. Thomas, Springfield, 1955.

28. Lepeschkin, E.: Modern Electrocardiography, Volume I, The Q-R-S-T-U- Complex. Wilkins Company, Baltimore,1951. p. 140.

29. Delange, F., and Ermans, A.M.: Further studies on endemic cretinism in Central Africa. Horm. Metab. Res. 3:431, 1971

30. Delange, F.; Hershman, J.M. and Ermans, A.M.: Relationship between the serum thyrotropin level, the prevalence of goiter and the pattern of iodine metabolism in Idjwi Island. J. Clin. Endocrinol. Metab. 33: 261-268, 1971.

31. Megevand, A.; Mathieu, H. and Royer, P.: Anomalies squelettiques et troubles du métabolisme du calcium dans les insuffisances thyroïdiennes de l'enfant. In: Les Hypothyroïdies. (F. Bamatter and A. Megevand, eds.). XVIIIème Congrès de l'Association des Pédiâtres de Langue Française. S. Karger, Berlin 1961. p. 205.

32. Caffey, J.: Pediatric X-ray Diagnosis. Year Book Medical Publishers, Berlin 1967.

33. Andersen, H.J.: Studies of hypothyroidism in children. Acta Paediatr. Suppl. 125, 1961.

34. Wilkins, L.: Epiphyseal dysgenesis associated with hypothyroidism. Amer. J. Dis. Child. 61:13-34, 1941.

35. Zondek, H.: The electrocardiogram in myxedema. Brit. Heart J. 26:227-232, 1964.

36. Nickel, S.N. and Frame, B.: Neurologic manifestations of myxedema. Neurology 8:511-517, 1958.

37. McGirr, E.M. and Hutchinson, J.H.: Dysgenesis of the thyroid gland as a cause of cretinism and juvenile myxedema. _J. Clin. Endocrinol. Metab._ 15:668-679, 1955.

38. Melot, G.J.; Jeanmart-Nichez, L.; Dumont, J.; Ermans, A.M. and Bastenie, P.A.: Les aspects radiologiques du crétinisme endémique. _J. Belg. Radiol._ 45:385-403, 1962.

39. Thilly, C.; Delange, F. and Ermans, A.M. Unpublished data.

40. Delange, F. and Ermans, A.M.: Role of dietary goitrogen in the etiology of endemic goiter on Idjwi Island. _Amer. J. Clin. Nutr._ 24:1354-1360, 1971.

41. Conn, E.E.: Cyanogenic glucosides. _J. Agr. Food. Chem._ 17:519-526, 1969.

42. Delange, F.; Ermans, A.M.; Vis. H.L. and Stanbury, J.B.: Endemic cretinism in Idjwi Island. _J. Clin. Endocrinol. Metab._ In press.

A NOTE ON IODINE DEFICIENCY AND THYROID FUNCTION IN "NEUROLOGICAL" CRETINISM IN HIGHLAND ECUADOR

Rodrigo Fierro-Benítez

Departamento de Radioisotopos

Escuela Politecnica Nacional, Quito, Ecuador

Studies on retarded children in two villages in highland Ecuador (La Esperanza and Tocachi) have shown no statistical relationship between mental developmental age and thyroid size. Cretins without goiter had mental ages ranging from two to four yr, whereas those with goiter of large size also had mental ages ranging from two to four.

Ten typical cretins were brought to a hospital in Quito for study of iodine metabolism. Prior to any treatment, a mean value of 10 μg of iodine per day was found in the urine. Only one of these 10 cretins had clinical characteristics suggestive of a hypothyroid state.

Cretins without goiter had high values for $PB^{131}I$, whereas those with goiter had somewhat lower values. The uptake of radioactive iodine was extremely high and the turnover rate of iodine in the thyroid was approximately 10 times normal. The quantity of iodine stored in the glands proved, on kinetic analysis, to be on average lower than normal, but the rate of loss of iodine from the thyroid was sharply elevated above normal.

Administration of thyrotropic hormone resulted in uniformly increased radioactive iodine uptake and either no change or an increase in the calculated quantity of iodine in the thyroid. These observations suggest that the thyroid was already well-stimulated by endogenous thyrotrophic hormone. In two instances

*Recording of the remarks made by Dr. Fierro, edited by the Editors.

a standard triiodothyronine suppression test was done, which proved to be positive in one and negative in the other. With only one exception, the T_3 resin uptake test was normal. Plasma proteins were normal in all, as were measurements of cholesterol. Low plasma levels of carotene were consistent with the limited vitamin A in the diet. Only one patient had a distinctly low value for protein bound iodine. This was 2.8 μg per 100 ml. This same patient had a retarded Achilles ankle relaxation time; those of the rest were normal.

Histological studies on skeletal muscle biopsies disclosed an absence of any disturbance in muscle fiber architecture. Slight to moderate atrophy with reduction of muscle fiber diameter was observed in seven of the 10 patients. These patients did not have the Hoffman syndrome, in that all seven had diminished diameter of the muscle groups. Some foci of degeneration were seen in longitudinal sections, but there is no reason to think ipso facto that these differed from other members of the community without evidence of retardation. Thus, the defectives of this region do not differ from the normal members of the community in terms of protein bound iodine concentration of the serum, triiodothyronine resin uptake or Achilles reflex, and muscle changes are minimal.

To emphasize this point we have studied in detail the three most severely affected patients in our series. These subjects had the most retarded speech, the most impaired motor coordination and one of these was clinically hypothyroid. Thus, there appeared to be little, if any, relationship between the actual and presently existing thyroid states and the classic manifestations of neurological endemic cretinism.

What is the relationship between the status of children and their mothers? In the present series 477 children were born of normal mothers, 23 defective children were born of normal mothers, i.e., five percent. Twenty-six normal children have been born of defective mothers, and 16 defective children of defective mothers. Thus, 50 percent of the children who are defective were born of defective mothers. Thus, there appears to be a very clear and important tendency for a mother who is a cretin to have a child who is defective.

DISCUSSION BY PARTICIPANTS

ERMANS: I am impressed with your figures of plasma $PB^{131}I$, which for several cases reached extremely high values. These are not the usual values found in endemic goiter in response to iodine deficiency. This implies marked reduction of the intrathyroid stores and also that these glands have been partially destroyed.

PRETELL: There is a significant difference in the data. With Fierro's subjects, the uptakes are significantly higher than the normal population.

ROSMAN: The muscle changes that Dr. Fierro showed, like those I showed this morning, can be due to a variety of disorders. They may represent disuse atrophy. It is critical to determine when they appear, if they are reversible and whether they are due to muscle or neurological disease. Small foci of atrophied fibers can occur in either situation. Muscle lesions in hypothyroidism have been of interest for many years. There exists a syndrome, called Kocher-Debré-Semelaigne, in which hypothyroid infants have very large muscles that appear normal histologically (1).

REFERENCES

1. Najjar, S.S. and Nachman, H.S.: Hypothyroidism with muscular "hypertrophy," (Kocher-Debré-Semelaigne Syndrome). J. Pediat. 66: 901, 1965.

SIMILARITIES AND DIFFERENCES BETWEEN SPORADIC AND ENDEMIC CRETINISM

Basil S. Hetzel

Department of Social and Preventive Medicine, Monash University, Alfred Hospital, Melbourne, Australia

There has until recently been confusion between the two types of cretinism - sporadic and endemic cretinism. A brief historical review helps to place the present position in perspective while comparing cretinism in the various areas.

The term "cretinism" was used in the latter half of the eighteenth century by European authors - and notably in Diderot's <u>Encyclopédie</u> (1754) to describe "an imbecile who is deaf, dumb, with a goiter hanging down to the waist," known to be widely prevalent in Switzerland, Southern France and Northern Italy - among people living in the valleys of the Alps and Pyrenees. Typical examples of the Alpine cretins are shown in illustrations to the Report of the Sardinian Royal Commission published in 1848 (1). Earlier this year, I had an opportunity to peruse this impressive report by courtesy of Dr. W. R. Trotter of London. I was struck by certain features of these illustrated Alpine cretins which are still noticeable today in New Guinea.

The constant association with endemic goiter led to use of the term "endemic cretinism". In fact, some did not have a palpable thyroid, though usually a goiter was present.

The condition known as "sporadic cretinism" dates from the recognition by the English clinicians Curling (2) and Fagge (3) of a condition of thyroid deficiency associated with retarded physical and mental development which is corrected by use of thyroid preparations. This condition may be associated with goiter as in the classical biosynthetic defects first recognized by Stanbury and Querido (9), without goiter when associated with a failure of development of the thyroid during fetal life, or with the presence of only a fragmentary thyroid at the base of the tongue. This condition of sporadic cretinism is widespread throughout the world - it exhibits no geographical localization.

Curling and Fagge assumed that sporadic cretinism was the same disease as endemic cretinism. Kocher followed this, and until recently most English and American authors have done the same (4). However, McCarrison in 1908 (5) clearly described two clinical pictures in Himalayan cretins. The first, "nervous cretinism" was characterized by mental deficiency, deaf-mutism, ataxia with spasticity, and included knock-knee without hypothyroidism. A second type "myxedematous cretinism" was characterized by hypothyroidism and some mental deficiency. Deaf-mutism was present in 87 percent of the 203 cretins he described.

In recent years, Costa and his colleagues (6) have studied cretins from the Alpine valleys of Northern Italy and have shown clearly that they differ from sporadic cretins. In general the Alpine cretins were clinically euthyroid, unlike the sporadic cretin. The alpine cretins were mentally retarded deaf-mutes with gross neurological deformities similar to those originally described by the Sardinian Commission from the same area.

DeQuervain and Wegelin (7), however, considered that some degree of hypothyroidism was present in the endemic cretins studied by them at Berne in Switzerland. Nevertheless, they were forced to admit that some of the manifestations, particularly deaf-mutism, could not be attributed to hypothyroidism because deaf-mutism as they pointed out, is not a manifestation of sporadic cretinism. More recent studies by Koenig (8) have confirmed that clinical hypothyroidism occurs only in a minority of cretins in Switzerland.

Stanbury and Querido (9) defined a cretin as suffering from "permanent retardation in development of the skeleton or central nervous system resulting from thyroid deficiency which existed during fetal or early neonatal life." Subsequently, Costa (10) reiterated the view that endemic cretins were not necessarily hypothyroid in the light of his own recent studies in the Alpine valleys of the Piedmont.

Since 1960, there has been a spate of studies made outside Europe - notably in the Congo, the Himalayas, New Guinea and South America. The main features of endemic cretinism reported from these areas will now be reviewed.

CRETINISM IN THE CONGO

Excellent detailed descriptions by the active Belgian group are now available from two areas - the Uele (11,12) and Idjwi Island (13).

The overall incidence of cretinism was 1.1 percent of the population of the Northern part of Idjwi Island, and was associated with a 54 percent goiter rate. 99 cretins were seen, of whom 11 were clinically euthyroid. Nine of the 11 were deaf-mute and seven had a spastic diplegia of the lower limbs. The remaining 88 showed gross clinical evidence of hypothyroidism including growth and mental retardation, failure of maturation of the features, dry scaly skin, prominent abdomen (often with an umbilical hernia), and delay in sexual development. There was a long relaxation time in the tendon reflex. Apart from slow movement, neurological signs were essentially normal. None of these hypothyroid cretins showed deaf-mutism. The clinical diagnosis of hypothyroidism was confirmed in 21 of these hypothyroid cretins by x-ray evidence of delayed bone maturation with epiphyseal and metaphyseal dysgenesis. The findings suggested that hypothyroidism had appeared around birth or during the first months of life. Electrocardiography showed low voltage QRS complexes and T waves which were significantly increased by administration of triiodothyronine for five days.

Serum PSIs were lower (1.3± 0.2 μg per 100 ml) than in euthyroid controls (3.7± 0.1 μg per 100 ml) in the same area. Very high blood TSH levels (mean 580± 125 μμ per ml) using immunoassay were observed consistent with gross hypothyroidism. Thyroid scannings suggested a small thyroid in the normal position.

The clinical and laboratory findings in these hypothyroid patients are entirely consistent with the clinical picture of sporadic cretinism. As pointed out by the authors, the condition in the Congo differs from that of all other endemic areas in the very high proportion of hypothyroid cretins seen. It is important to note that the hypothyroid picture was not associated with deaf-mutism or spastic diplegia. These features were only observed in euthyroid subjects.

The condition appears to have arisen at or in the first few months after birth, and the authors suggest that it may well be due to a toxic substance from the food. A thiocyanate - possibly a goitrogen - is produced by detoxication of cyanide resulting from the hydrolysis of linamarin, a major constituent of cassava which is consumed in large quantities in the diet.

CRETINISM IN NEW GUINEA

Descriptions available from both East and West New Guinea reveal an identical clinical picture (14,15,16). In contrast to the Congo, clinical hypothyroidism was not seen in these cretins. However, varying degrees of mental deficiency, deaf-mutism and spasticity were noted in both areas, with a smooth skin. Squint also occurred. X-rays of the hips revealed normal femoral heads in 23 cretins in East New Guinea and no evidence of electrocardiograph abnormalities associated with myxedema. An overall incidence of 2.5 percent was noted in one area of Eastern New Guinea (16), similar to rates observed elsewhere (4).

Plasma PBIs were lower (1.8 ± 1.4 μg per 100 ml) in goitrous cretins than in goitrous subjects without neurological signs (2.9 ± 1.7 μg per 100 ml). Radioactive iodine uptake was also lower in the goitrous cretins. The lack of discharge of ^{131}I following perchlorate administration excluded an organification defect.

The picture described in New Guinea is therefore characterized by multiple neurologic defects. Detailed studies have revealed both perceptive and conductive components in the deafness (15). The spastic diplegia produces a characteristic gait and stance with hypotonia which enables these subjects to be readily spotted by the experienced observer (15,16). Short stature was noted only in a minority of these subjects [26 percent of 254 cases seen in Eastern New Guinea (10)] and may well have been due to malnutrition. In only one instance (an infant aged one year seen just before death) was a clinically hypothyroid subject seen in Eastern New Guinea. Adult hypothyroidism is seen in Eastern New Guinea but it is uncommon and not geographically associated with endemic goiter. The possibility of severely hypothyroid subjects being missed in the surveys can be excluded, but it is possible that they would not survive long in the rigorous environment of the Highlands of New Guinea (16). The clinical picture observed is therefore in marked contrast to that described in the Congo.

CRETINISM IN SOUTH AMERICA

Detailed descriptions are available from Brazil (17,18) and Ecuador (19,20). In Brazil in 1963, Lobo *et al.* reported 24 neurologic cretins and two hypothyroid cretins of 26 studied in Goias. Subsequently, a more extensive survey of Mato Grosso State revealed 0.17 percent cretinism and 0.33 percent deaf-mutism in a sample of 1,525 families (18). This was associated with goiter rates of 61 percent in females and 35 percent in males.

Lobo *et al.* (18) comment on the similarity of the picture seen in Brazil to that observed in New Guinea and in Switzerland.

In Ecuador, studies in two separate areas (19,20) revealed significant and usually severe neurological damage in cretin subjects with mental retardation, imparied hearing, and spastic diplegia of variable severity. The subjects were usually not clinically hypothyroid although they had large goiters with low levels of circulating thyroid hormone. A few clinically hypothyroid subjects were seen with low serum PBI and grossly elevated TSH levels (20). There were many other people in the same communities with lesser degrees of neurological damage with mental deficiency, deaf-mutism or short stature. The predominant picture was therefore that of neurological damage, although clinical hypothyroidism was seen in a small minority of cases. Administration of triiodothyronine to a series of neurologic cretins had no effect on their clinical state (20) or laboratory findings in contrast to the effects on the Congo cretins (13). This further indicates a clinical picture distinct from hypothyroid cretinism.

CRETINISM IN THE HIMALAYAS

The original observations of McCarrison in 1908 of two types of cretinism were confirmed in 1934 by Stott and Gupta (21). Stott *et al.* (22) reported variable rates of deaf-mutism ranging from 150 per 10,000 in the Himalayan region to 50 per 10,000 further south. Srinivasan *et al.* (23) described 20 subjects with deaf-mutism and varying degrees of mental retardation without clinical hypothyroidism in the state of Bihar in the Himalayan foothills.

In a recent extensive study in Nepal, Ibbertson *et al.*(24) found a similar clinical pattern of cretinism and deaf-mutism to that described by McCarrison in Gilgit. The Sherpa population of Nepal have an ethnic origin entirely different from the Indian population. Cretinism and deaf-mutism were noted in 5.9 percent (28) and 4.7 percent (22) respectively of a group of 475 Sherpas. The incidence of cretinism was higher in one village (Porche) which had a much higher goiter rate. All cretins were considered to be clinically hypothyroid while 50 percent with deaf-mutism alone were also judged to be hypothyroid. Hearing loss was perceptive in type; 19 of the 28 cretins were deaf-mutes. Six cretins had upper motor neuron lesions with increased tendon reflexes. These findings are somewhat at variance with the previous reports from other areas. The association of deaf-mutism and upper motor neuron lesions was not observed with gross hypothyroidism in the Congo and yet in these "myxedematous cretins" in Nepal these features were often associated. Convincing objective evidence of hypothyroidism in these Nepalese cases is not provided in the published report, although observations were made of serum cholesterol, ECG voltage and ankle reflex time. Final assessment of these findings must await such evidence, including serum TSH levels, as the Belgian group provided for the Congo (13).

In reviewing their findings, Ibbertson _et al_. (24) refer to the two types of cretinism but emphasize the continuing spectrum of physical, mental and functional abnormality. The higher incidence of cretinism in the village of Porche might have been associated with higher altitude, more inter-marriage or a mild goitrogen in the form of buckwheat.

DISCUSSION

This review of cretinism in the four different areas reveals two distinct clinical pictures - one similar to that of sporadic cretinism and characterized by classical hypothyroidism with growth retardation, the other characterized by multiple neurological defects including deaf-mutism and spastic diplegia _without_ clinical hypothyroidism. The first pattern is characteristic of the Congo, being observed in 90 percent of cases seen in the northern part of Idjwi Island (13). The second is characteristic of East and West New Guinea where varying degress of it are observed without any evidence of clinically hypothyroid subjects (14,15,16). In South America, the neurological picture predominates, with a minority of hypothyroid cretins (19,20). In the Himalayas, the predominant clinical picture also appears to be predominantly one of neurological damage as described in earlier reports (5,21,22,23). The recent study from Nepal (24) suggests a higher incidence of hypothyroidism but further data are needed to substantiate this finding.

The question that arises is whether these two clinical varieties are related or not in their cause and pathogenesis. They are both clearly associated with endemic goiter and iodine deficiency in the Congo and New Guinea. However, it does appear from the recent studies that the two clinical pictures do not overlap. The same patient does not usually show both gross clinical hypothyroidism and the neurologic lesions of deafness and spastic diplegia. This contrasts with McCarrison's original description and also with the recent report from Nepal. At this stage, McCarrison's criteria for diagnosis of hypothyroidism cannot be verified. Further data are required substantiating the association of clinical hypothyroidism and deafness in Nepal.

In the first condition, as seen in the Congo, reversal of certain hypothyroid features following administration of triiodothyronine has been demonstrated. In neurologic cretinism, the clinical picture has been unaffected by triiodothyronine, a finding to be expected in view of the euthyroid clinical state. The association of euthyroidism with gross lowering of the level of circulating thyroid hormones can possibly be explained by secretion of increased amounts of triiodothyronine. This can be presumed from the only slightly elevated levels of TSH (25) in the face of extremely low levels of circulating thyroid hormones usually associated with gross clinical hypothyroidism and gross excess of TSH outside of endemic goiter areas. Evidence of this increase in T_3 secretion is available from the Uele studies (26) and also from Nepal (24) using chromotographic procedures. More data are being obtained from Eastern New Guinea using the recently developed immunoassay of T_3. Increase in secretion of T_3 in experimental animals fed iodine deficient diets has also been shown (27,28).

The development of gross clinical hypothyroidism, notably in the Congo and to a minor extent elsewhere, indicates failure of the adaptive thyroid secretory mechanism which is usually adequate to maintain clinical euthyroidism under conditions of severe iodine deficiency. This failure may occur because of loss of thyroid tissue from various destructive processes, because of a goitrogen or possibly from the severity of the iodine deficiency itself. In the Congo, decrease in thyroid size has been observed. There is also some evidence of the presence of a goitrogen from the diet, which may account for the gross discrepancy between the clinical appearance there and elsewhere (13). Such a factor might operate in other endemic goiter areas as an adjuvant to the primary factor of iodine deficiency and account for a low incidence of hypothyroidism. The clinical picture of hypothyroid cretinism in the Congo is consistent with the occurrence of hypothyroidism around birth or during the first few months of life (13), which would be consistent with the possibility of goitrogen.

The lack of clinical overlap between the two types of cretin observed in the Congo and elsewhere makes it difficult to resist the view that the neurologic euthyroid cretin represents an entirely different entity with a distinct pathogenesis, as suggested by Dumont (29). The possibility of fetal hypothyroidism has been discussed extensively in previous papers (9,15). However, recent investigations (30) fail to reveal evidence of fetal hypothyroidism under conditions of severe iodine deficiency in Peru.

The question of whether severe iodine deficiency itself produces fetal damage has been examined in Eastern New Guinea (31). The opportunity to set up a controlled trial was provided by iodized oil administration by injection of alternate families in a population of 8,000 living in an area where neurologic cretinism was known to occur. Subsequent follow-up over four years revealed 26 "neurologic cretins" out of 534 children born to mothers who had not received iodized oil - the mothers of five of these retarded infants were noted to be pregnant at the start of the trial. In comparison, seven cases of neurologic cretinism occurred among 498 children born to mothers who had been treated with iodized oil - in six of these seven cases the mother was noted to be pregnant when the trial began. The clinical diagnosis of neurologic cretinism was made in these infants if there was delay in reaching motor milestones together with deafness or squint. The diagnosis was made without knowledge of whether a mother had received iodized oil or saline. Detailed findings on these infants are presented elsewhere (31,32). These results suggest that correction of iodine deficiency with iodized oil is effective in the prevention of neurologic cretinism if given before conception. The findings suggest that severe iodine deficiency in the mother produces neurological damage during fetal development which results in the clinical entity of neurological cretinism.

There is a great dearth of information regarding the neuropathology of neurologic cretinism. Clinical studies (33) suggest that cerebral cortical and eighth nerve damage are responsible for mental retardation and deafness. The frequent presence of squint suggests associated brain stem damage. None of these features occurs in sporadic hypothyroid cretinism. They cannot be attributed to clinical hypothyroidism. Rather they appear to represent a distinct entity, "iodine deficient embryopathy". This condition may eventually be found to occur under other circumstances than in association with endemic goiter.

Endemic cretinism therefore includes two distinct clinical entities with different etiology and pathogenesis. The common entity, neurological cretinism, predominates in the Himalayas, New Guinea and South America. The less common entity is hypothyroid cretinism which is indistinguishable clinically from sporadic cretinism and predominates in the African Congo.

SUMMARY

Sporadic cretinism is a condition of thyroid gland deficiency associated with retarded physical and mental development. It can be corrected by use of thyroid hormone preparations. It is not geographically localized.

Endemic cretinism is geographically associated with endemic goiter and iodine deficiency. It disappears following correction of iodine deficiency. It includes two clinical entities - neurologic cretinism characterized by mental retardation, deafness, disorders of gait and stance, with absence of clinical hypothyroidism, and hypothyroid cretinism which is indistinguishable clinically from sporadic cretinism.

DISCUSSION BY PARTICIPANTS

STANBURY: Would Dr. Fierro comment on hypothyroidism among the Ecuadorean cretins? I have been impressed at the change which occurs with many of them when they are given thyroid medication. That is the acid test.

FIERRO: The problem remains very complex to me after checking the results of thyroid treatment on early diagnosed defective children. There were three types of behaviors. The first, those deficient infants whose DQ's (Development Quotients), in spite of early diagnosis and continued treatment, remain severely retarded. Secondly, subjects whose DQ's rose slightly as a consequence of merely an increment of motor maturation. There was not any increment of the other neuromotor functions with the treatment, i.e. speech or intellectual capacity. The third type, children whose DQ's rose to close to the low normal range, because all the neuromotor functions were improved. In the first type the major problem was irreversible neurological damage. In the second the improvement could be explained because there was a hypothyroid component besides some less severe neurological damage. In the third type, the major problem was the hypothyroid component.

The different severity of neurological damage and the response to thyroid treatment could be attributed to several factors besides the hypothyroid component, i.e. protein malnutrition, vitamin A deficiency, etc.

ERMANS: On Idjwi Island where prophylaxis with iodized oil was introduced five years ago, no more cretins have been born.

HORNABROOK: One of the things that seems to be obscuring the picture is a clinical conclusion based on an epidemiological procedure. The question of how the series was selected is very important. In Eastern New Guinea, and I think I speak for everyone working there, the series was selected by the community being asked to produce people with a deficiency, so there is a bias toward deaf-mutism or mental defect. Some of the other series may be similarly biased.

QUERIDO: The figures from Western New Guinea are an exception. There each hut has been investigated.

BUTTFIELD: The same thing is true in the case of our first 254 patients. We looked in every village and at every person.

HORNABROOK: I am sure that you did not examine every individual in a thorough neurological way. It would not be possible to detect defects in near-normal people in the time that was taken for that study.

HETZEL: I do not think that this affects the point i.e., that clinical hypothyroidism, as it is usually recognized, does not appear to occur in New Guinea in relation to endemic goiter. There are, of course, sporadic instances of this in Eastern New Guinea. We have admittedly only done 30-odd TSH assays. They are nowhere near the levels in Zaire; we have seen them up to 50 or 70 μμg.

STANBURY: But if you treat these people, a lot of them do change, which is important.

BUTTFIELD: Not to the extent they did in Zaire. When the group in the original description was given thyroxine they did not improve. I have seen at least two who were hypothyroid and died.

DELANGE: First, as to the diagnosis of hypothyroidism in cretins on Idjwi Island Dr. Stanbury and I tried to find later, by looking into the huts, if cretins who could not walk were missed in the survey. We did not find any. Secondly, in field surveys it may be difficult to make a clinical diagnosis of hypothyroidism. On the best days, we saw around 600 people a day. If we missed some, the prevalence of hypothyroidism would only increase.

PITTMAN: What is needed is a reliable chemical marker. Even if one uses a clinical trial, what he ends up with is a vague impression of change. It seems to me that high serum TSH is a marker for hypothyroidism, although I know there is argument about this.

HETZEL: We do have some data that indicates that from 10 or 20 to 100 is borderline. Some myxedematous cretins go up to 900.

QUERIDO: We agree that the picture in both sides of New Guinea and in Ecuador is one entity. The Zaire people come up with another clinical picture, and Ibbertson reports 60 percent clinical hypothyroidism and dwarfs. One can put the question whether the picture seen in Zaire is indeed endemic cretinism. If one reads the McCarrison 1908 paper in Lancet (5) and compares the histology of the thyroid gland with Wydler's description on the Swiss endemia (34) it is identical. In the Swiss endemia many cretins were seen with thyroid atrophy, identical to those described by McCarrison. Therefore in certain endemias destruction of the thyroid occurs. One has to assume that what Dr. Ibbertson observed in Nepal is identical to McCarrison's observations. This suggests that the Zaire picture is also present in other endemias, but occurs in the Zaire in an isolated form. Dr. Koenig, does atrophy of the thyroid disappear with iodine prophylaxis?

KOENIG: All I can say is that the few cretins who have died showed some type of fibrous atrophy as described by A. Wydler (34).

QUERIDO: You stated that no new cretins were born in the past twenty years in Switzerland. This suggests that thyroid atrophy has also disappeared with iodine prophylaxis. The question then is, will the Zaire abnormalities also disappear with iodine prophylaxis?

HETZEL: You are saying that the endemics in the Himalayas, New Guinea, and Switzerland can be reconciled. The outstanding thing is that Zaire is different.

BUTTFIELD: In the early group in New Guinea, there was no difference between the saline-treated and iodine-treated groups in death rate and in hypothyroidism. The only thing is that those people who had a goiter which disappeared after iodine therapy were in a better condition to work. Also in those people who had T_3-resin uptakes performed, we consistently found the means within the normal range. Dr. Delange told me that his T_3-resin uptakes were below the normal range in Zaire. With all its imperfections, to me this is the one test that gives the information we need about thyroid status. TSH does not.

PITTMAN: But the T_3-resin uptake can be normal in subjects with advanced myxedema; it is really a very gross and insensitive test. I think the main use is to rule out thyroxine-binding globulin deficiency in patients with low hormone levels. Serum TSH is the first hormonal or other abnormality to show up as a patient begins to develop primary hypothyroidism, even before circulating T_4 levels become very low.

IBBERTSON: Our T_3-resins were below the normal range. This indicated thyroxine deficiency, but a significant metabolic contribution from triiodothyronine is not excluded.

KOENIG: Smith *et al.* (35) in Baltimore in 1957 described the picture in severely hypothyroid children with oligophrenia, severe mental retardation, spasticity, and practically everything the neurologic picture in New Guinea shows. We have since seen in our department about six severely-invalidized people with congenital hypothyroidism in whom bone age would be below eight months of pregnancy. When we examined them at age two to 10, they had the same kind of motor neuron deficiency described in endemic cretinism. That is why I think there is a similarity, to say the least. They are never deaf.

HETZEL: I think it is fairly obvious that there is a great difference between this entity - a rare neurological complication of gross hypothyroidism - and what we are talking about in endemic goiter areas.

ROSMAN: The Smith _et al_. paper, to which Dr. Koenig referred, reported 128 patients. A number showed neurological signs but these were not well detailed. There subsequently was a study of institutionalized cretins in Michigan (36); again, the neurological signs were not well described. I have personally examined about two dozen cretins at the Fernald State School in Waverley, Massachusetts. Many showed minor abnormalities on neurological examination. All of the patients had been treated with thyroid hormone, however, and many of them were in their 50's and 60's, ages when minor neurological abnormalities are not unusual. In summary, there has been no good study of the neurology of sporadic cretinism in the United States.

ERMANS: In answering Dr. Querido's question, what is now seen in Zaire is identical to what was seen by McCarrison in Switzerland, and by Ibbertson, and it will probably disappear with iodine prophylaxis. In the region of Idjwi in which we have been giving iodized salt therapy for five years, no more cretins are born.

IBBERTSON: An important implication from that observation is that the thyroid atrophy is dependent on elemental iodine deficiency.

HETZEL: In Zaire have you given iodized oil to a cretin and observed improvement in function? That is what you have to show.

DELANGE: We did not treat them with iodized oil, because we know that large doses of iodine given to someone who has a small pool of iodine in the thyroid may block iodine organification. We have shown that with only two mg of iodine given to euthyroid Idjwi subjects one may block the thyroid

KOENIG: In the work of Wydler (34) quoted by Professor Querido, 111 thyroid glands of cretins were studied. The author ended by saying the same thing that De Quervain and Wegelin in a book published in 1936 (37), said - there is no such thing as a typical cretinous gland. The thyroid gland in endemic cretins in Switzerland can be anything from almost total atrophy to a huge goiter with parenchymatous, colloid, partially cystic, partially atrophic tissue.

DEGROOT: The discussion is moving toward the point that there are different causes between endemic and sporadic cretinism, and that iodide deficiency may play a role in endemic cretinism. I don't think anyone has presented evidence so far which allows this to be more than pure speculation. Everything presented can fit with the concept of fetal hypothyroidism as a cause of cretinism. The difference in the clinical syndrome of sporadic and endemic cretinism doesn't mean much, because none of us has seen an athyreotic cretin, sporadic cretin born of a hypothyroid mother, which would be the required test case. The degree of hypothyroidism in the sporadic cretin in utero is probably very different from that of the endemic cretin, whose mother may also be hypothyroid. Further, none of us has seen an endemic cretin who received treatment within the first three months. We also have the experiments which we will hear about later, in which antithyroid drugs were put into the chick embryo and produced otic lesions typical of hypothyroidism without iodine deficiency. We also know that the fetal rat can be made to look like a bizarre cretin by giving it methimazole in utero. It seems to me that the burden of proof is still on someone who suggests that there is a difference between severe fetal thyroid hormone deficiency and what we see in endemic cretinism.

REFERENCES

1. Relazione della Commissione di S.M. il Re di Sardegna "Studiare il cretinismo". Stamperia Reale, Turin, 1848.

2. Curling, T.B.: Med. Chir. Trans. 32:303, 1850.

3. Fagge, C.H.: Sporadic cretinism occurring in England. Medico-chir. Trans. 54:155-170, 1871.

4. Trotter, W.H.: The association of deafness with thyroid dysfunction. Br. Med. Bull. 16:92-98, 1960.

5. McCarrison, R.: Observations on endemic cretinism in the Chitral and Gilgit Valleys. Lancet 2: 1275-1280, 1908.

6. Costa, A.; Coltino, F.; Mortara, M. and Vogliazzo, V.: Endemic cretinism in Piedmont. Panminerva Med. 5:250-259, 1964.

7. DeQuervain, F. and Wegelin, C.: Der endemische Kretinism. Springer, Berlin, 1936.

8. Koenig, M.P.: Die kongenitale Hypothyreose und der endemishe Kretinismus. Springer, Berlin, 1968

9. Stanbury, J.B. and Querido, A.: Genetic and environmental factors in cretinism: Classification. J. Clin. Endocrinol. Metab. 16:1922, 1956.

10. Costa, A.: Has endemic cretinism any relation to thyroid deficiency? J. Clin. Endocrinol. Metab. 17:801, 1957.

11. Bastenie, P.A.; Ermans, A.M.; Thys, O.; Beckers, C.; Van den Schrieck, H.G. and deVisscher, M.: Endemic goiter in the Uele region. III. Endemic cretinism. J. Clin. Endocrinol. Metab. 22:187-194, 1962.

12. Dumont, J.E.; Ermans, A.M. and Bastenie, P.A.: Thyroidal function in a goiter endemic. IV. Hypothyroidism and endemic cretinism. J. Clin. Endocrinol. Metab. 23:325-335, 1963.

13. Delange, F.: Ermans, A.M.; Vis, H.L. and Stanbury, J.B.: Endemic cretinism in Idjwi Island. In: Endemic Cretinism (B.S. Hetzel and P.O.D. Pharoah, eds.). Institute of Human Biology, Papua, New Guinea, 1971. pp. 33-53.

14. McCullagh, S.F.: The Huon Peninsula endemic: IV. Endemic goitre and congenital defect. Med. J. Aust.1:884-890, 1963.

15. Choufoer, J.C.; Van Rhijn, M. and Querido, A.: Endemic goiter in Western New Guinea. II. Clinical picture, incidence and pathogenesis of endemic cretinism. J. Clin. Endocrinol. Metab.25:385-402, 1965.

16. Buttfield, I.H. and Hetzel, B.S.: Endemic cretinism in Eastern New Guinea. Aust. Ann. Med. 18:217-221, 1969.

17. Lobo, L.C.G.; Pompeu, F. and Rosenthal, D.: Endemic cretinism in Goiaz, Brazil. J. Clin. Endocrinol. Metab. 23:407-412, 1963.

18. Lobo, L.C.G.; Quelce-Salgado, A. and Freire-Maia, A.: Studies on endemic goiter and cretinism in Brazil. 1. Epidemiological survey in Mato Grosso. In: Endemic Goiter. Report of the meeting of the PAHO Scientific Group on Research in Endemic Goiter held in Mexico, 1968. (J.B. Stanbury, ed.). Scientific Publication No. 193, Washington, 1969. pp. 85-89.

19. Fierro-Benítez, R.; Penafiel, W.; DeGroot, L.J. and Ramirez, I.: Endemic goiter and endemic cretinism in the Andean Region. New Eng. J. Med. 280:296, 1969

20. Fierro-Benítez, R.; Stanbury, J.B.; Querido, A.; DeGroot, L.J.; Alban, R. and Cordova, J.: Endemic cretinism in the Andean region of Ecuador. J. Clin. Endocrinol. Metab. 30:228-236, 1970.

21. Stott, H. and Gupta, S.P.: Distribution of goitre in United Provinces. 4. Further notes on the aetiology of goiter in super-endemic areas of the Gonda and Gorakhpur Districts. 5. Further clinical notes on endemic goitre, sub-thyroidism, cretinism, and deaf-mutism in super-endemic areas of the Gonda and Gorakhpur Districts. Ind. J. Med. Res. 21:649-654, 1934.

22. Stott, H.; Bhatia, B.B.; Lal, R.S. and Rai, K.C.: The distribution and cause of endemic goitre in the United Provinces. Ind. J. Med. Res. 18:1059-1086, 1931.

23. Srinivasan, S.; Subramanyan, T.A.V.; Sinha, A.; Deo, G. and Ramalingaswami, V.: Himalayan endemic deaf-mutism. Lancet 2: 176-178, 1964.

24. Ibbertson, H.K.; Pearl, M.; McKinnon, J.; Tait, J.M.; Lim, T. and Gill, M.B.: Endemic cretinism in Nepal. In: Endemic Cretinism Monograph Series No. 2. (B.S. Hetzel and P.O.D. Pharoah, eds.). Institute of Human Biology, Papua, New Guinea, 1971. pp. 71-88.

25. Buttfield, I.H.; Hetzel, B.S. and Odell, W.D.: Effect of iodized oil on serum TSH determined by immunoassay in endemic goiter subjects. J. Clin. Endocrinol. Metab. 21:175, 1961.

26. deVisscher, M.; Beckers, C.; Schrieck, M.; deSmet, M.; Ermans, A.M.; Galperin, H. and Bastenie, P.A.: Endemic goiter in the Uele Region (Republic of Congo). I. General aspects and functional studies. J. Clin. Endocrinology. Metab. 21:175, 1961.

27. Querido, A.; Schut, K. and Terpstra. J.: Hormone synthesis in the iodine-deficient thyroid gland. Ciba Colloq. Endocrinol. 10:124, 1957.

28. Karmakar, M.G.; Kochipillai, N.; Deo, M.G. and Ramalingaswami, V.: Adaptation of thyroid gland to iodine deficiency. Life Sci. 8:1135, 1969.

29. Dumont, J.E.; Delange, F. and Ermans, A.M.: Endemic cretinism. In: Endemic Goiter. Report of the meeting of the PAHO Scientific Group on Research in Endemic Goiter held in Mexico, 1968 (J.B. Stanbury, ed.). Scientific Publication No. 193. Washington, 1969, pp. 91-98.

30. Pretell, E.A. and Stanbury, J.B.: Effect of chronic iodine deficiency on maternal and fetal thyroid hormone synthesis. In: Endemic Cretinism (B.S. Hetzel and P.O.D. Pharoah, eds.). Institute of Human Biology, Papua, New Guinea, 1971. pp. 117-124.

31. Pharoah, P.O.D.; Buttfield,I.H. and Hetzel, B.S.: Neurological damage to the fetus resulting from severe iodine deficiency during pregnancy. Lancet 1: 308-310, 1971.

32. Pharoah, P.O.D.: Epidemiological studies of endemic cretinism in the Jimi River Valley in New Guinea. In: Endemic Cretinism (B.S. Hetzel and P.O.D. Pharoah, eds.). Institute of Human Biology, Papua, New Guinea, 1971, pp. 109-116.

33. Hornabrook, R.W.: Neurological aspects of endemic cretinism in Eastern New Guinea. In: Endemic Cretinism (B.S. Hetzel and P.O.D. Pharoah, eds.). Institute of Human Biology, Papua, New Guinea, 1971, pp. 105-107.

34. Wydler, A.: Die Histologie der Kretinenstruma (G. Fischer, ed.). Jena, 1926.

35. Smith, D.W.; Blizzard, R.M. and Wilkins, L.: The mental prognosis in hypothyroidism of infancy and childhood. Pediatrics 19:1011-1022, 1957.

36. Beierwaltes, W.H.; Carr, E.A.; Raman, G.; Spafford, N.R.; Aster, R.A. and Lowrey, G.H.: Institutionalized Cretins in the State of Michigan. J. Mich. State Med. Soc. 58:1077-1095, 1959.

37. DeQuervain, F. and Wegelin, C.: Der endemische Kretinism. Springer, Berlin, 1936.

SECTION 2
IDENTIFICATION AND ASSESSMENT OF CRETINISM

INTELLECTUAL ASSESSMENT IN PRIMITIVE SOCIETIES, WITH A PRELIMINARY REPORT OF A STUDY OF THE EFFECTS OF EARLY IODINE SUPPLEMENTATION ON INTELLIGENCE

Frederick L. Trowbridge

Center for Disease Control

Atlanta, Georgia

Mental deficiency is perhaps the most tragic aspect of endemic cretinism. Yet, little has been done to define the nature and extent of intellectual deficiency in areas where endemic cretinism is widely seen. The mental deficiency of a typical cretin is obvious, but it is not known whether iodine deficiency or other factors which may lead to endemic cretinism can also cause variable and less obvious intellectual deficits in individuals who are not cretins. Another important question relates to time factors in the effects of iodine deficiency on intellectual development. It has been presumed that the most critical period is in early development. However, one reported study suggested that iodine supplementation as late as four to eight years of age might have some effect on measured intelligence (1). This finding is theoretically difficult to interpret, but indicates the need for further study of this important problem.

MEANS OF INTELLECTUAL ASSESSMENT

Perhaps the reason that so little has been done in the assessment of intelligence in areas of endemic cretinism is that the tools for assessing intelligence in primitive societies are poorly developed. Intelligence is an elusive entity, and intelligence tests under any conditions are no more than estimates of mental ability. When tests are applied outside of the culture in which they were developed, additional problems arise. Most fundamentally, these stem from the different way in which reality is perceived, the different manner of interpreting problems, and the different modes of thought which characterize each culture. Because of these differences tests designed to assess intelligence as defined by one culture may be invalid in another.

Many extrinsic factors can affect test results when tests are inadequately adapted to the local culture. The novelty and strangeness of the test situation may be frightening or upsetting. Motivation to perform well can be culturally determined and highly variable. Instructions may be misunderstood. Materials may seem foreign and meaningless or may hold unintended meanings or associations leading to incorrect evaluation of responses.

Broad biological and social factors also affect test scores. Poor nutrition, infection, crowding, lack of intellectual stimulation, inferior language experience, and other environmental factors can influence the results of any intelligence assessment. In underdeveloped areas such conditions may be starkly evident, but their specific effect on intellectual development is extremely difficult to quantify. This reality confounds attempts to identify or test specific causal factors as they relate to intellectual development.

The many hazards encountered in attempting intellectual assessment in different cultures has emphasized the need for tests less affected by cultural "bias." Important progress has been made in this direction. In general the attempt has been to minimize language-dependent items and to eliminate materials which would be familiar in one culture but unfamiliar in another. There are many examples of these so-called "culture-fair" tests. Among the more widely used are tests of "inter-sensory modalities" developed by Birch and Lefford (2, 3). This testing technique evaluates the integration of perception through visual, kinesthetic, and "haptic" modalities. The haptic modality refers to the perception of the shape of an object which the subject feels but cannot see. In testing kinesthetic perception the subject's hand holds a stylus which is guided around the outline of an object to be identified. Application of inter-sensory testing techniques has been made by Cravioto in assessing the interaction of nutrition and mental development in Mexican school-age children (4). Klein has adapted inter-sensory techniques for application to a rural Guatemalan culture (5).

Other tests which utilize materials that can be administered cross-culturally are Raven's Progressive Matrices (6) and Kohs Blocks. These tests present non-verbal figurative problems in the form of objects or designs which must be correctly aligned or rearranged to complete a prescribed pattern. There are numerous other tests of this type which have analogous format. An adaption of Kohs Block Designs has been made by Ord for use in New Guinea with subjects who have had very little exposure to Western culture (7).

Despite the important advantages of tests which avoid culture-bound features, the most fundamental problems of cross-cultural testing are not eliminated. All persons live within a cultural context, and responses to any testing situation will be molded by that culture. The so-called "culture-fair" tests may reliably demonstrate individual differences within a culture, but the significance of what is measured may vary from one culture to another.

When testing is to be done within a culture rather than between different cultures it may be practical to aim not at developing a culture-free test, but rather to adapt a standard test or develop new test procedures within that cultural context. In either case it is obvious that materials, instructions and test conditions must be suited to the local environment. Tests must also be standardized for a particular culture by the criteria of reliability and validity. Reliability is a measure of within-test and the test-to-test consistency. Items which are assigned a given level of difficulty must be passed or failed by appropriate percentages of children of various ages. The test should not be sensitive to extrinsic factors in the conditions of testing, so that tests given at different times will be comparable.

Another obvious criteria which must be applied is that of validity. For a test to be valid within a culture there must be a relationship between test results and external correlates of intelligence such as school performance or occupational achievement.

The limitations of whatever testing method is used must be recognized. When properly applied, intelligence tests can be used to measure differences in mental ability within a culture. It is always far more hazardous to attempt to compare the results obtained in one culture with those obtained in another.

EVALUATION OF INTELLIGENCE AFTER IODINE SUPPLEMENTATION: REPORT OF A STUDY

Having discussed an approach to intellectual assessment in primitive societies, a specific application of intelligence testing in an endemic goiter area is now presented. This study involved the mental assessment of children after iodine supplementation, comparing children who were exposed to supplemented levels of iodine at various times in gestation or infancy with non-supplemented control groups.

METHOD

Two populations of rural Ecuadorean children were tested. One population was drawn from a village in which iodine supplementation was given in March, 1966, by depot intramuscular injection. Supplementation was given to approximately 90 percent of individuals in the village, from newborns to aged persons. The control population was drawn from a nearby village similar in social, cultural, and economic makeup, but in which no iodine supplementation was given. Details of this iodine supplementation program and of ongoing studies in the same villages have been reported elsewhere (8).

In each village the children were divided into three groups. Group I consisted of children born in the nine-month period before the iodine was given. In the test village this group received the iodine injection some time between birth and nine months of age. Group II consisted of children born in the nine-month period immediately after iodinization. In the test village these children were born of mothers receiving the iodine injection during the gestational period. They were, therefore, exposed to supplemented levels of iodine for from less than one month to the full nine months of gestation. Group III consisted of children born from nine to 18 months after iodinization. In the test village the mothers had iodine supplementation prior to their conception. Therefore, these children experienced supplemented levels of iodine during their entire gestational period.

The ages of the children at the time of testing varied from a mean age of five years four months for Group I to a mean age of three years 10 months for Group III. Exact ages for the purpose of scoring were determined primarily from baptismal records kept by the parish priest.

In the test village all surviving children born within the dates specified for each group and who could be found and identified were tested. A slightly larger number of children in each group from the other village were tested to serve as controls. They were selected to give a roughly even distribution throughout the age range of each group. The children called to be tested each day were of mixed ages representing a sampling of all groups, and the group identification of the child was unknown to the physician administering the test. Also, testing was changed from one village to the other every two to four days to prevent any inadvertent changes in testing conditions or procedure from affecting relative performance.

The test used was an adaptation of the Stanford-Binet Intelligence Scale. The tests for ages two through eight years were translated into Spanish, employing words and phrasing judged to be most easily understood by these rural Ecuadorean children. The translation was made by an Ecuadorean physician who had lived in the test village for two years and had a thorough knowledge of the terminology and manner of speaking used by the people. The test was administered according to this translation by a North American physician with a good working knowledge of Spanish. To insure that the presentation was clear and that responses were interpreted correctly, an Ecuadorean medical student observed all tests and participated when necessary. The simplicity of the terminology used in the questions for the age levels tested was such that the children had no difficulty understanding the questions or instructions. The guidelines for giving the tests were adhered to closely. The manner of scoring also followed the standard form. New materials were substituted in a number of questions because the standard Stanford-Binet items were obviously not pertinent to the rural South American culture. Substituted material was chosen to maintain the intent of the original item. A listing and description of all substitutions and modifications is available from the author.

Although the children tested were all at least three and one half years of age, some of them failed to complete successfully all of the Stanford-Binet at the two year level. Therefore, in some cases items from the Catell Infant Intelligence Scale were used to establish a baseline at which all items were completed successfully. Once established, this baseline was used for scoring purposes in the same manner as a baseline established with the Stanford-Binet items.

The tests were carried out in a single room in each village set up for the purpose. The examiner sat across a small table from the child. To one side, behind a desk, sat an assistant who recorded the responses to each question. The Ecuadorean medical student sat slightly behind the child in order to be able to hear and observe all responses. The children in these villages were often shy, and it was found important to have the mother of the child in the room to provide a reassuring presence. The mother was seated to the rear of the child so that she could not give visible clues to the child. No verbal assistance from the mother was permitted.

Several minutes were spent initially playing "catch" with a plastic ball or playing with a doll to give the child a chance to accomodate to the new surroundings. Subsequently, testing was begun with playful items at the three year level; stringing beads on a shoestring and building a block tower and bridge. The picture vocabulary was given next since performance on this item served as an indicator of the child's verbal baseline. Testing was then continued at the level at which the picture vocabulary was successfully passed. As defined in the Stanford-Binet method testing was continued from the baseline where all items were passed, to the ceiling level at which all items were failed. The child's mental age was then calculated by adding up credit for the items completed successfully between these two levels. An IQ was then determined from the standard tables in the Stanford-Binet manual.

After testing was completed results were excluded if circumstances were encountered which would invalidate test results. Exclusions were made for the following reasons:

1. If the child was uncooperative and resistant to the testing situation to the point of being unscorable.

2. If the child was recognized as mentally deficient by the parents and others in the village.

3. If the child displayed behavior abnormalities such as excessive nervousness or hyperactivity.

4. If the score was so strikingly low as to suggest that the child was an unrecognized deficient or that he grossly failed to understand what was required by the test.

A pilot study was conducted to standardize instructions, materials and procedures. Twenty-two children from the control village were tested. These pilot-phase children were excluded from participation in the actual study.

RESULTS

A total of 125 children were tested (Table 1), 59 in the test village (Tocachi) and 66 in the control village (La Esperanza). After testing, some scores were excluded for the reasons outlined above. A total of 14 exclusions were made (Table 2). These exclusions were distributed throughout the test groups. After exclusions, the remaining total of 111 children were included in final tabulations, 51 from Tocachi and 60 from La Esperanza (Table 3).

Table 1. Children tested

Group	Tocachi	La Esperanza	Total
I	16	19	35
II	21	23	44
III	22	24	46
Total	59	66	125

Table 2. Exclusion of scores

Reason:	Tocachi I	II	III	La Esperanza I	II	III	Total
Unscorable	0	2	1	0	0	2	5
Mental Deficient	0	0	2	0	0	1	3
Behavioral Abnormality	1	0	0	0	2	0	3
Score Below 50	2	0	0	1	0	0	3
Total	3	2	3	1	2	3	14

The number of children in each group varied from 13 to 21. There was also some variation in the proportion of male and female subjects in each group. However, the total number of male and female subjects tested was not greatly different.

Social data tabulations indicated some differences between the villages (Table 4). In Tocachi there was a higher reported literacy rate and a higher percentage of fathers who worked as farmers. A lower percentage of families in Tocachi reported cretins among their close relatives.

Anthropometric data were generally comparable between the two villages. However, children in Group I in Tocachi were generally shorter and weighed less than their counterparts in Group I in La Esperanza.

Table 3. Composition of test groups - after exclusions

	Tocachi			La Esperanza			Total		
Group	M	F	Total	M	F	Total	M	F	Total
I	10	3	13	11	7	18	21	10	31
II	11	8	19	9	12	21	20	20	40
III	6	13	19	7	14	21	13	27	40
Total	27	24	51	27	33	60	54	57	111

Table 4. Social data

Literacy	% Tocachi	% La Esperanza
Mother	56.3	36.4
Father	86.4	77.4
Both	42.6	33.3
Neither	4.3	21.2
Ownership		
House	60.4	68.1
Land	39.1	45.5
Radio	45.3	48.4
Father's Occupation		
Farmer	95.0	72.2
Other	5.0	27.8
Cretins Among Relatives		
	33.3	46.0

Mean IQ scores for all groups showed no significant difference between the test and control villages (Table 5). Also, within the control village there was no significant difference between the mean IQ score of the three groups. However, within the test village there was a progressive increase in mean IQ score from Group I to Group III (Table 6). Children in Group III in Tocachi, whose mothers were iodized before conception, had a mean IQ score which was significantly greater than the mean IQ score of children in Group I, who received iodine supplementation after birth (p=.005). Similarly, Group II children, whose mothers received iodine during the gestational period, showed a mean IQ score which was significantly higher than that of Group I in the same village (p=.05). Mean IQ scores for all groups are presented in Table 5. The excess in mean IQ scores of Group II and Group III is indicated. The difference between the mean IQ values of Group II and Group III in Tocachi was not significant.

Within the test groups in Tocachi there were fairly wide but not statistically significant differences between the mean IQ scores of male and female subjects. Comparing female scores within Tocachi showed a striking progression from a mean score of 61 for females in Group I, to 68 in Group II, to 78 in Group III. The difference between Group I and Group II and between Group II and Group III were statistically significant. Mean IQ scores for males in Tocachi showed a significant difference between a mean score of

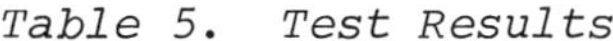

Table 5. Test Results

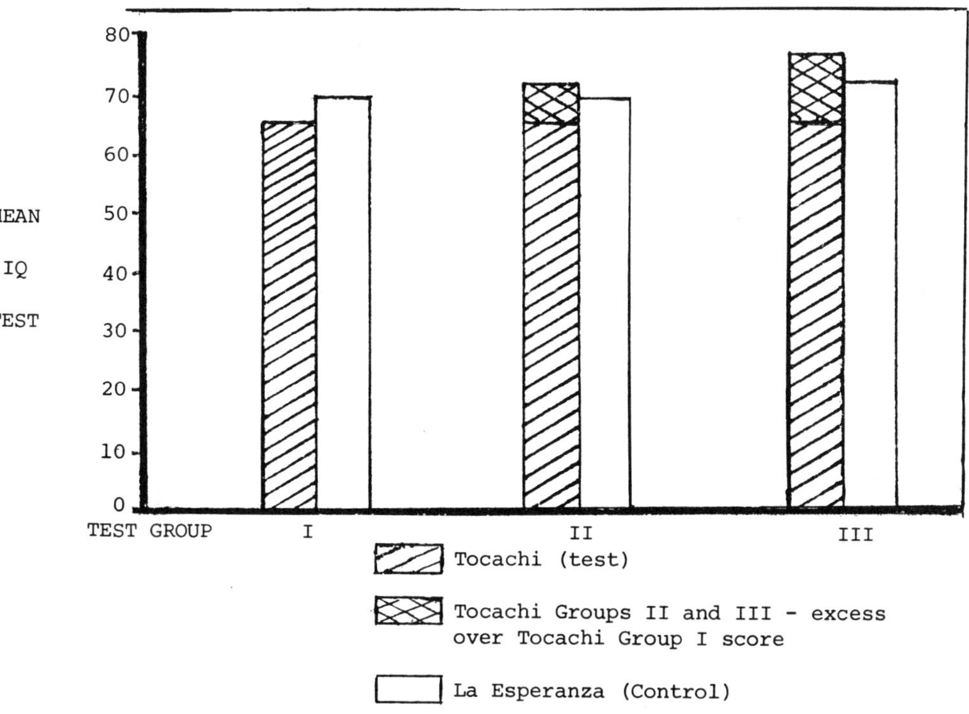

66 in Group I and a mean score of 75 in Group II. A mean score for group III of 73 showed a slight trend in the opposite direction from the rest of the data.

Table 6. Mean I.Q. Scores

	Toacachi			La Esperanza		
GROUP	M	F	TOTAL	M	F	TOTAL
I	66	61	65.2	69	70	69.9
II	75	68	72.3	66	70	69.0
III	73	78	76.8	72	72	72.4
TOTAL			72.2			70.4

Inclusion of scores which were excluded for the reasons outlined did not substantially affect the trend or the significant implications of the data.

DISCUSSION

The most significant implications of the data relate to the mean IQ scores of Group I in Tocachi. Because this is a critical group it is important to outline some atypical characteristics which it displayed. It was the smallest group and contained an unequal sex distribution of 10 males and 3 females. As a group its height and weight values were smaller than its control group in La Esperanza. The difference stemmed predominantly from the small stature and low weight of the 3 females in this group. The irregularities in the composition of this group are interesting to note but do not negate the implication of the low mean IQ score of the group as a whole.

The mean IQ score of Tocachi Group I was distinctly although not significantly lower than the corresponding group in the control village. This lower IQ value may reflect a real difference in IQ between the two villages. It is possible that Tocachi's basal level of measurable intelligence was lower than that of La Esperanza prior to iodine supplementation, and that the improvement seen in test scores in Group II and Group III children resulted from the provision of iodine at a critical stage in gestation. Unfortunately, no pretest of intelligence in the two villages was performed. Therefore this possibility can only remain in the realm of conjecture.

The six children whose scores were excluded because of behavioral abnormalities or because of excessively low scores form an interesting group which deserves further comment. As a group these children were below the mean for their age for height, weight, and head circumference. Some were strikingly small for their age and might have been children with severe nutritional inadequacy. Perhaps of greatest significance are the extremely low scores in children who were not known mental deficients. Some children displayed behavioral abnormalities which might explain their poor score. However, other children seemed to participate well in the testing but still scored in the same range as children who were recognized as mental deficients. These children may have been unrecognized mentally retarded children.

Further statistical work is required to evaluate the within-test and the test-to-test reliability of the modified Stanford-Binet Scale used. Also, it would be valuable to further validate the tests through comparison of scores with the results of other testing and with other criteria such as future school performance.

Longitudinal studies of development using Gesell Scales have been carried out in both villages since iodine supplementation was given. Comparison of results from the Gesell Scales with those from the present study on an individual and group basis would be a valuable validation tool.

It is important to note that subjects recognized as mentally deficient did score at the extreme low end of the scale. At the opposite end of the scale, the four-year-old daughter of an Ecuadorean physician who was tested but was not part of the study had an IQ score of 125. This correspondence of test scores at both extremes with anticipated performance levels provides some rough validation of the testing.

Despite all attempts to adapt the Stanford-Binet to the local culture and to apply the test consistently, the study has obvious weaknesses. The test used has significant cultural bias. The reliability and validity of the test has not been demonstrated. While the implications of the data may be significant, it must be stressed that they are preliminary in nature and are based on data which has important qualifications and limitations.

SUMMARY

The factors which cause severe mental deficiency in cretins may also cause variable and more subtle mental deficits in individuals from the same environmental and genetic background. The extent of mental deficiency in areas of endemic cretinism and the effects of iodine prophylaxis on intellectual development have been little studied, in large part because of methodological difficulties in making valid intellectual assessments in primitive societies.

An approach to intellectual assessment is outlined, and a study is reported on the effects of iodized oil prophylaxis at different stages of gestation and early infancy. Results are preliminary and qualified but suggest that iodine prophylaxis of mothers before conception or during gestation may improve subsequent intelligence test performance of their children when compared with the performance of children who were not exposed to iodine supplementation until after birth.

Validity of testing increases with age. It would be advantageous to retest the same groups as the children grow older. This would provide data for comparison with the findings of the present study.

Comparison of scores with the results of ongoing longitudinal studies in the same villages would provide additional validation.

Further delineation of the interaction of iodine prophylaxis and mental development is required. It is proposed that future programs of iodine prophylaxis in areas of endemic goiter should include intellectual assessment of children in both preliminary and follow-up evaluation. The need to establish pre-treatment norms for intelligence test performance is stressed.

ACKNOWLEDGEMENTS

The author wishes to acknowledge the assistance of Dr. John Stanbury and Dr. Philip Dodge in formulating the study, and the collaboration of Dr. Rodrigo Fierro-Benitez and Dr. Ignacio Ramirez, in adapting the study for use in Ecuador. Mrs. Jane Trowbridge and Mr. Jose Suarez assisted in the testing procedure. Miss Mary Shepherd assisted by typing the manuscript.

This study was supported in part by U. S. Public Health Service Training Grant No. AM05618.

DISCUSSION BY PARTICIPANTS

PRETELL: We have been doing similar studies in Peru. We have tested by two different groups of psychologists and by different tests, and there was good correlation among the groups.

BALÁZS: I would like to point out that iodine supplementation was left out during a crucial period of the development of the CNS, that is during the immediate postnatal period.

STANBURY: Don't you think that there was supplementation in the sense that there would be enough transplacental transfer to build up quite adequate stores in the newborn?

PRETELL: We were able to test urinary excretion of iodine from control children and children born to iodine-injected mothers about two years after birth. In children born to non-treated mothers the iodine excretion for 24 hours was about 20 μg. In children born to treated mothers, it was about 67 μg. That probably was due to transfer during gestation, but also after birth by lactation. We also measured iodine excretion in milk and found it was much higher in the treated mothers.

REFERENCES

1. Dodge, P.R. et al.: Effect on intelligence of iodine in oil administered to young children. A preliminary report. In: Endemic Goiter. Report of the meeting of the PAHO Scientific Group on Research in Endemic Goiter held in Mexico, 1968 (J.B. Stanbury, ed.). PAHO Scientific Publication No. 193, Washington, 1969. pp 378-380.

2. Birch, H.G. and Lefford, A.: Intersensory development in children. Monogr. Soc. Res. Child Dev. Serial No. 89:1-48, 1963.

3. Birch, H.G. and Lefford, A.: Visual differentiation. Intersensory integration and voluntary motor control. Monogr. Soc. Res. Child Dev. Serial No. 110:1-77, 1967.

4. Cravioto, J.; Delicarde, E.R. and Birch, H.G.: Nutrition, growth and neurointegrative development: An experimental and ecological study. Pediatrics. 38:319-372, 1966.

5. Klein, R.E. Unpublished. Address requests for information to Dr. Robert Klein, Director, Human Development Division, Instituto de Nutricion de Centro America y Panama, Guatemala City, Guatemala.

6. Birch, H.R.: Raven's progressive matrices. J. Genet. Psychol. 93:199-228, 1958.

7. Breshuvel, S., ed.: Methods for the measurement of psychological performance. International Biological Programme, Blackwell Scientific Publications, Oxford, 1969. pp. 87-93

8. Fierro-Benítez, R.; Ramirez, I.; Estrella, E.; Jaramillo, C.; Diaz, C. and Urresta, J.: Iodized oil in the prevention of endemic goiter and associated defects in the Andean region of Ecuador. In: Endemic Goiter. Report of the meeting of the PAHO Scientific Group on Research in Endemic Goiter held in Mexico, 1968 (J.B. Stanbury, ed.). PAHO Scientific Publication No. 193, Washington, 1969. pp. 306-394.

A BIBLIOGRAPHY - INTELLECTUAL ASSESSMENT IN PRIMITIVE SOCIETIES

Anastasi, A.: _Psychological Testing_. Macmillan, New York, 1968.

Birch, H.G. and Lefford, A.: Intersensory development in children. _Monogr. Soc. Res. Child Dev._ Serial No. 89:1-48, 1963.

Birch, H.G. and Lefford, A.: Visual differentiation. Intersensory integration and voluntary motor control. _Monogr. Soc. Res. Child Dev._ Serial No. 110:1-77, 1967.

Birch, H.G.: Raven's progressive matrices. _J. Genet. Psychol._ 93:199-228, 1958.

Breshuvel, S., ed.: Methods for the measurement of psychological performance. In: _International Biological Programme_. Blackwell Scientific Publications, Oxford, 1969. pp 87-93.

Cravioto, J.; Delicarde, E.R. and Birch, H.G.: Nutrition, growth and neurointegrative development: An experimental and Ecologic Study. _Pediatrics_. 38:319-372, 1966.

Dodge, R.R. _et al._: Effect on intelligence of iodine in oil administered to young children. A preliminary report. In: _Endemic Goiter_. Report of the meeting of the PAHO Scientific Group on Research in Endemic Goiter held in Mexico, 1968 (J.B. Stanbury, ed.). PAHO Scientific Publication No. 193, Washington, 1969. pp. 378-380.

Fierro-Benítez, R.; Ramirez, I.; Estrella, E.; Jaramillo, C.; Diaz, C. and Urresta, J.: Iodized oil in the prevention of endemic goiter and associated defects in the Andean region of Ecuador. In: _Endemic Goiter_. Report of the meeting of the PAHO Scientific Group on Research in Endemic Goiter held in Mexico, 1968 (J.B. Stanbury, ed.). PAHO Scientific Publication No. 193, Washington, 1969. pp. 306-394.

Vernon, P.E.: _Intelligence and Cultural Environment_. Methuen, London, 1969.

INTELLIGENCE: IMPLICATION OF AND FOR DEAFNESS

James Youniss

Center for Research in Thinking and Language

Catholic University of America, Washington, D.C.

The patient with endemic cretinism is often deaf, and in the same communities there are often deaf persons who do not share the other clinical attributes of endemic cretinism. The field investigator may be confronted with the problem of assessing the intelligence of these patients in a situation of social and intellectual deprivation and across cultural and language barriers. In this paper two issues are addressed concerning nonverbal intelligence. The first concerns the meaning of non-verbal intelligence, and the second deafness, both as a problem in itself and as it provides implications for concepts of development. The central task at issue from the practical point of view is how can one best proceed when assessing intelligence in children who cannot hear and therefore do not know language well enough to be tested with standard verbal instruments. If the task were simply to find a good nonverbal test, there would be no difficulty. There are a number of such instruments available, including Raven's Matrices, Porteus Mazes, the Goodenough-Harris Draw-A-Man, the nonverbal scale of the WISC, and so on. All of these are accompanied by validating research data which indicate their respective usefulness and each could be applied to deaf children with slight modification.

But obviously there are several problems involved, and psychologists are only now beginning to gain awareness of the need to solve them before arriving at a choice among instruments. When assessing intelligence in a deaf child, the evaluator has to answer several questions prior to the moment he selects a particular test. First, he must clarify his concept of deafness: Is it a physical handicap alone? Are there psychological entailments of deafness? What is the implication of hearing loss for language? If language is affected, then are there other consequents such as in the area of thinking? Second, he must clarify his concept of intelligence: Shall intelligence be operationally defined as the results on certain tests? Or, should it be defined in developmental terms? Is intelligence a capacity which eventuates in measurable skills? Or, is it a set of factors which can be separately identified and assessed? Third, he must ask himself the purpose of the whole diagnostic procedure : Will the results be used to plan the child's educational program? Will they be used simply to be included in the child's record as an identifying piece of general information? Will they be used, as is often the case, to confirm what is already suspected about the child?

DEAFNESS IN A PSYCHOLOGICAL PERSPECTIVE

These and other questions seem obvious enough, but are presented here in order to introduce a new perspective on deafness, intelligence, and the issues which confront any sensible assessment. The argument which follows is based on the past 12 years of research from the Center for Research in Thinking and Language.

In 1960 we approached these general problems in the context of a psychological literature which (a) closely identified thinking with language, and (b) characterized the deaf person as "perceptually bound," "rigid," "suspicious," "perservative," and "concrete." When put together (a) and (b) were mutually reinforcing. Without the benefit of the societal natural language, the deaf person should be and apparently was limited in his thinking. For example, in order to break out of the concrete restrictions of incoming physical stimulation it was presumed that a cognitive tool like language with its arbitrary referential function was required. Without this, how could the deaf person ever hope to achieve the level of intelligence attained by normal language users?

When we looked into the matter further we found that this description and the line of reasoning behind it were only partially accurate.

First, it was true that, in the main, profoundly deaf children did indeed spend their early years in the absence of a social symbol system. Most deaf children are born to hearing parents, and most hearing parents are advised to speak but never gesture to their deaf offspring. Consequently the deaf children typically spend their early home life not comprehending oral speech, not producing sentences, but gesturing as best they can in idiosyncratic symbols. In school often there is continuation of this pattern. Until recently, almost every school for the deaf in the

United States adhered formally to the "oral method" of teaching, a method which denied use of the deaf adult person's manual language of signs and held out oral speech and speech (lip) reading as the main means of communication. Further, written speech also fits this same pattern. Deaf children do not read well. If one takes a grade four reading level as a measure of mature reading ability, then perhaps only 10 to 20 percent of all deaf children ever achieve this level even after 14 to 16 yr of schooling.

The picture on language is clear up to a point. Up until the time the child enters the secondary grades he is told to use a language which he is unable to comprehend or produce and he is not given a substitute symbol system. Now, according to psychological theories we ought to observe some profound effects in thinking, adjustment, and motivation. It was a surprise then that surveys of the living patterns of deaf adults showed that they are productively employed patriotic citizens who are concerned parents, live a rich social life, know how to cooperate in a community, know when and where to seek help when required, and generally can only be described as normal adults. These surveys taken in New York State and Frederick County, Maryland (1,2) dealt with complete samples, were not selective, and hence, are quite powerful in their implications. These data could be considered a close approximation to the so called <u>crucial experiment.</u> A natural condition, deafness, which coupled with arbitrary policy, prevents children from acquiring a social language at least up to age seven or later. This <u>deprivation</u> should have clear consequents if language is a necessary factor in psychological development. The finding, however, is that the absence of this factor does not prevent development to normal maturity. The conclusion, therefore, seems inevitable: Language can be neither sufficient nor necessary for intelligence.

This conclusion is not easy to accept, and indeed several arguments are consistently raised against it. It is said that while the deaf may not acquire the societal language, they have some kind of "language," meaning some kind of interior symbol system. Or, it is said that the little bit of speech they achieve is sufficient to allow thinking to proceed. Or it is said that speech is only one manifestation of language, while language in a cultural sense is part and substance of all we experience and do. These and several other redefinitions of "language" may be just so much evasion away from the point that the deaf child develops during his formative years without competence in written, spoken, speech or manual languages and yet without severe negative consequences to his intelligence or personality.

Further examples from our own research may be considered before going into the problem of theory. Deaf students from ages eight to 16 yr were presented 20 problems of the following type (3). The subject was given several balls, e.g., six yellow and four green, which he put individually into a covered box. He was then asked to draw the balls out one at a time and to predict before each draw which color he was most likely to draw out. This was meant to be an assessment of the child's concept of probability. The measure was complex enough to assure that probability and not something else was being observed since in order to succeed the child had to keep a running count of his draws, calculate whether he had just been correct or incorrect, and estimate anew each time a draw produced a new set of odds.

The results were clear. Deaf children showed the same developmental pattern as normal, middle class hearing subjects in terms of sensitivity to different odds, sure-thing predictions determined by keeping track of previous draws, and in a sex differences favoring boys, dropping of alternation choices in favor of selection by ratios, etc. Although the deaf lagged behind the hearing in terms of chronological age at which each new turn was observed, the deaf showed the same developmental shifts and arrived at the same levels of maturity ("catching up") as their hearing counterparts.

Deaf and hearing children were asked to imagine and draw liquid in a bottle as the bottle was covered with a stocking and rotated 45 degrees, 90 degrees, 135 degrees, etc., up to 235 degrees. Each time the bottle was rotated the child was to draw the liquid on a paper on which the outline of the bottle corresponded to the rotated position. The correct production was in each case a line corresponding to the horizontal plane parallel to the table top, irrespective of the position of the bottle. This problem of imagery had been studied by Piaget previously and there were expected developmental patterns in terms of kinds of errors and age changes. It was found that both deaf and hearing subjects matched Piaget's expectations (4,5). A developmental shift was observed from ages eight and nine to ages 11 and 12. Performance was ordered so that success varied in order from vertical to horizontal to diagonal rotations. When given additional training, both deaf and hearing subjects showed limited improvement to the next more difficult transformation, neither gaining more information than that.

These are but two specific cases of some 80 published studies which have attempted comparisons between deaf and hearing subjects on problems measuring thinking (6). The data in general show more often comparability than differences and, importantly, when developmental analyses allow, they show rather detailed qualitative similarities which give the statistical results a new meaning (7).

LANGUAGE AND THINKING

Why should the thinking of deaf children develop in a manner comparable to language-using children who hear? For a complete answer a new concept of intelligence is required. The system offered by Piaget appears to be an adequate beginning point (5). This is the only modern developmental theory which would allow deaf children to be normal, all others putting the burden of thinking on a causal mechanism which is either language itself or a derivative from language. In this theory, the basis of intelligence is the child's actions and his reflection on these actions which yield intelligent organizations or structures. These structures are neither imposed by physical reality nor outcomes of language nor innately given. Rather, they are *constructions* on the child's part. Concepts of probability, or knowledge of major spatial planes, or of classification hierarchies, or understanding the necessity of logical inferences are, thus, not to be found available in the outside world to be made known to the child through the vehicle of language, but conceptions which describe the products of the organization of action. Deaf, blind, "culturally deprived," children reared in agricultural societies, etc., are no more prevented from gaining intelligent organizing structures than their own actions allow. There are now several cross-cultural studies which bear out this point and demand that we at least give the old language-thinking relation a new airing.

With regard to language as a symbol system, Piaget's theory asserts that symbols *per se* are not the instruments which carry intelligence forward. Symbols are only as good as or as poor as the intelligence which they serve. This is true because the referential meaning of symbols is the structure from which they emanate. While symbols obviously aid thinking, they cannot produce structures, no matter how sophisticated the symbols might be.

Piaget has called this the "awkward problem" because there seems to be so much evidence to pare away before one gets to the core of the issue. In the first place, children use symbols liberally as if they understood the adult reference. Moreover, symbols by definition seem to have characteristics which are essential to thinking, such as abstraction, arbitrariness, and flexibility. Finally, when we look at our own thinking, we observe linguistic symbols in our personal introspections.

Piaget responds to these points in turn. As to the last, he agrees with current theorists [e.g., Miller, (8)] that we are never aware of thinking processes but only their results. The symbols we see in introspection are outcomes of thinking and not thinking itself. As to characteristics of verbal symbols, Piaget asserts that those cited above can indeed be achieved in the adult thinker's intelligence; but they come from structures rather than symbols *per se*. This is shown when we probe children's thinking carefully and find that at different developmental stages the same symbols are used but in entirely different ways to refer to structures currently available. There is nothing inherent in symbols which dictate their effects on thinking. As to children's use of symbols, Piaget cautions against identifying symbols with what they are supposed to represent. The child who counts to ten may have a conception of number which is yet so elementary that he cannot see the equivalence and necessity in the fact that (3+2)=(2+3)=(3+1+1). What it means to understand *number* is more than word-reference; structures are required and will come when the child's own actions show him that *order* and *recombination* (analysis), for example, must of necessity be irrelevant to numerical results. That is, several discrete actions continue to yield the same result; hence *number* objects are constructed.

This, of course, is not the place to recapitulate Piaget's theory or to defend it. What is at stake, however, is a critical point. Psychology historically has been committed to the argument that thinking is language which has become internalized. Speech is prior and causal to thinking. The facts of thinking in deafness were incompatible with this theory. The results with deaf children show that this cannot be the case. They show that Piaget's position describes well and in detail their development. Thus it has been essential to abandon the former position and explore Piaget's theory. The results have been more than satisfactory up to this point in time.

NONVERBAL INTELLIGENCE

Historically nonverbal intelligence has been accorded secondary status in psychology. Verbal intelligence correlates more highly with other achievements than does nonverbal intelligence. Moreover, nonverbal intelligence is a substitute for verbal measures only when the latter cannot be used. That is, when one has a population which is *de facto* deprived, nonverbal tests are required: future infantry soldiers from the rural South; brain damaged persons; culturally "deprived" children; people from "underdeveloped" cultures; etc. In order to give these populations a fair chance to show capability, one drops language - in which sophisticated people could be tested - and turns to a secondary medium. Notice the circular nature of this reasoning.

This reasoning has been applied to deafness. For example, until five years ago, scientists regularly argued that the manual language of the deaf adult was inferior to our verbal system because it was concrete by definition. Signs, because they pictorially depicted objects which they represented, could not be the stuff from which abstract thinking flowed. Here we see a misunderstanding of what symbols are and can do. But the symbol is not concrete or abstract; it is _the symbol user who can employ a symbol concretely or abstractly_. Nonverbal actions likewise are not concrete or abstract _in themselves_. They can be used in several ways and, in Piaget's terms, they are the stuff from which intelligence grows. At the same time, like symbols, they also reflect the structures which have already been achieved. Verbal is not to be identified with what is best. Especially with intelligence and symbols it is necessary to be overly cautious before adopting value judgments without considering the problem thoroughly.

The distinction between verbal and nonverbal intelligence is a poor substitute for answering the question of what intelligence is or what it can do for the individual. To maintain the separation does not conform to Piaget's observations. In order to avoid further confusions, it may be suggested that the term _intelligence_ include development in both verbal and nonverbal realms. Further, a developmental model should be a means for seeing the nonstatic character of symbols and actions as well as the organization from which both gain their psychological meaning.

DISCUSSION

To return to the problems posed as essential in any diagnostic effort, we can expand their meaning and implications more precisely. _A clear conception of deafness_ means distinguishing among the audiological problem, its attendant physical associates, and potential psychological issues. It also means knowing the deaf person and the extent to which he is pursuing a productive and full life. Pediatricians, speech pathologists, and audiological educators do not do this regularly. They mix objective diagnosis of deafness with an outmoded theory of thinking which misleads the parent and puts arbitrary barriers between the child and society. More enlightened programs in recent years have begun with the premise that communication can only benefit both parent and child. Finger spelling or sign language is then made available instead of the skimpy promise that if the parent only speaks and never gestures, the deaf child will silently pass into the hearing world.

Clarification of one's concept of intelligence obviously means that the diagnostician must do more than keep his catalogue of tests up to date. There is no end to available instruments, once a clear concept begins to dictate one's choice. The old excuse that research does the conceptualizing and the diagnostician the application, requires a kind of schizophrenic approach from which the deaf child reaps only ill consequences. Piaget's theory at least should be given a try. Further, the data insist that the reconception of the role of language puts thinking first and subordinates verbal skills.

Many examples are available to illustrate this point. A practical case comes from a recent seminar in which the writer was asked to help experienced teachers of the deaf think for two weeks about thinking. A first revelation was that these teachers who saw the child behave and act every day were in fact observing his thinking. It became immediately obvious that these teachers had more information about that child's thinking than the expert who had given a 45 minute protocol on one day in the child's life. A second revelation was that their data, based on the child's behavior, fitted a concept of intelligence which put its generation at the doorstep of experience. One teacher explained this clearly with the following illustration. His class of six students had just been tested and found to be mildly retarded on a test of spatial knowledge. He did not believe the results and to prove his case he took the children outside the school campus to various locations in town and told them to find their ways back to school. Needless to say, even on unfamiliar terrain these youngsters were able to utilize their intelligent spatial structures to make quick returns.

<u>The purpose of the diagnosis</u> is no less important than the above points and obviously flows from them. While the aim varies from case to case clear conceptions of deafness and intelligence will dictate how far one must carry out observations to arrive at a useful description of the child. Indeed, without these, there is no way to tell when one has stopped short or gone too far. Perhaps this is why we see so often justification for a certain test to be, "It's a good test." When we ask, "For What?" we are told, "For intelligence," as if it were an entity like weight and tests were scales.

In this paper the precise relation of Piaget's theory to intelligence and deafness has only been highlighted. Because of the importance of the problem and the need to reanalyze our concepts regarding language, several references to a relevant literature are provided for those who would pursue the matter more fully (6,7,9).

SUMMARY

The research of the past decade has opened up several new problems concerning the relation of language to thinking and verbal to nonverbal intelligence. The beginnings of a reconception process in which both deafness and intelligence can be seen more clearly are emerging. The impact of deafness on the development of capacity to perform many tasks previously thought to require verbal skills has been overemphasized. The fact that deaf persons perform so adequately and "intelligently" is testimony to this.

REFERENCES

1. Rainer, J.D., Altshuler, K.Z. and Kallmann, F.J., eds.: *Family and Mental Health Problems in a Deaf Population.* C.C. Thomas, Springfield, Illinois, 1969.

2. Furfey, P.H. and Harte, J.: *Interaction of Deaf and Hearing in Frederick County, Maryland.* Final Report of SRS project No. RD 1012-s. Studies from the Bureau of Social Research No. 3. Catholic University of America, 1964.

3. Ross, B.M.: Probability concepts in deaf and hearing children. *Child Dev.* 37:917-927, 1966.

4. Robertson, A. and Youniss, J.: Anticipatory visual imagery in deaf and hearing children. *Child Dev.* 40:123-135, 1969.

5. Piaget, J. and Inhelder, B.: *The Psychology of the Child.* Basic Books, New York, 1969.

6. Furth, H.G.: Linguistic deficiency and thinking: research with deaf subjects 1964-1969. *Psychol. Bull.* 76:58-72, 1971.

7. Miller, G.A.: *Psychology: The Science of Mental Life.* Harper and Row, New York, 1962.

8. Furth, H.G.: *Thinking Without Language; Psychological Implications of Deafness.* Free Press, New York, 1966.

9. Furth, H.G. and Youniss, J.: Formal operations and language. *Int. J. Psychol.* 6:49-64, 1971.

THYROID FUNCTION TESTS IN ENDEMIC CRETINISM

Jerome M. Hershman

Metabolic Research Laboratory, Birmingham Veterans Administration Hospital, and Division of Endocrinology and Metabolism, Department of Medicine, University of Alabama, Birmingham, Alabama

In the past decade several groups have carried out comprehensive studies of thyroid function in patients with endemic cretinism. In general, these studies supported the clinical impression of either (1) a euthyroid state with altered parameters of iodine metabolism reflecting the severe iodine deficiency of the population or (2) hypothyroidism which was obvious clinically. As has been made abundantly clear in this symposium, the definition of endemic cretinism has varied. In this review, I have accepted the investigators' criteria for classifying their patients as cretins. The review will not deal with thyroid function tests in the sporadic cretin in whom thyroid function is clearly abnormal due to thyroid dysgenesis (cryptothyroidism), or to specific defects in the biosynthesis of thyroid hormone in the sporadic goitrous cretin, or to defects recently described in the biologic effect of TSH (1) or in the secretion of thyrotropin (2).

THYROID FUNCTION STUDIES

Table I is a characterization of the population of cretins in the various reports. The patients from the Uele and Idjwi regions of the Congo were uniformly hypothyroid; in contrast, the other groups of patients were generally euthyroid by clinical assessment but had the abnormalities of the central nervous system and sometimes in the development of the bones characteristic of the endemic cretin. The distribution between males and females was nearly equal. The Swiss cretins were an older group because the number of endemic cretins in Switzerland has decreased greatly in recent years. The urinary iodine reflects the iodine deficiency of the various populations, which was most severe in

Table 1: Characterization of endemic cretins who had studies of thyroid function

Area	Ref.	Year	No. of Patients	Female Percent	Age Range	Hypothyroid Percent	Urine I µg/day	Thyroid Size
Switzerland	3	1968	31	55	46-93	29	---	None large
Congo	4,5	1963	36	50	8-32	100	9	28/36<25 g
Brazil	6,7	1963,69	26	73	14-62	8	44-77[3]	69% nodular goiter
Ecuador	8	1970	10	60	12-40	0	10.4	4/10 not goitrous
W.New Guinea	9	1965	17[1]	50	1-18	0	2.5	usually no goiter[4]
E.New Guinea	10	1969	61[2]	49	---	0	---	74% no visible goiter

[1] 17 of a group of 80 had study of iodine metabolism
[2] 61 of a group of 254 had study of iodine metabolism
[3] In non-cretins
[4] 12/58 over age six years not palpable

New Guinea. Many of the cretins in Switzerland and especially in the Congo had small thyroids; those in South America and New Guinea had goiters similar in character and size to those of the rest of the goitrous population.

Table II shows the results of thyroid function tests in the endemic cretins. The serum protein-bound iodine (PBI) in hypothyroid cretins of the Congo was low. Euthyroid cretins of Brazil had PBI values that were generally normal in Goiaz; the PBI (and thyroid uptakes) were lower in cretins of Matto Grosso where goiter endemicity is more severe than in Goiaz (7). Cretins in Ecuador had a lower PBI and their mean T_4I was only 2.2 μg per 100 ml (8). The very low PBI in western New Guinea cretins was similar to that of the non-defective natives. The normal resin uptake of T_3 in cretins of eastern New Guinea and Ecuador excluded low thyroxine-binding globulin as the basis for the low PBI. Presumably a relatively high concentration of T_3 which is not measured in the PBI was responsible for the euthyroid state.

The thyroid uptakes of radioiodine were high in the cretins but tended to be less than that of the normal populations of the region; in the Congo, the thyroid uptakes of the cretins were much lower than the rest of the population. Elevated $PB^{131}I$ indicated rapid turnover of thyroidal iodine, even in the myxedematous cretins of the Congo.

The response to exogenous TSH was normal in the South American cretins, absent in the Congo, and present in 59 percent of the Swiss cretins. Suppression tests with T_3 were reported in only a few subjects. Normal suppression was found in Brazil but in none of four Congolese cretins. The latter finding suggests that the intense endogenous stimulation of thyroid function was not under normal feedback control. Thyroid antibodies were not found in Brazilian cretins (6) nor in 16 cretins of the Congo (11) nor in 10 mothers of cretins in western New Guinea (10). This tended to refute the concept that chronic thyroiditis or transmission of maternal thyroid antibodies was responsible for endemic cretinism.

Tests with perchlorate or thiocyanate to uncover defects in organic binding of iodine were usually normal, as were most of the limited studies for detection of iodotyrosine deiodinase defects. However, two of five Swiss cretins excreted significant amounts of diiodotyrosine in their urine (3). The serum cholesterol of the cretins was not strikingly abnormal (3,4,8).

In the cretins of the Congo, thyroid hormone secretion

Table 2: Thyroid function studies in endemic cretins. Figures in parenthesis show the values for the normal population. References same as in Table 1.

Area	PBI µg/100 ml Mean	PBI µg/100 ml Range	Thyroid Uptake %/24 hr Mean	Thyroid Uptake %/24 hr Range	$PB^{131}I$ 48 hr %/L	Normal Response To TSH	Normal T_3 Suppression	Serum TBG^{1}	Abnormal Perchlorate Test	Abnormal DIT Test^{2}
Switzerland	3.3	1.0-6.1 (3.5-8.0)	34.5^{4}	7-68 (20-60)^{4}	0.48	10/17^{5}	1/1		3/17	2/5
Congo	0.5 (3.5)	0-2.2	30 (87)		1.16	0/6	0/4		0/4^{6}	0/5
Brazil	5.5^{3}		32.6^{3} (38)			6/6	6/6			
Ecuador	4.0^{6}	2.8-5.4	69	47-87	1.29	Yes	1/2	Normal		
W.New Guinea	1.5 (1.9)	0.5-4.3 (0.3-4.8)	78 (87)	60-92 (65-100)	>1.0 (>1.0)					
E.New Guinea	2.6 (4.1)		63 (70)					Normal	1/11	

1 Thyroxine-binding globulin (TBG); elevated by T_3 resin-uptake
2 Deiodination of diiodotyrosine (DIT)
3 Excludes two hypothyroid cretins who had PBI of 2.0 and thyroid uptake of nine percent
4 Maximum uptake at various time intervals
5 Normal responses/subjects tested
6 After thiocyanate

proceeded at a fast rate but involved only minute amounts of iodine. The absolute uptake of iodine was 5.7 μg per day and thyroxine degradation was only 8μg per day (5). Failure of these thyroids to suppress or stimulate showed that they were already functioning at their highest level of activity.

Study of the iodoproteins of nodular goiters in seven cretins of Goiaz, Brazil,showed an increase in a 4.2 S iodoprotein. This was probably iodoalbumin which has been found in other subjects with thyroid hyperplasia (12).

In the patients who were euthyroid based on clinical evaluation at the time of the study of thyroid function, it is obvious that the tests could not indicate the status of thyroid function in the fetus or mother during the period of development of the abnormalities characteristic of cretinism.

SERUM THYROTROPIN (TSH)

The studies of Studer and Greer on experimental iodine deficiency in rats suggest that increased TSH secretion is the most important factor in producing the thyroidal response to iodine deficiency (13). Measurement of serum TSH by radioimmunoassay has become a useful tool for clinical investigation of factors which regulate thyroid function (14,15). This assay provides a practical method for assessing the role of TSH in goitrogenesis. Table III lists values for immunoreactive TSH in studies of endemic goiter. The subjects of these studies were considered euthyroid. While the results are comparable because the serum TSH was reported in terms of the same International Human Reference Standard A; variation of the technique between laboratories permits only tentative conclusions. In general, the values were highest in those regions with the severest deficiency of iodine.

Buttfield and his colleagues studied the serum TSH in eastern New Guinea in a population on very low iodine intake (16). Thirteen of 25 subjects had values which exceeded 12 microunits per ml, the upper limit of normal for a euthyroid American population. None of them was reported to be an endemic cretin. Three months following injection of iodized oil the serum TSH fell in 20 of the 25 subjects. Only limited studies of the serum TSH in endemic cretins have been reported. Adams *et al.* (21) found that the serum TSH estimated by bioassay in four euthyroid cretins in western New Guinea was no different from

Table 3: Immunoreactive TSH in endemic goiter

Area	Ref.	Iodine µg/day*	Serum TSH+ µU/ml
E. New Guinea	16	2.5	18 (4.8-79)
Congo-Idjwi	17	15	9.6 (2.5-123)
Egypt, New Valley	18	36	6.9 (4.5-11)
Argentina, Neuquen	19	30	4 (2.4-7.2)
Colombia, Cauca Valley	20	254	3.3 (1.0-10.6)

* Estimated mean daily urine excretion or intake of iodine
\+ Mean; range in parentheses

the elevated serum TSH of goitrous non-defectives in this population. Table IV lists the values of serum TSH in 10 hypothyroid cretins in the Congo (17). These values were 10 to 100 times higher than those observed in euthyroid inhabitants of the same area. Clearly, more data on TSH in "euthyroid" cretins are badly needed.

What is the significance of an elevated serum TSH? Although elevation of serum TSH occurs in primary hypothyroidism, it also occurs in patients with reduced thyroid reserve consequent to chronic thyroiditis or after partial thyroidectomy in the absence of clinical evidence of hypothyroidism. One interpretation of the significance of an elevated serum TSH is that it indicates the pituitary-hypothalamic receptors are activated by a low concentration of circulating thyroid hormone and that hypothyroidism exists in relation to these receptors. This implies that the hypothalamus or pituitary or both are exquisitely sensitive to the effects of thyroid hormone in comparison with other tissues.

Table 4: Serum TSH in 10 myxedematous cretins (17)

Patient	Sex	Age	Goiter Stage	24-Hr. ^{131}I Thyroid Uptake % Dose	$PB^{127}I$ µg/100 ml	Serum TSH µU/ml
1	M*	20	0	29.1	0.6	475
2	F	17	0	23.4	1.0	1175
3	F	15	0	57.4	1.0	410
4	M	15	0	20.3	0.3	412
5	M	21	0	27.5	0.6	378
6	F	25	0	30.6	0.5	465
7	F	21	0	24.1	0.4	1440
8	F	21	0	30.0	0.6	220
9	F	11	0	--	1.0	495
10	M	15-20	0	--	0.5	332

*M= Male, F= Female

Perhaps the developing neurologic structures of the fetus and newborn are also exquisitely sensitive to thyroid hormone so that an amount which is insufficient to affect development of function of other tissues can produce irreversible detrimental changes in the brain. The elevated serum TSH in the myxedematous patient falls to normal with the usual replacement dose of thyroid hormone (22,23). The author supports the contention that an elevated serum TSH is the most sensitive indicator of hypothyroidism and that a distinctly elevated serum TSH can be used to establish the diagnosis of hypothyroidism in a region of endemic goiter.

SUMMARY

Reports of studies of thyroid function in endemic cretins of six regions showed no substantial differences from the goitrous population when the cretins were euthyroid; in general there was rapid turnover of iodine. In hypothyroid cretins of the Congo, the PBI and thyroid uptake were reduced. Serum TSH levels in different regions of endemic goiter tended to be elevated in presumably euthyroid individuals in an inverse relation to the iodine intake. Myxedematous Congolese cretins of Idjwi Island had serum TSH levels 10 to 100 times greater than the euthyroid population of the region. A distinctly elevated serum TSH may be useful to establish the diagnosis of hypothyroidism in endemic cretins.

ACKNOWLEDGEMENTS

This work was supported by USPHS Research Grant HD05487 from the National Institute of Child Health and Human Development and VA Research Funds.

DISCUSSION BY PARTICIPANTS

BUTTFIELD: How is elevated TSH defined in a region of endemic goiter?

HERSHMAN: It has not been adequately defined in a region of endemic goiter. In our population of patients in Alabama, the values go up to 10 microunits per ml, which includes three standard deviations. Patients with hypothyroidism customarily have values which exceed 20 microunits per ml. There are patients with mild or equivocal hypothyroidism with values between 10 and 20, but the correlation between the level of hypothyroidism and the elevation of the serum TSH is not good. We have had patients with obvious severe myxedema with levels that were 40 to 100 microunits, and patients with levels of several hundred microunits who were obviously hypothyroid, but in whom the myxedema was not severe. When the levels go to twice that of a clearly euthyroid population, perhaps to about 20, that is distinctly abnormal. It might be used as an indication of hypothyroidism, at least in relation to what the pituitary and hypothalamus are recognizing - the amounts of circulating thyroid hormone they are responding to.

BECKERS: I wish to support very strongly the idea that TSH determination is an excellent procedure for detecting hypothyroidism. We have had the same experience as Dr. Hershman. I would like to add (as we will discuss later) that by using TRH, one can explore the pituitary-thyroid axis, more-or-less as one makes a glucose tolerance test to detect chemical diabetes. It appears indeed that at times TSH may be apparently normal, while the TSH response to TRH is not. I also have another question related to the Zaire studies. You said that in the endemic cretins of the Uele, thyroid function was not suppressed by T_3 administration. I thought that some of them were suppressed by T3.

DELANGE: No. In the four Uele cretins tested, uptake was not depressed by T_3 in any one of the patients. We tried to depress uptake in eight Idjwi cretins. We gave very low doses of T_3, 25 µg per day for five days (they weighed 25 kilos). We had to stop the treatment in two of them after two or three days because of tachycardia. In one who could continue the treatment there was no decrease in uptake. In some of them there was even an increase in uptake. We would not interpret this to mean that they cannot be suppressed, because when you see that the TSH level can rise over 1,000 microunits per ml, it is possible that such small doses over a short time would not be sufficient.

HETZEL: We did half a dozen who suppressed perfectly well.

DEGROOT: Is TSH eleveation a _sine qua non_ of hypothyroidism? Is it conceivable that a person with severe iodine deficiency might be in "balance" with euthyroidism maintained by a high TSH? Secondly, I wonder whether people who are iodine deficient for a long term with high TSHs, or with destroyed thyroid glands, could get TSH-producing tumors? Some people who are myxedematous after ^{131}I therapy have nonsuppressible high TSH. This suggests that they might have developed pituitary tumors which are non-suppressible.

HERSHMAN: The second point is interesting. I have not done methodical studies of patients with hypothyroidism after radio-iodine, but, in several patients we have studied, the serum TSH comes down to normal with replacement. It may be a matter of how long the patient is hypothyroid, but I do not think that autonomous TSH-producing adenomas have been confirmed in patients with longstanding hypothyroidism. In regard to the first point, I think that we are reaching a semantic impasse. It is not widely accepted that one can define hypothyroidism on the basis of an elevated serum TSH. If the elevated serum TSH is in contradiction to clinical judgment it generally is not accepted.

STANBURY: In support of Dr. DeGroot's point, engineering is full of feedback loops which bring the system back to the state it was originally. We are dealing with feedback loops here, and I see no inconsistency with the concept that the patient can be back to normal with an elevated TSH.

HERSHMAN: I think the physiological data suggests that what the pituitary responds to is the level of thyroid hormone that reaches it. Increased TSH secretion is a compensatory mechanism to get the diseased thyroid to work harder. However, if a thyroid that is inefficient for some other reason, such as lack of substrate, is truly able to make normal amounts of thyroid hormone which reaches the pituitary, the pituitary would be turned off. On that basis, I think that the elevated TSH means that the thyroid hormone reaching the pituitary is insufficient.

ERMANS: Severe iodine deficiency has been reported in a part of Idjwi in which the prevalence of goiter is almost normal. The PBI of these patients is quite normal and they have no clinical signs of hypothyroidism; their growth is normal. The organic iodine content of the thyroid of these subjects is only about one-half mg. In order to secrete 100 μg of hormonal iodine per day a marked acceleration of iodine turnover must be ensured by an increased TSH stimulation. Elevated TSH levels were indeed found in the serum of these patients. I am not sure ,therefore,that high TSH levels necessarily mean actual hypothyroidism.

HERSHMAN: But these levels of TSH in the Idjwi region, with few exceptions, were less than 20. They tended, as a population, to be definitely higher in the goitrous region. There was progression from the Belgian controls, to the iodine-deficiency region, to the goitrous region. The point I am making is that when the levels are definitely high, it is an indication of hypothyroidism.

MOSIER: It seems to me better to reserve the term "hypothyroidism" for patients in whom there is evidence of a deficiency of circulating thyroid hormone, with clinical signs of hypometabolism. Although a definition of hypothyroidism based on a high TSH level might be satisfactory in endemic cretinism, it could not be applied across the board. As examples of exceptions there are the forms of hypothyroidism in which TSH release is affected because of hypothalamic dysfunction or pituitary pathology. In addition, certain other metabolic functions, including glucocorticoid function, may influence TSH release.

HERSHMAN: In experimental animals, stress seems to suppress TSH but that has not been demonstrated in man. TSH is not labile, like growth hormone and ACTH, in response to stress.

PITTMAN: I would like to ask Dr. DeGroot,if everything is fine at a new steady state, what is the signal that maintains the TSH at the higher level?

DEGROOT: One "signal" could be the same amount of thyroid hormone that signals release of the normal amount of TSH, the amount just below that which would turn TSH off. A second possibility could be a T_4 level a small percentage below normal, which might be all it takes to turn TSH on.

HERSHMAN: This is in conflict with data recently presented by Gorman, Cotton, and Mayberry (23). They reported that elevated TSH's in myxedematous individuals were suppressed with stepwise increments of replacement doses of thyroid hormones. At conventional replacement doses, 0.2 milligram T_4 or 0.1 milligram T_3 , TSH was suppressed to normal levels. It seems as if exogenous thyroid hormone readily turns off TSH.

REFERENCES

1. Stanbury, J.B., Rocmans, P., Buhler, U.K. and Ochi, Y.: Congential hypothyroidism with impaired thyroid response to thyrotropin. N. Engl. J. Med. 279:1132-1136, 1968.

2. Miyai, K., Azukizawa, M. and Kumahara, Y.: Familial isolated thyrotropin deficiency with cretinism. N. Engl. J. Med. 285:1043-1048, 1971.

3. Koenig, M.P.: Die kongenitale Hypothyreose und der endemische Kretinismus. Springer, Berlin, 1968.

4. Dumont, J.E., Ermans, A.M. and Bastenie, P.A.: Thyroidal function in a goiter endemic. IV. Hypothyroidism and endemic cretinism. J. Clin. Endocrinol. Metab. 23:325-335, 1963.

5. Dumont, J.E., Ermans, A.M. and Bastenie, P.A.: Thyroid function in a goiter endemic. V. Mechanism of thyroid failure in the Uele endemic cretins. J. Clin. Endocrinol. Metab. 23:847-860, 1963.

6. Lobo, L.C.G., Pompeu, F. and Rosenthal, D.: Endemic cretinism in Goiaz, Brazil. J. Clin. Endocrinol. Metab. 23:407-412, 1963.

7. Rosenthal, D., Lobo, L.C.G., Rebello, M.A. and Fridman, J.: Studies on endemic goiter and cretinism in Brazil. 3. Thyroid function studies. In: Endemic Goiter. Report of the meeting of the PAHO Scientific Group on Research in Endemic Goiter held in Mexico, 1968 (J.B. Stanbury, ed.), Pan American Health Organization Scientific Publication No. 193, Washington, 1969. pp. 217-226.

8. Fierro-Benitez, R., Stanbury, J.B., Querido, A., DeGroot, L.J., Alban, R. and Cordova, J.: Endemic cretinism in the Andean region of Ecuador. J. Clin. Endocrinol. Metab. 30:228-236, 1970.

9. Choufoer, J.C., Van Rhijn, M. and Querido, A.: Endemic goiter in western New Guinea. II. Clinical picture, incidence and pathogenesis of endemic cretinism. J. Clin. Endocrinol. Metab. 25:385-402, 1965.

10. Buttfield, I.H., Hetzel, B.S.: Endemic cretinism in eastern New Guinea. Australas. Ann. Med. 18:217-221, 1969.

11. Bastenie, P.A., Ermans, A.M., Thys, O., Beckers, C, Van den Schrieck, H.G. and De Visscher, M.: Endemic goiter in the Uele region. III. Endemic cretinism. J. Clin. Endocrinol. Metab. 22:187-194, 1962.

12. Lobo, L.C.G., Da Silva, M.M., Hargreaves, F.B. and Couceiro, A.M.: Thyroidal iodoproteins in endemic cretins. J. Clin. Endocrinol. Metab. 24:285-293, 1964.

13. Studer, H., Greer, M.A.: A study of the mechanisms involved in the production of iodine-deficiency goiter. Acta Endocrinol. (Kbh.) 49:610-628, 1965.

14. Hershman, J.M., Pittman, J.A., Jr.: Utility of the radio-immunoassay of serum thyrotrophin in man. Ann. Intern. Med. 74:481-490, 1971.

15. Hershman, J.M., Pittman, J.A., Jr.: Control of thyrotropin secretion in man. N. Engl. J. Med. 285:997-1006, 1971.

16. Buttfield, I.H., Hetzel, B.S. and Odell, W.D.: Effect of iodized oil on serum TSH determined by immunoassay in endemic goiter subjects. J. Clin. Endocrinol. Metab. 28:1664-1666, 1968.

17. Delange, F., Hershman, J.M. and Ermans, A.M.: Relationship between the serum thyrotropin level, the prevalence of goiter and the pattern of iodine metabolism in Idjwi Island. J. Clin. Endocrinol. Metab. 33:261-268, 1971.

18. Coble, Y.D., Jr., Kohler, P.O.: Plasma TSH levels in endemic goiter subjects. J. Clin. Endocrinol. Metab. 31: 220-221, 1970.

19. Pisarev, M.A., Utiger, R.D., Salvaneschi, J.P., Altschuler, N. and DeGroot, L.J.: Serum TSH and thyroxine in goitrous subjects in Argentina. J. Clin. Endocrinol. Metab. 30: 680-681, 1970.

20. Wahner, H.W., Mayberry, W.E., Gaitan, E., and Gaitan, J.E.: Endemic goiter in the Cauca Valley. III. Role of serum TSH in goitrogenesis. J. Clin. Endocrinol. Metab. 32:491-496, 1971.

21. Adams, D.D., Kennedy, T.H., Choufoer, J.C., and Querido, A.: Endemic goiter in western New Guinea. III. Thyroid-stimulating activity of serum from severely iodine-deficient people. J. Clin. Endocrinol. Metab. 28:685-692, 1968.

22. Odell, W.D., Wilber, J.F. and Utiger, R.D.: Studies of thyrotropin physiology by means of radioimmunoassay. Recent Progr. Horm. Res. 23:47-78, 1967.

23. Cotton, G.E., Gorman, C.A. and Mayberry, W.E.: Suppression of thyrotropin (h-TSH) in serums of patients with myxedema of varying etiology treated with thyroid hormones. N. Engl. J. Med. 285:529-533, 1971.

A SURVEY OF THE CLINICAL AND METABOLIC PATTERNS OF ENDEMIC CRETINISM

F. Delange, A. Costa, A.M. Ermans, H.K. Ibbertson, A. Querido and J.B. Stanbury

CEMUBAC Medical Team. Department of Pediatrics and Radioisotopes, School of Medicine, St. Peter Hospital. University of Brussels, Belgium. IRSAC, Zwiro, Zaire Republic. Mauriziana Hospital, Turin, Italy. Department of Endocrinology, School of Medicine, Auckland, New Zealand. Department of Medicine, University of Leiden, Holland. Department of Nutrition and Food Science, Massachusetts Institute of Technology, Cambridge, Massachusetts.

Since the work of McCarrison (1) and that of De Quervain and Wegelin (2), a large number of articles have been devoted to the description of the clinical and metabolic characteristics of endemic cretinism (3-19). Yet the definition of the term "endemic cretin" has continued until very recently (20, 21) to constitute the subject of passionate discussion, especially between the respective defenders of neurological (22) and of hypothyroid endemic cretinism (7).

As Querido has pointed out (22),: "A definition in medicine can be based on etiology, on a basic morphological or physiological lesion common to all defects, or it can be purely of a descriptive nature." The definition of the syndrome of endemic cretinism rests essentially on a description of the disease, because its causes are still unknown (20, 23) or hypothetical (19, 24) (see also Ermans *et al.*, chapter of the present volume) and because the reports on the histological lesions of endemic cretinism are few and incomplete (2, 25).

The purpose of the present paper is to compare the essential clinical and biological characteristics observed in subjects labelled "endemic cretins" in various regions of the world and to try to fit them into coherent patterns. This recapitulation could serve as a basis for proposing a more comprehensive and general definition of endemic cretinism.

The principal symptoms of endemic cretinism encountered in varying combinations are mental retardation, neurological defects, deaf-mutism, hypothyroidism and dwarfism (20, 21). The symptoms are accompanied in some cases by biologic signs of thyroid failure (7, 18,19).

The distribution frequencies of these different symptoms and signs in the forms of endemic cretinism reported in New Guinea (12, 14,), Ecuador (15, 16), Brazil (6), Italy (11), Nepal (18) and Congo [Rep. of Zaire (5, 7, 8, 19)], were compared with the aid of data from the literature. The results of this comparison are shown in Fig. 1. For the purpose of this analysis, only the patients with obvious mental retardation were considered as endemic cretins. Mental retardation is often difficult to establish with accuracy in remote regions because of the lack of standardized psychomotor tests for the populations in question and difficulties of communication.

We have grouped under the term "neurological defects" a series of anomalies associated in varying degrees of severity: these are first motor defects, most often characterized by paresis or paralysis of pyramidal origin, sometimes accompanied by extra-pyramidal signs; serious impairment of muscular tonus, ranging from hypo- to hypertonia; and abnormal gait, which is either spastic or ataxic. The criteria on which the clinical diagnosis of hypothyroidism is based are retarded linear growth and maturation of body proportions; myxedematous, thickened, puffy, dry, and scaly skin; and marked delay in sexual development. The criteria of normality for thyroid function are the results obtained for uptake and PBI in clinically euthyroid adults living in the same region as the cretins. Height is compared with that of the local population used as a control. Epiphyseal malformation typical of hypothyroidism is always accompanied by very considerable retardation of bone maturation.

The frequency of distribution of these different symptoms has been considered on the basis of their presence in all (100 percent), most (over 50 percent) or some (10-15 percent) of the cretins living in a particular region. Fig. 1 shows that the patients described as endemic cretins actually exhibit extremely different clinical, biological and radiologic symptoms from one region to another. Two very pronounced types are recognizable: myxedematous and nervous endemic cretinism. The most typical example of nervous cretinism is encountered in New Guinea (12, 14): the subjects show extreme mental deficiency with major neurological defects and deaf-mutism in almost all. Goiter prevalence is comparable to that of the rest of the population and thyroid

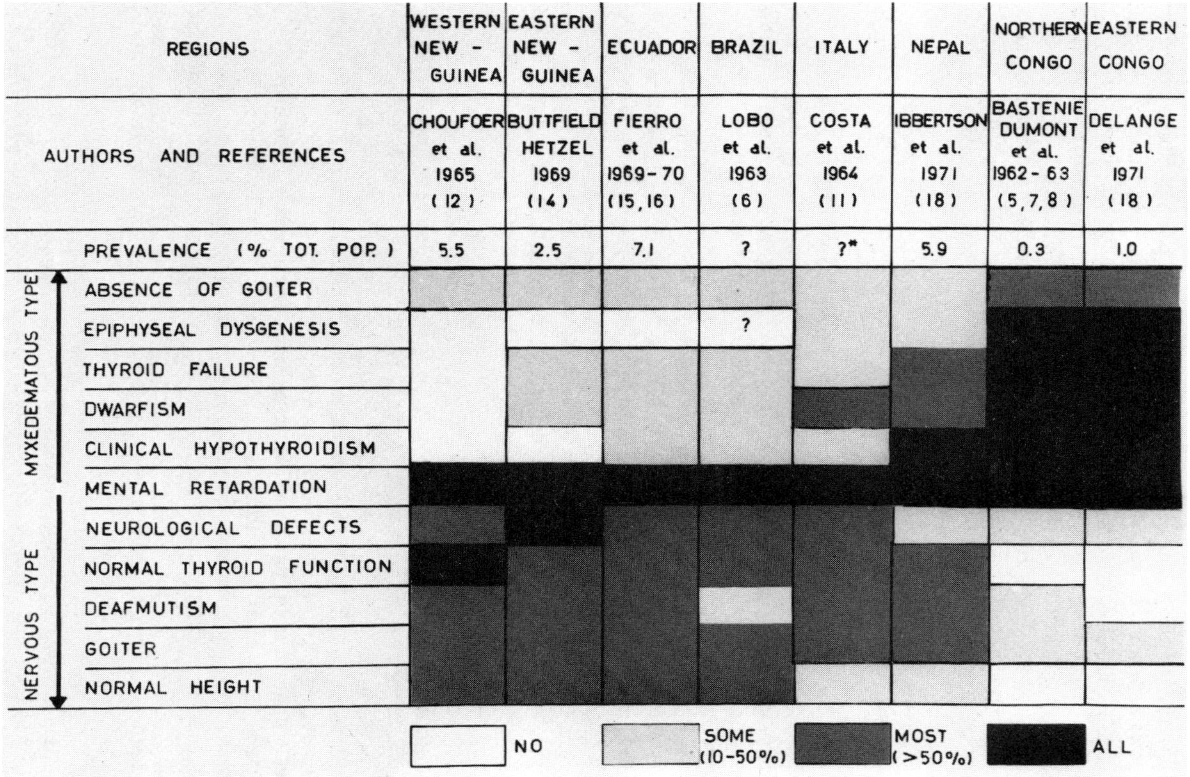

	REGIONS	WESTERN NEW - GUINEA	EASTERN NEW - GUINEA	ECUADOR	BRAZIL	ITALY	NEPAL	NORTHERN CONGO	EASTERN CONGO
	AUTHORS AND REFERENCES	CHOUFOER et al. 1965 (12)	BUTTFIELD HETZEL 1969 (14)	FIERRO et al. 1969-70 (15,16)	LOBO et al. 1963 (6)	COSTA et al. 1964 (11)	IBBERTSON et al. 1971 (18)	BASTENIE DUMONT et al. 1962-63 (5,7,8)	DELANGE et al. 1971 (18)
	PREVALENCE (% TOT. POP.)	5.5	2.5	7.1	?	?*	5.9	0.3	1.0
MYXEDEMATOUS TYPE	ABSENCE OF GOITER								
	EPIPHYSEAL DYSGENESIS				?				
	THYROID FAILURE								
	DWARFISM								
	CLINICAL HYPOTHYROIDISM								
	MENTAL RETARDATION								
NERVOUS TYPE	NEUROLOGICAL DEFECTS								
	NORMAL THYROID FUNCTION								
	DEAFMUTISM								
	GOITER								
	NORMAL HEIGHT								

NO — SOME (10-50%) — MOST (>50%) — ALL

Fig. 1. Comparison of the distribution frequencies of the main clinical and metabolic characteristics observed in endemic cretins in New Guinea, South America, Italy, Nepal and the Zaire Republic. The prevalence of 0.03% reported in Italy is not mentioned because it might have been modified critically by recent changes in socio-economic and nutritional conditions.

metabolic status is apparently normal. Most of the subjects are normal in height. At the other extreme are myxedematous cretins, typified by those encountered in Zaire (7,19). These subjects are less mentally retarded than the preceding type, all are dwarfs, with thyroid insufficiency and extremely retarded bone maturation. Most of these cretins have no goiter. The clinical pictures reported in other regions are situated between these two extreme forms. Thus, for instance, the majority of cretins in South America (6, 15, 16) show predominantly neurological defects, but certain of them exhibit clear signs of hypothyroidism. The same situation has been reported in Italy by Costa et al. (11) and in Switzerland by Koenig (13). Finally, in Nepal (18), cretins who represent almost six percent of the population of some regions show definite signs of thyroid insufficiency, associated in most with deaf-mutism and in some with other neurological defects.

In view of the diversity of criteria used for defining the fundamental characteristics of cretinism, one of us (F.D.) has tried to clarify the question by inviting various investigators with personal experience of the problem to complete a stardardized form designed to assemble systematically as much as possible of the data currently available. The standardized form covered schematically all the epidemiologic, clinical and biological aspects of endemic cretinism which have been quantified so far. The form consisted of two separate parts: the first concerned the criteria used by each of the authors for making a diagnosis of endemic cretinism; the second concerned detailed description of the clinical signs, and the results of the biological, radiologic and other tests made on the cretins studied.

The criteria used by the teams of Leiden, Brussels and Auckland to diagnose endemic cretinism are: mental retardation associated with one of the following signs: irreversible neuromuscular disorders, irreversible anomalies in hearing and speech extending in certain cases to deaf-mutism, impairment of somatic development, and hypothyroidism. The Turin team added the complementary concept of anomalies of behavior and, in addition, the word hypothyroidism was not associated with the concept of retarded development, for the low stature of most cretins does not always refer to hypothyroidism.

The epidemiologic and clinical data collected by the authors on endemic cretinism in New Guinea, Italy, Nepal, and the Zaire Republic are summarized in Table 1. The prevalence of cretinism observed in these different regions is very variable: it rises from one percent in regions of Zaire to almost six percent in goitrous districts in Nepal (8). Furthermore, as stated earlier, the clinical symptoms exhibited by the cretins in these regions are very different from one region to another. On the basis of the descriptions furnished by each of the authors, four categories can be

*Table 1. Comparison of the clinical patterns of endemic cretinism in Western New Guinea, Italy, Nepal, and the Zaire Republic. The figures indicate the prevalence of cretinism expressed in percent of the total population of the region studied. *See comment on Fig. 1.*

Regions Surveyed	Mulia Valley Western New Guinea	Northern Italy (Cuneo Province)	Khumbu Region Nepalese Himalayas	Idjwi Island Kivu - Zaire
Total population	1,500	550,000	±2,000	9,000
Authors	Querido et al. 1965	Costa et al. 1964	Ibbertson et al. 1971	Delange et al. 1971
TYPES OF CRETINISM				
Major neurological defects only	5.5	0.03* (both rows)	-	(0.1)
Neurological defects ± slight hypothyroidism	-		(4.6)	-
Hypothyroidism ± slight Neurological defects	-	-	5.9	-
Major hypothyroidism only	-	-	-	1.0

defined according to the severity of the signs of thyroid insufficiency or neurological defects. The cretins of New Guinea show neurological damage only; those of Italy show neurological signs and minor, but sometimes clear, manifestations of thyroid insufficiency; those of Nepal show mainly signs of hypothyroidism, associated in some cases with neurological defects; and finally the cretins of Zaire exhibit major signs of thyroid insufficiency almost exclusively. The 4.6 percent of subjects observed in Nepal who show deaf-mutism and slight signs of hypothyroidism are indicated in brackets because their mental retardation is not very apparent. The deaf-mute cretins of Idjwi are indicated in brackets also because their prevalence does not exceed that observed in the non-goitrous populations (26).

Table 2 compares goiter prevalence, radioiodine uptake, and PBI in the four types of endemic cretinism with the corresponding values obtained for control subjects in the same regions. Goiter prevalence and thyroid function in endemic cretins of New Guinea are comparable to those of the control subjects. In contrast, a considerable drop in uptake and PBI is observed in the cretins of Zaire. Furthermore, the prevalence of goiter is only half as high as in the controls. Evidence of some degree of clinical hypothyroidism in endemic cretins in Italy and Nepal is associated with a decrease of PBI.

The diversity of the clinical and biological pictures displayed by the cretins in the goiter endemics studied is illustrated in Figs. 2-5.

Thus, subjects labelled "endemic cretins" exhibit patterns which are extremely variable, depending on the goiter endemic which is studied. The dominant symptom is severe mental retardation. It is accompanied by a series of clinical and metabolic signs reflecting varying degrees of impairment of the nervous system and thyroid function.

The principal task of this review is to emphasize that the forms of nervous cretinism and myxedematous cretinism, as distinguished earlier by McCarrison (1) and more recently by Dumont, *et al.* (20), in fact constitute the extreme aspects of a continuous spectrum of developmental anomalies between which there are numerous intermediate forms. An overall definition of the disease must take this situation into account.

*Table 2. Comparison of the biological patterns of endemic cretinism in western New Guinea, Italy, Nepal, and Zaire**

Regions surveyed	New Guinea	Italy	Nepal	Zaire
Controls	G = ± 60% U_{max} = 87.2 ± 7.8 PBI = 1.9 ± 1.2	G = 15%** U_{24h} = 39.0 ± 9.3 PBI = 6.3 ± 0.8	G = 92% U_{48h} = 64.5 ± 16.8 PBI = 2.9 ± 1.6	G = 54% U_{24h} = 79.5 ± 13.6 PBI = 3.7 ± 1.7
TYPES OF CRETINISM				
Major neurological defects only	G = 60% U_{max} = 78.1 ± 9.9 PBI = 1.5 ± 0.8	-	-	-
Neurological defects ± slight hypothyroidism	- -	G = 71% U_{24h} = 49.7 ± 7.0 PBI = 5.6 ± 0.4	- - -	- - -
Hypothyroidism ± slight neurological defects	-	-	G = 68% U_{48h} = 72.6 ± 18.2 PBI = 1.8 ± 1.9	-
Major hypothyroidism only	-	-	-	G = 25% U_{24h} = 40.0 ± 20.0 PBI = 1.3 ± 0.9

*G = Prevalence of goiter in percent of the total population (controls) or in the cretins.
U = Thyroid uptake of radioiodine in percent of the dose.
PBI = Level of the plasma protein-bound iodine in μg per 100 ml.
Mean values ± standard deviation

**The figure reported for controls in Italy concerns male school children of the province of Cuneo.

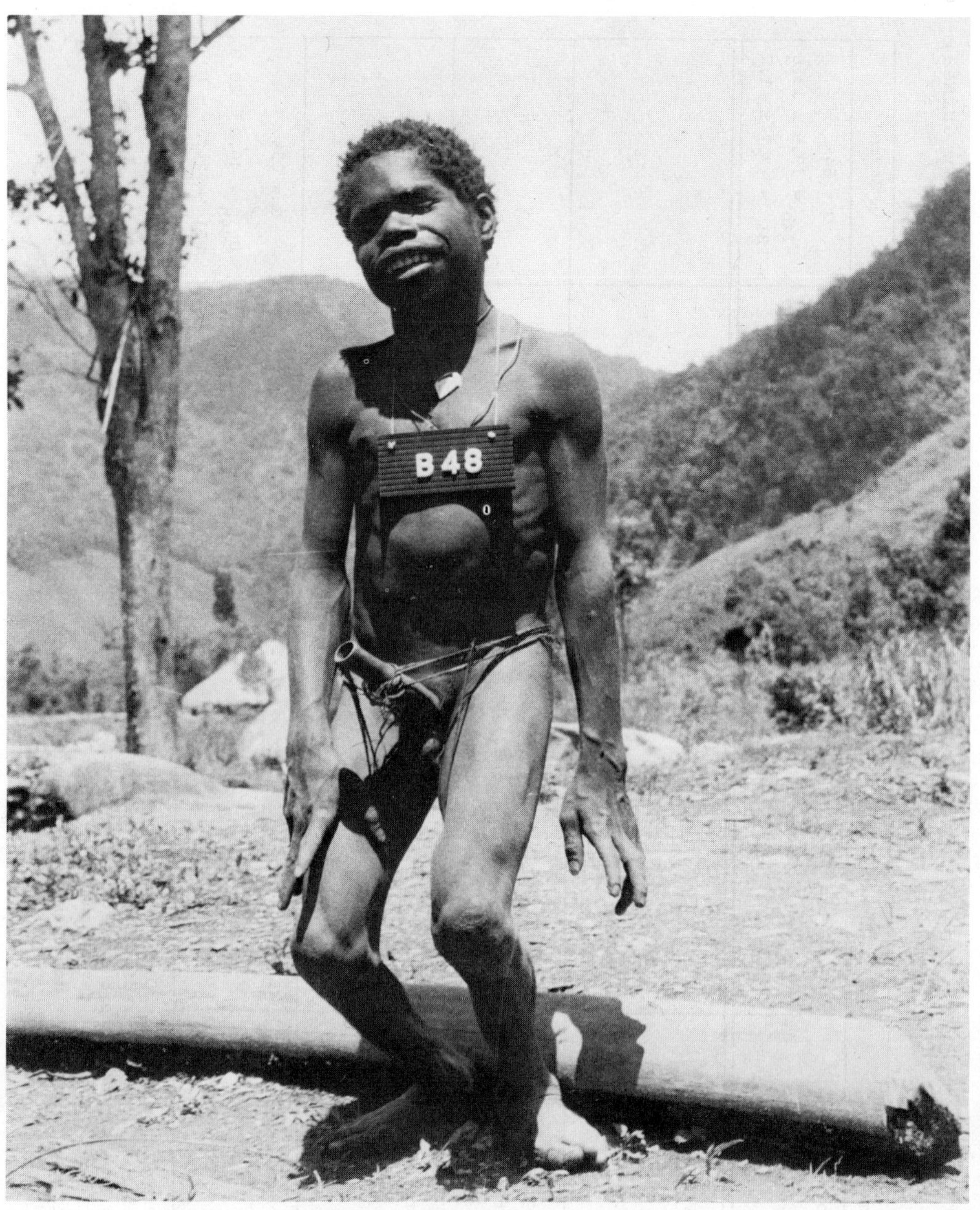

Fig. 2. Endemic cretin in Western New Guinea: boy, 14 yr old, thyroid twice normal size with one nodule palpable. Deaf-mutism, amentia, neuromotor disability, squinting - $PB^{127}I$: 1.7 µg per 100 ml, 6 hr neck uptake: 92%. Normal development of femoral epiphyses.

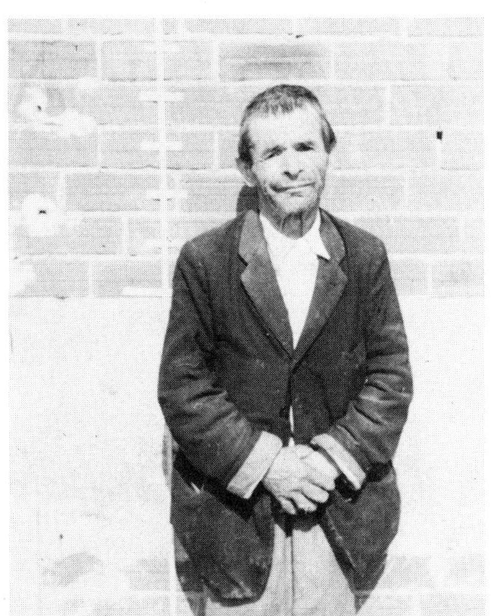

Fig. 3. Endemic cretin in Italy (Piedmont): male, 50 yr old, mental deficiency, height 152 cm (92% of normal), no goiter. $BP^{127}I$: 4.6 μg per 100 ml, 24 hr ^{131}I thyroid uptake: 57%.

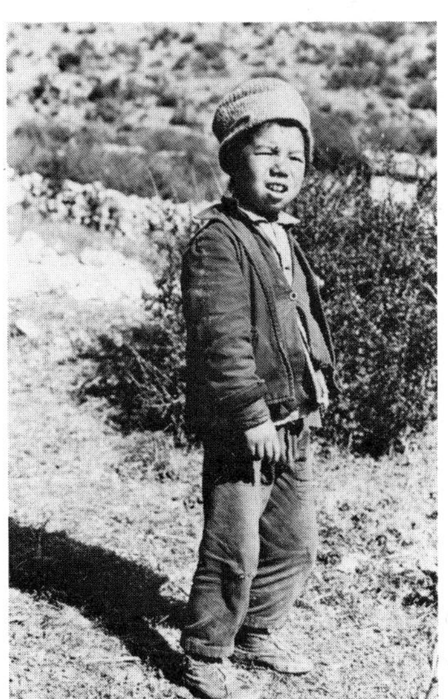

Fig. 4. A typical Sherpa hypothyroid cretin with ataxic gait and spasticity of the legs. Age 17 yr, ^{131}I neck uptake at 4 hr: 46%. Serum $PB^{127}I$, 1.2 μg per 100 ml.

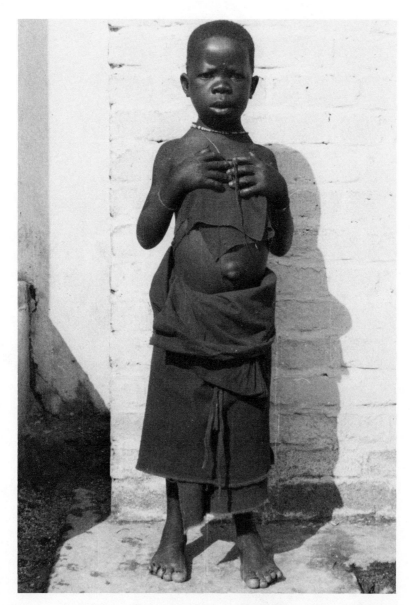

Fig. 5. Endemic cretin in Zaire Republic (Idjwi Island): female, 20 yr old, mental deficiency, height 109 cm (69% of normal), no goiter, dry skin, umbilical hernia, primary amenorrhea. Clinically hypothyroid. $PB^{127}I$: 1.3 µg per 100 ml, 24 hr ^{131}I thyroid uptake: 23%. Bone age: 8 yr. TSH: 1,440 µu per ml.

SUMMARY

The main clinical and metabolic characteristics observed in subjects labelled "endemic cretins" in various endemic goiter areas of the world have been compared. The comparison is based partly on data obtained from the literature and partly on personal observations made by the authors in New Guinea, Italy, Nepal, and the Zaire Republic.

The picture of endemic cretinism, as illustrated by the cretins studied, is extremely polymorphous. It is characterized essentially by irreversible mental retardation and by an almost continuous spectrum of clinical and metabolic signs, reflecting varying degrees of impairment of the nervous system and thyroid function.

ACKNOWLEDGEMENTS

*Supported in part by the "Fonds de la Recherche Scientifique" (Belgium) by Euratom, Universities of Pisa and Brussels, and by USPH Grant No. AM 10992.

REFERENCES

1. McCarrison, R.: Observation on endemic cretinism in the Chitral and Gilgit Valleys. Lancet 2:1275-1280, 1908.

2. De Quervain, F. and Wegelin, C.: Der endemisch Kretinismus. Springer-Verlag, Berlin, 1936.

3. Stanbury, J.B.; Brownell, G.L.; Riggs, D.S.; Perinetti, H.; Itoiz, J. and Del Castillo, E.B.: Endemic goiter, the adaptation of man to iodine deficiency. Harvard University Press, Cambridge, 1954.

4. Kicic, M.; Milutinovic, P.; Djordjevic, S. and Ramzin, S.: Endocrinological aspects of an endemic focus of cretinism. In: Advances in Thyroid Research (R. Pitt-Rivers, ed.). Pergamon Press, London, 1961. pp. 301-306.

5. Bastenie, P.A.; Ermans, A.M.; Thys, O.; Beckers, C.; Vandenshrieck, H.G. and De Visscher, M.: Endemic goiter in the Uele Region. III. Endemic cretinism. J. Clin. Endocrinol. and Metab. 22:187-194, 1962.

6. Lobo, L.C.G.; Pompeu, F. and Rosenthal, D.: Endemic cretinism in Goiaz, Brazil. J. Clin. Endocrinol. and Metab. 23: 407-412, 1963.

7. Dumont, J.E.; Ermans, A.M. and Bastcnie, P.A.: Thyroidal function in a goiter endemic. IV. Hypothyroidism and endemic cretinism. J. Clin. Endocrinol. and Metab. 23:325-335, 1963.

8. Dumont, J.E.; Ermans, A.M. and Bastcnie, P.A.: Thyroidal function in a goiter endemic. V. Mechanism of thyroid failure in the Uele endemic cretins. J. Clin. Endocrinol. and Metab. 23: 847-860, 1963.

9. McCullagh, S.F.: The Huon pensinsula endemic. IV. Endemic goiter and congenital defects. Med. J. Austr. 50:884-890, 1963.

10. Srinivasan, S.; Subramanyan, T.A.V.; Sinha, A.; Deo, M.G. and Ramalingaswami, V.: Himalayan endemic deaf-mutism. Lancet 2:176-178, 1964.

11. Costa, A; Cottino, F.; Mortara, M. and Vogliazzo, U.: Endemic cretinism in Piedmont. Panminerva Medica 6:250-259, 1964.

12. Choufoer, J.C.; Van Rhijn, M. and Querido, A.: Endemic goiter in Western New Guinea. II. Clinical picture, incidence, and pathogenesis of endemic cretinism. J. Clin. Endocrinol. and Metab. 25:385-402, 1965.

13. Koenig, M.P.: Die kongenitale Hypothyreose und der endemische Kretinismus. Springer-Verlag, Berlin, 1968.

14. Buttfield, I.H. and Hetzel, B.S.: Endemic cretinism in Eastern New Guinea. Austral. Ann. Med. 18:217-221, 1969.

15. Fierro-Benítez, R.; Penafiel, W.; DeGroot, L.J. and Ramírez, I.: Endemic goiter and endemic cretinism in the Andean region. New Eng. J. Med. 280:296-302, 1969.

16. Fierro-Benítez, R.; Stanbury, J.B.; Querido, A.; DeGroot, L.; Alban, R. and Cordova, J.: Endemic cretinism in the Andean region of Ecuador. J. Clin. Endocrinol. and Metab. 30:228-236, 1970.

17. Mortara, M. and Rubino, R.: Cretinismo Endemico - La malattia I suoi aspetti neurologici. Roma, Consiglia Nasionale delle Richerche (Quaderni de la Ricerca Scientifica No. 62):1-59, 1970.

18. Ibbertson, H.K.; Pearl, M.; McKinnon, J.; Tait, J.M.; Lim, T. and Gill, M.D.: Endemic cretinism in Nepal. In: Endemic Cretinism. Monogr. Series No. 2 (B.S. Hetzel and P.O.D. Pharoah, eds.) Institute of Human Biology, Papua, New Guinea 1971. pp. 71-88.

19. Delange, F.; Ermans, A.M.; Vis, H.L. and Stanbury, J.B.: Endemic cretinism in Idjwi Island. In: Endemic Cretinism Mongr. Series No. 2, (B.S. Hetzel and P.O.D. Pharoah, eds.). Institute of Human Biology, Papua, New Guinea 1971. pp. 33-53.

20. Dumont, J.E.; Delange, F. and Ermans, A.M.: Endemic cretinism In: Endemic Goiter. Report of the meeting of the PAHO Scientific Group on Endemic Goiter held in Mexico, 1968 (J.B. Stanbury, ed.). PAHO Scientific Publication No. 193, Washington, 1969. pp. 91-98.

21. Querido, A.: Definition of endemic cretinism. In: Endemic Cretinism Mongr. Series No. 2, (B.S. Hetzel and P.O.D. Pharoah, eds.). Institute of Human Biology, Papua, New Guinea 1971. pp. 132-133.

22. Querido, A.: Endemic cretinism: a search for a tenable definition. In: Endemic Goiter. Report of the meeting of the PAHO Scientific Group on Endemic Goiter held in Mexico, 1968 (J.B. Stanbury, ed.). PAHO Scientific Publication No. 193, Washington, 1969. pp. 85-90.

23. Anonymous: The etiology of endemic cretinism. Nutr. Rev. 29: 227-230, 1971.

24. Pharoah, P.O.D.; Buttfield, I.H. and Hetzel, B.S.: Neurological damage to the fetus resulting from severe iodine deficiency during pregnancy. Lancet 1:308-310, 1971.

25. Vickery, A.L.; Fierro-Benitez, R. and Kakulas, B.A.: Skeletal muscle structure in endemic cretinism. Amer. J. Path. 49: 193-202, 1966.

26. Friedmann, I.: The pathology of deafness. In: Sensorineural Hearing Loss (G.E.W. Wolstenholme and J. Knight, eds.). Churchill, London, 1970. pp.41-68.

SECTION 3
PREVENTION OF CRETINISM

HISTORY OF IODINE PROPHYLAXIS WITH REGARD TO CRETINISM AND DEAF-MUTISM

A. Querido

Department of Medicine, University of Leiden, Holland

The literature on the prevention of endemic goiter through iodine prophylaxis is extensive, starting with the classic studies by Marine and Kimball from 1917 to 1919 (1). While endemic cretinism is found only in areas with severe endemic goiter and iodine deficiency, in this chapter we will be concerned with the evidence that iodine prophylaxis is also effective in the prevention of endemic cretinism.

The significance for health of endemic goiter is essentially different from that of endemic cretinism. If severe endemic goiter leads to complications, these can be effectively treated. Endemic cretinism, on the other hand, with manifestations such as mental deficiency and deaf-mutism, **is irreparable.** It is a true public health problem of mental health in a community and therefore deserves more attention than it has hitherto received. Endemic cretinism may not affect health statistics in a considerable way, but it may profoundly affect the potential for development of a community.

In order to assess the efficacy of iodine prophylaxis, it is clearly necessary to use indicators to establish the frequency of endemic cretinism. This is a complicated problem. It is not difficult to recognize the most severe cases of endemic cretinism, with severe mental deficiency, growth retardation, neuromotor abnormalities and deaf-mutism. There exists, however, a whole spectrum of these abnormalities varying from slight to severe. The techniques for collecting data are also difficult. The frequency cannot be measured, for instance, by studying school populations (where cretins will not be found) but only by visiting each home in a community. It is therefore not surprising that few studies are available on the frequency of endemic cretinism before and after iodine prophylaxis.

Some authors have indicated (2) that endemic cretinism in some areas has disappeared spontaneously before iodine prophylaxis was instituted. Improvement of socio-economic conditions and of communications such as railroads were considered as possible explanations. Elsewhere (3) we have discussed the confusing issues of poor socio-economic conditions, such as undernutrition and illiteracy, with the description of the epidemiological manifestations of endemic cretinism. Improvement of communications will bring foods from other areas, which may improve the iodine intake. Even a small increase of iodine intake can be highly significant because endemic cretinism only occurs in the presence of most severe iodine deficiency (4), with urinary iodine excretions below 15 μg per 24 hr, and even then only in a small percentage of the newly born. Even under conditions of severe iodine deficiency the situation is marginal. Thus the most reasonable explanation for the "spontaneous" disappearance of endemic cretinism is a slight increase of iodine intake. Since endemic cretinism has never been reported from areas with an average urinary iodine excretion of more than 20 μg per 24 hrs, those who relate the appearance of endemic cretinism to factors other than iodine deficiency are obligated to reinforce their contention with studies on iodine excretion before they can be taken seriously.

Apart from the reports elsewhere in this volume, of which some recently appeared elsewhere as preliminary communications, few studies are available on the effect of iodine prophylaxis on the prevention of endemic cretinism. From Switzerland, the country where the conditions before and after iodine prophylaxis were most thoroughly studied, Koenig (2) reported in 1968 that no cretins had been born in the past 20 years. This observation is important because Switzerland is a highly developed country with obligatory schooling and extensive medical services. Koenig based his conclusions on careful examinations in institutions in Canton Bern, and in the village of Blumenstein, where Eugster made his detailed observations in 1937 (5). The criteria used were the presence of at least three of the following symptoms: oligophrenia, deaf-mutism or deafness, and stunted growth or neuromuscular disorders. Information obtained from health workers in Canton Wallis also indicated that no cretins were born in the past 20 years.

The only report in which the same investigators studied a community before and after iodine prophylaxis appeared in 1960 from Yugoslavia, by Kičič and coworkers (6). The criteria used for endemic cretinism were those given by de Quervain and Wegelin (8) which are based on social adaptation. The observations were done in the village Gornja Josanica, which had a goiter prevalence of 84 percent. In the period (preceding iodized salt prophylaxis) before 1930 the incidence of cretinism among the newborn was 13 percent. After the economic standard of the village was raised it was about seven percent. This level was maintained until 1954, when iodine prophylaxis (1 part potassium iodide in 100,000 parts NaCl) was started. During the succeeding 14 years no cretins, "cretinoids" or deaf-mutes were born (7). Kičič *et al.* also suggested a positive effect of iodine prophylaxis on stature of children in their population (6).

In 1945, Wespi (9) reported on the reduction of deaf-mutism in Switzerland following introduction of iodized salt. Endemic deaf-mutism, which only occurs in areas with severe endemic goiter, can be used as a marker for the presence of endemic cretinism for all endemias which have been recently studied, such as in West and East New Guinea, Ecuador and Nepal. The exception is the Zaire Republic where deaf-mutism is not a part of the syndrome. Wespi collected his data through three Swiss organizations which for many years have provided care and education for deaf-mutes and deaf persons. The sources provided information about nearly all individuals who needed speech education in a period before, during and after iodine prophylaxis in the different cantons. Fig.1 presents the overall results in Switzerland between 1915 and 1932. From the studies done in detail in each canton, there was always a correlation (with one exception) between time of introduction and amount of iodized salt used and the disappearance of deaf-mutism. The only exception was Canton Wallis, for which different explanations were considered, such as more hereditary forms of deaf-mutism, the question whether indeed the centers with cretinism were reached and so on. The data are convincing because two correlations were used: the *time* of introduction of iodized salt, and an approximation of the *amount* used. Furthermore, studies were available on the classification of the deaf-mutism in Canton Zurich, which had a high level of affected individuals, and Canton Waadt, with a low frequency. The difference between these cantons was found to be only in the congenital form of deaf-mutism, which was much higher in Zurich.

Wespi's study with deaf-mutism as a marker for endemic cretinism offers up until the present the best evidence supporting the *effect* of iodine prophylaxis. It should not be forgotten however, that more reasons exist to link endemic cretinism with iodine deficiency. *Endemic* cretinism occurs only in areas with

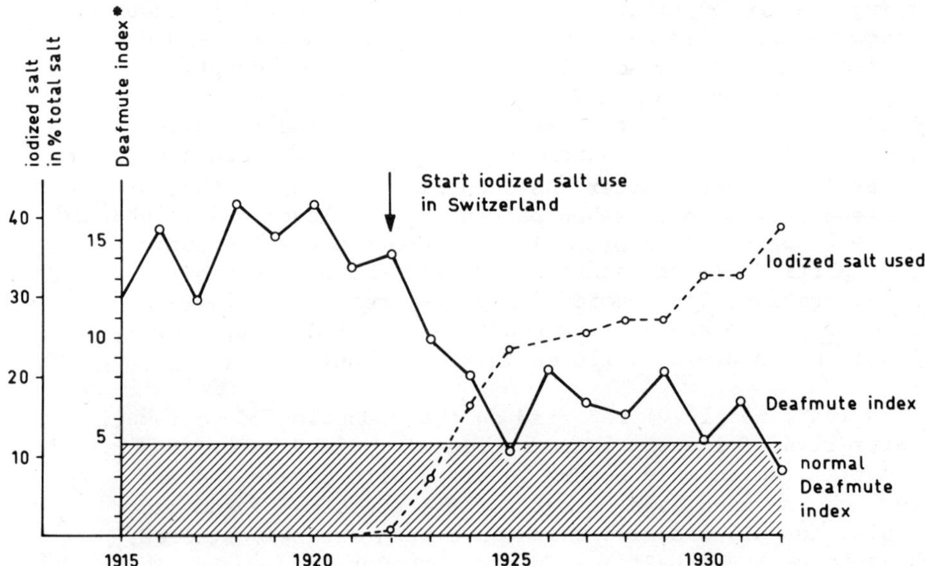

Fig. 1. Deaf-mutism and the use of iodized salt in Switzerland 1915 - 1932. From Wespi (9). *Deaf-mute index = Deaf-mute school children per 10,000 live births of the same year.

severe endemic goiter and is limited to those with an extremely low iodine intake (4,10). From the viewpoint of public health measures, the overall evidence is more than strong enough to underscore the necessity of iodine prophylaxis for areas with endemic cretinism.

In conclusion it seems appropriate to raise the question whether iodine prophylaxis in an area with severe iodine deficiency and cretinism does more than only prevent overt cretinism. Penrose (11) refers to a definition of a mentally defective individual as "one who by reason of incomplete mental development is incapable of independent social adaptation." This makes the definition for a mentally defective flexible and related to the level of development of the community. In a rural community scholastic defect is much less of a handicap than in an urban and developed society. In those communities where endemic cretinism has been recently studied, many individuals with low mental capacity must have been unnoticed. Dingman (12) calculated for the United States that the normal distribution of intelligence has a standard deviation of 16 points, which leads to three percent individuals in a population with IQ between 50 - 70. In the IQ group below 50, more individuals prevail than fits with the Gaussian curve. This indicates skewing. Do cretins only fit in this extreme group, or are the number of individuals with IQ's between 50 - 100 also increased above expectations? This is a very difficult question to answer because of the testing techniques involved. Be this as it may, there is no doubt that iodine prophylaxis for affected areas is an important step towards improvement of mental health.

SUMMARY

Endemic cretinism is primarily a problem of mental health in the affected communities. Strong evidence exists that it is prevented through iodine prophylaxis, because it only occurs in areas with extreme iodine deficiency, with 24 hour urinary iodine excretion values below 15 µg. Objective data available from the period before 1960 are scarce because of the technical difficulties of assessing frequencies in epidemiological studies. It is likely that iodine prophylaxis, besides preventing overt cretinism, also may improve the average mental capacity in communities with severe iodine deficiency and cretinism.

ACKNOWLEDGEMENTS

Figure 1 reprinted by permission of the publishers of *Schweizerische Medizinische Wochenschrift*.

DISCUSSION BY PARTICIPANTS

KOENIG: I agree entirely with Dr. Querido's statement that asking local authorities is absolutely no help. When we did field studies in Austria, we asked the Steyermark health department and every local health officer how many cretins they had. Their responses went from, "We have in our community approximately twelve cretins" to, "We have none", or, "We think there may be some in some social institutions." If we asked physicians, they said, "We have a great many." So we went to the social workers, who must by law keep records of every child who does not attend school. We found that in 1936 this area had a very severe encephalitis epidemic and there were a great number of postencephalitic idiots there. Of course for an untrained physician a child with postencephalitic idiocy and goiter is a "cretin." The same holds true for deaf-mutism in Switzerland. Wespi's work (9) is in part the basis of De Reynier's studies (13). De Reynier gave a certain figure for endemic deaf-mutism in Switzerland in 1953. Questioned on what basis he made the diagnosis he answered, "These were people for whom we had no other explanation for deaf-mutism and they had a goiter, so we thought this must be deaf-mutism of the endemic type." In the last 12 years I have talked with Eugster repeatedly. He often claimed that Michaelis showed already around 1850 how endemic cretinism regressed in Switzerland and southern Germany even before railways came. All this is to say that it is very difficult for us in Central Europe to get "hard" data on the true incidence of endemic deaf-mutism and cretinism. Wespi (9) and Kičič (14) are among the few who have done systematic work.

QUERIDO: Perhaps only 90 percent of the data were available for Wespi's study. That does not change the evidence of this figure, which is based on trend. It shows that there is a tendency toward a strong relationship between the intake of iodized salt and the decrease of deaf-mutism. One must have strong data to refute the paper of Wespi.

KOENIG: I agree that the tendency is strong. I just want to point out that the European data need to be considered with some reservation.

ERMANS: I suppose that your statement about the role of iodine deficiency in the etiology of cretinism is solid enough to require consideration from the public health point of view. However, it might be dangerous to give too much proof. I am not convinced that your data show differences in goiter prevalence in relation to iodine urinary excretion. Excretion rates from about 4 μg per day are unbelievable from a kinetic point of view. Considering a thyroid uptake of 80 percent, this would mean a general turnover of iodide of about 20 μg; this is evidently too low. I think that other factors than iodine deficiency have to be considered to explain the difference of incidence of goiter and cretinism.

STANBURY: In the Kičič study, the diagnosis was said to have been made in newborns, which raises the whole question of whether a diagnosis of endemic cretinism can be made in newborns. In my limited experience, one must wait a year or more to be sure. There was an expectation of seven cases of cretinism out of 106, and none was found during the six years' observation period. The probability of this is only about 0.1. [Since Discussion, new data from the Yugoslavian group has become available, which extended the period of observation from 6 yr to 14 yr (7)].

GARDNER: I think it is virtually impossible to diagnose athyreotic cretinism in the newborn. It will rarely be diagnosed within two months.

MOSIER: I would think the earliest signs are poor sucking and lethargy. These might appear as early as 24 to 48 hours; but unfortunately they are non-specific signs in the newborn.

DELANGE: Lowrey has published the frequency distribution of the symptoms in congenital hypothyroidism as a function of age (15). The first symptom in the newborn is usually difficulty in drinking. As to deaf-mutism as a uniform tracer for endemic cretinism, this was discussed at length at the Goroka meeting (16) and the consensus was that it was not. One of the reasons is that deaf-mutism is exceptional in myxedematous cretinism. Also, as recently extensively reviewed by Fraser from a personal study of 3,534 cases (17), the causes of profound deafness in childhood are very numerous and remain unknown in about 30 percent of the cases. So I think that deaf-mutism is not a specific tracer.

QUERIDO: Yes. I have to state that deaf-mutism is a marker for cretinism as it is seen in Switzerland, New Guinea, Ecuador, the Himalayas, but not for Zaire.

DELANGE: I agree.

COSTA: I would like to comment about the relation between the excretion of iodine and the frequency of cretinism. In some provinces of Piedmont the iodine urinary excretion of the school-boys is 30-40 μg per gm of creatinine. Nevertheless in these places endemic cretinism has never been observed. In the Aosta valley the urinary excretion of the school-boys is today 70 μg per gm of creatinine and endemic cretinism has not yet totally disappeared. A point that is missing in your study is the localization of cretinism: endemic cretinism and endemic deaf-mutism are always localized at some places. This localization was so recognized that the bishop of Chambery told people to marry away from places where cretinism was endemic if they did not want cretin children. Napoleon ordered that all the population be taken from these endemic zones.

QUERIDO: I agree completely about location. This is the strong point of the Mulia (New Guinea) study, where the people that moved into Mulia had abnormal children, after previously having normal children elsewhere. There was also a difference in iodine excretion between the locations.

KOENIG: We have told the people in charge of the neonatal units that they should do a total thyroxine and a bone age of the knee of any child that has a prolonged icterus (hyperbilirubinemia after the eighth day), umbilical hernia, and poor sucking.

PITTMAN: Again I would like to sell the idea of doing a serum TSH. It is specific. TSH will be normal within 72 hours if the child is not cold.

DEGROOT: Do you think your data support the idea that there is a general lowering of IQ in areas of endemic cretinism? Does this open the door to the idea that mental deficiency may occur in areas where there is no endemic cretinism, but where endemic goiter is present?

QUERIDO; I suspect that the distribution of mental deficiency in an area with endemic cretinism is unimodal because extensive observations during a long period in Leiden on treated patients with sporadic cretinism disclosed that the IQs varied anywhere from 50 to 110 (18). In sporadic cretinism, as in endemic cretinism there is insufficient production of thyroid hormones prenatally, and therefore some resemblance in the two types of mental deficiency will exist.

REFERENCES

1. Marine, D. and Kimball, O.P.: Prevention of simple goiter in man. Fourth paper. Arch. Intern. Med. 25:661-672, 1920.

2. Koenig, M.P.: Die kongenitale Hypothyreose und der endemische Kretinismus. Springer, Berlin, 1968.

3. Querido, A.: Endemic cretinism: a search for a tenable definition. In: Endemic Goiter. Report of the meeting of the PAHO Scientific Group on Research in Endemic Goiter held in Mexico, 1968 (J.G. Stanbury, ed.). PAHO Scientific Publication No. 193, Washington, 1969. pp.85-89.

4. Querido, A.: Epidemiology of cretinism. In: Endemic Cretinism (B.S. Hetzel and P.O.D. Pharoah, eds.). Inst. Human Biology, Monogr. 2, Papua, New Guinea, 1971. pp. 9-18.

5. Eugster, J.: Arch. Julius Klausstiftung: 13:383, 1938.

6. Kičič, M.; Milutinović, P.; Djordjević, S. and Ramzin, S.: Endocrinological aspects of an endemic focus of cretinism. In: Advances of Thyroid Research (R. Pitt-Rivers, ed.). Pergamon Press, London, 1961. pp. 301-306.

7. Ramzin, S.; Kičic, M.; Dordević, S. and Todorović, M.: The results of years-long preventive iodine treatment of endemic goitre. Acta Med. Iugosl. 22:77-90, 1968.

8. DeQuervain, F. and Wegelin, C.: Der endemische Kretinismus. Springer, Berlin, 1936.

9. Wespi, H.J.: Abnahme der Taubstumnheit in der Schweiz als Folge der Kropfprophylaxe mit iodiertem Kochsalz. Schweiz. Med. Wochenschr. 75:625-629, 1945.

10. Eggenberger, H.: Das Vollsalz zur Prophylaxe von Kropf und Kretinismus. Bircher, Bern, 1924.

11. Penrose, L.S.: The Biology of Mental Defect. Sidgwick and Jackson, London, 1963.

12. Dingman, H. F. and Tarjan, G.: Am. J. Ment. Defic. 64:991-994, 1960.

13. De Reynier, D.: La surdi-mutite en Suisse en 1953. Fortschr. HNO Heilkd. 5:1-73, 1959.

14. Kičič, M.; Milutinović, P.; Djordjević, S. and Ramzin, S.: Endocrinological aspects of an endemic focus of cretinism. In: Advances of Thyroid Research (R. Pitt-Rivers, ed.). Permagon Press, London, 1961. pp. 301-306.

15.. Lowrey, G.H.; Aster, R.H.; Carr, E.A.; Raman, G.; Beierwaltes, W.H. and Spafford, N.R.: Am. J. Dis. Child. 96:131, 1958.

16. Hetzel, B.S. and Pharoah, P.O.D. (Eds.): Endemic Cretinism. Proceedings of a symposium held at Institute of Human Biology, Goroka, T.P.N.G. January 27-29, 1971. Inst. Human Biology Mongr. 2, Papua, New Guinea, 1971.

17. Fraser, G.R.: In: Sensorineural Hearing Loss (G.E.W. Wolstenholme and J. Knight, Eds.). Churchill, London, 1970.

18. Gemund, J.J. van, and Laurent de Angulo, M.S.: Normal and abnormal development of brain and behaviour. University Press, Leiden, 1971. pp. 299-313.

THE EFFECT OF IODINE PROPHYLAXIS ON THE INCIDENCE OF ENDEMIC CRETINISM

P.O.D. Pharoah, I.H. Buttfield, and B.S. Hetzel

Institute of Human Biology, Goroka, Papua, New Guinea
Department of Nuclear Medicine, Queensland Radium Institute, Brisbane, Australia. Monash Medical School, Brahran, Victoria, Australia

It is generally accepted that dietary iodine deficiency is the major factor in the etiology of endemic goiter in most areas of the world. The effectiveness of iodine prophylaxis for endemic goiter was firmly established by Marine and Kimball (1) in a controlled trial in Ohio and has subsequently been confirmed by programs of salt iodization (2,3), iodization of bread and water supplies (4) and the intra-muscular administration of iodized oil. (5,6,7) Other factors are also known to influence the incidence of endemic goiter, e.g. dietary goitrogens (8), hardness of water supplies (9,10) and also perhaps water pollution (11). These factors are almost always superimposed on a dietary iodine deficiency.

The association between endemic cretinism and endemic goiter is a geographical one in that endemic cretinism is only found in areas where goiter is endemic. This fact is incorporated in the definition of endemic cretinism as given by the Pan American Health Organization (12). An endemic cretin was defined as an individual with irreversible changes in mental development, _born in an endemic goiter area_ and exhibiting a combination of some of the following characteristics not explained by other causes:

1. Irreversible neuromuscular disorders
2. Irreversible abnormalities in hearing and speech leading in certain cases to deaf-mutism;

3. Impairment of somatic development
4. Hypothyroidism.

The correlation between dietary iodine deficiency and endemic goiter and the geographical association of endemic cretinism with endemic goiter has naturally led to the postulate that dietary iodine deficiency is of importance in the etiology of endemic cretinism. The main support for this postulate has been the remarkable disappearance of endemic cretinism when iodine prophylaxis is introduced to an area. This was well documented by Wespi (13), who correlated the incidence of deaf-mutism in the various cantons of Switzerland with the quantity of iodized salt consumed. More recently Buttfield and Hetzel (14) following up the work of McCullagh (5), reported that eleven endemic cretins were found who had been born since iodine prophylaxis was introduced into the Huon Peninsula in New Guinea, but none were born to women who had received depot iodine injections.

Opponents of the iodine deficiency hypothesis have pointed to the fact that endemic cretinism was on the decline in certain countries prior to the introduction of any form of iodine prophylaxis. Costa _et al._ (15) report such a decline in the Piedmont in Italy. The census figures from the Argentine Republic reported by Greenwald (16) show a striking decrease between the years 1869 and 1914 in every province. Koenig and Veraguth (17) state that the disappearance of cretinism predated by 10 years the introduction of iodine prophylaxis. Norris in 1847 (18) documented an endemic of cretinism in the village of Chisleborough, England, yet by 1871 he stated that cretinism in Chisleborough had almost died out (19). It appears that social and economic development in any country leads to the disappearance of endemic cretinism; Trotter (20) has criticised the study of Wespi on this ground. He points out that the negative correlation between the incidence of deaf-mutism and iodized salt consumption occurred at a time of active social change, so that other factors may have been responsible for the decline in deaf-mutism.

Until 1966 no controlled trial of iodine prophylaxis on the incidence of endemic cretinism had been carried out. Difficulties in controlling the use of measures such as iodized salt or iodide tablets were paramount. The introduction by McCullagh (5) of a single intramuscular injection of iodized oil and its proven effectiveness over a period of years (6) made a controlled trial more feasible. As a result, such a trial was instituted in the Jimi Valley of New Guinea where a high incidence of endemic cretinism had been reported. A preliminary report on the results has already appeared (21).

SUBJECTS AND METHODS

The Jimi is a remote valley in the western highlands of New Guinea which had its first contact with Europeans in 1953. Until 1970 this valley could only be reached by light aircraft or on foot. Some villages are now connected by vehicular roads, but access to the majority is still by walking tracks only.

The population of the valley is about 24,000. Individual villages have between 250 - 1,000 people, and lie at altitudes between 800 to 2,000 meters above sea level. The people live as homesteaders with houses and gardens scattered throughout the valley. Each village group has its own central meeting place.

Until very recently the economy of the people has been a subsistence one only.

In 1966 a controlled trial to determine the effectiveness of iodized oil as a prophylactic measure against endemic cretinism was commenced. From August to October, a patrol was carried out in conjunction with the local administration who were conducting a census. It covered 27 villages in the upper and middle valley with a population of 16,500. At each village all the people were assembled and a record made of their names and an estimate of each person's age. Women of childbearing age were asked if they were pregnant. If so, this was recorded but no formal confirming examination was made.

Goiter size was assessed as reported previously (21). Grade 0 is no enlargement. Grade 1 is a palpable but not visible enlargement with the head in the normal position and Grade 2 is a visible enlargement of the thyroid with the head in a normal position. The prevalence of Grade 1 plus Grade 2 gives the goiter rate (GR) and the prevalence of Grade 2 alone gives the visible goiter rate (VGR).

Alternate families were injected with either iodized oil or normal saline, each member of the family receiving four ml if aged 12 years or over and two ml if under the age of 12 years. The nature of the injection given was recorded on the census sheet. Each milliliter of iodized oil contains approximately 400 mg of elemental iodine.

Follow-up patrols were carried out in July, 1967; November, 1969; January, March and November, 1970 and January, May, August, November, December, 1971. Due to the remoteness of the region only thirteen of the original twenty-seven villages, with a population of 8,000, have been followed up. On each occasion all mothers and children in each village were assembled and checked against the census sheets. Infants born since 1966 were identified, their names and birth dates recorded. Birth dates were obtained from a variety of sources, from mission infant welfare records, from administration council records and from records kept by indigenous Aid-Post Orderlies stationed in some of the villages.

Each child was examined initially without knowledge of whether the mother had received oil or saline, primarily for evidence of motor retardation. The milestones assessed were those of sitting, standing and walking. Motor retardation was assumed to be present if these milestones were not attained by the ages of 12, 18 and 24 months respectively. In addition, the parents of all children were questioned as to whether they thought hearing and speech were normal. If they thought there was any abnormality of hearing or speech or if there was any motor retardation, a more formal attempt to assess deafness was made by having the child's attention distracted and noting if there was any response to a tuning fork, a snapping of fingers, or a hand clap. Auroscopic examination of the ear drum was also carried out to exclude otitis media.

A squint if present was noted. A more careful assessment of the extra-ocular movements was made in those children who were retarded in their motor milestones or had abnormalities of speech and hearing.

RESULTS

Table 1 gives the comparative goiter rates and visible goiter rates in the oil injected and the control groups. There were no significant differences in the numbers of males and females or in the goiter rates in these two groups.

Table 1. Goiter incidence in the population group studied for effect of iodized oil prophylaxis

	IODIZED OIL			SALINE		
Goiter Size	Total Population 3180	Males 1535	Females 1645	Total Population 3063	Males 1476	Females 1587
Grade 0	2540	1383	1157	2463	1355	1108
Grade 1	249	79	170	257	74	183
Grade 2	391	73	318	343	47	296
G.R.*	20.1%	9.9%	29.7%	19.6%	8.2%	30.2%
V.G.R.**	12.3%	4.8%	19.3%	11.2%	3.2%	18.7%

* Goiter rate
** Visible goiter rate

The number of children born to mothers who had oil or saline and the numbers of children who had died are given in Table 2. The latter figures are not accurate, particularly for the period July, 1967 to November, 1969 when the villages were not visited. Many of the children who were born and died during this time would not have been recorded.

Table 2. Birth data in relation to prophylaxis programs

Mother's Status	Total Births	Living Children	Deaths
Iodized Oil	687	577	110
Saline	626	495	131
Nil	62	48	14

For the purposes of the trial, affected children have been divided into four groups, as shown in Table 3. Group I are those presenting with the full syndrome of hearing or speech abnormality, abnormality of motor development and strabismus (Fig. 1).

Table 3. Classification of defective children in relation to administration of iodized oil

GROUP	TREATED			UNTREATED		
		Conception			Conception	
	Total	Before Trial	After Trial	Total	Before Trial	After Trial
I	3	2	1	18	3	15
II	3	3	0	13	2	11
III	2	2	0	4	2	2
IV	1	1	0	1	0	1

Group II includes those with abnormalities of hearing or speech and motor development (Fig. 2). Group III includes those with a hearing or speech defect only. Group IV includes those with motor retardation with an abnormal gait.

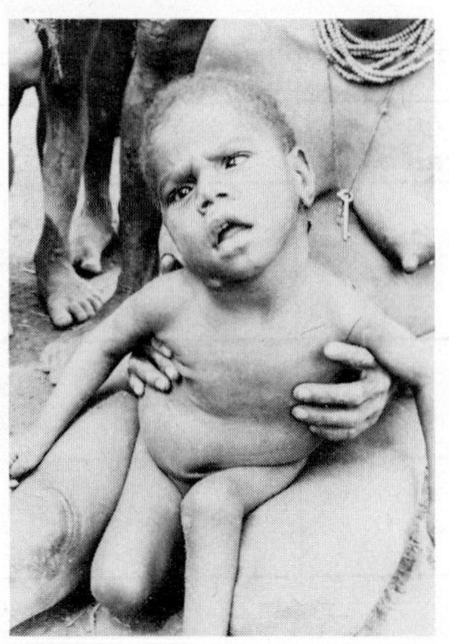

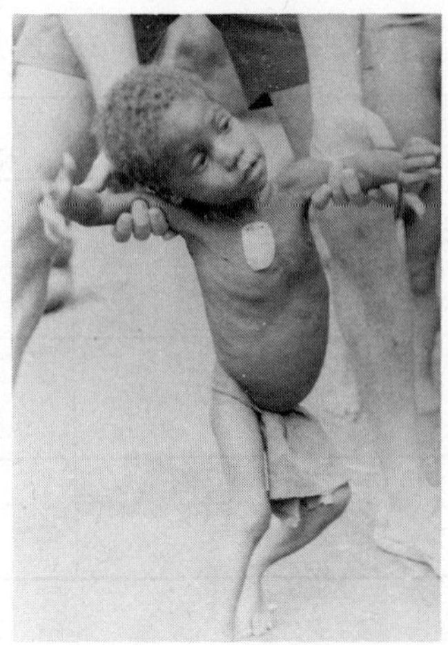

Figure 1. Patient classified as Group I in Table 3
Figure 2. Patient classified as Group II in Table 3.

An appendix is attached in which a brief resume of the history and clinical features of each affected child is given.

The lack of consensus on the definition of endemic cretinism gives rise to some difficulty in assessing the results of the trial. If, for epidemiological purposes, those patients in Groups I and II can be considered endemic cretins, then there have been six cretins born to women who have had iodized oil out of a total 687 children; in five of these six cases, conception had occurred prior to the iodized oil injection. In the sixth case, the mother received the injection on October 6, 1966 and the birth-date of the infant is recorded at August, 1967, i.e. approximately 42-46 weeks later. However, the lack of precision regarding the birth-date raises the possibility that conception had occurred prior to treatment in this instance also.

In the untreated group there have been 31 endemic cretins out of a total 688 children born since that trial commenced. In five of these 33, conception had occurred prior to the saline being given. It is concluded that the neurological syndrome of endemic cretinism has occurred in the untreated group and in six instances in the treated group in five of which conception had already occurred at the time of injection.

DISCUSSION

A number of authors have drawn attention to the possibility that McCarrison's (22) "nervous" type of endemic cretinism is a congenital defect. McCullagh (23) went so far as to call the syndrome "Goiter-associated congenital defect". Eggenberger and Messerli (3) stated that the deaf-mutism has its origin in the fourth month of fetal life although no evidence is presented for this statement. Costa *et al*. (15) remarked that endemic cretinism seems to develop during intra-uterine life.

The trial of iodized oil as a prophylactic measure against endemic cretinism described here lends support to the view that the neurological damage of endemic cretinism is an intra-uterine event possibly occurring during the first trimester of pregnancy. In this time relationship it resembles the defect produced by maternal rubella infection, and it is perhaps significant that deaf-mutism is common to both syndromes. It may be that the developing auditory apparatus is peculiarly susceptible to damage during this particular period.

Evidently administration of iodine as a depot injection is effective in preventing this damage, but how iodine exerts its prophylactic effect is not clearly understood. The view most widely held is that iodine deficiency leads to maternal hypothyroidism which is responsible for the fetal damage (24, 25), yet the evidence for this is not at all convincing. Clinical hypothyroidism is rarely seen in an endemic goiter area, and the fecundity precludes hypothyroidism of any magnitude since it is uncommon for a hypothyroid female to become pregnant. Table 1 discloses that the number of infants born to the oil injected group was not significantly different from the number born to the group that did not receive iodine. It has been suggested that subclinical biochemical hypothyroidism might exist in these women. Support for this comes from those studies reporting high serum TSH levels (26) and low serum PBI or serum thyroxine levels in some areas where iodine deficiency is severe (27, 28). It is possible therefore that a subclinical maternal hypothyroidism during a critical stage of fetal development leads to neurological damage to the fetus. This postulate seems not convincing because cases have been recorded of clinically hypothyroid women becoming pregnant and being delivered of normal children. The report by Hodges _et al_. (29) describe a woman with juvenile myxedema who had six pregnancies from which four infants survived. These four infants included a moron unable to talk at the age of four years nine months, a normal child, a mongolian idiot, and the fourth only seven months old when assessed which appeared normal. Only the first of these could possibly be said to resemble the syndrome of endemic cretinism. Lister and Ashe (30) reported a patient with myxedema untreated during the first four months of gestation who delivered a normal child.

Fetal hypothyroidism secondary to insufficient iodine is also postulated as the cause of endemic cretinism (31). However, congenitally athyreotic infants do not have the clinical features of endemic cretinism. Furthermore, there is a considerable body of evidence indicating that the human fetal thyroid commences functioning at about the 12th or 13th week of gestation whereas the damage characteristic of endemic cretinism appears from our epidemiologic observations possibly to occur before this time (32, 33).

If neither maternal nor fetal hypothyroidism can adequately account for the syndrome of endemic cretinism, how does iodine administration effectively prevent the disease? It is of course possible that a mild degree of maternal hypothyroidism coupled with fetal hypothyroidism resulting from severe iodine deficiency may be sufficient to cause the syndrome. It is also possible that elemental iodine, apart from its role in thyroid hormone synthesis, may be necessary for fetal neurological development. In this context it is perhaps significant that the mammalian ovary concentrates iodine in the developing ovum (34). If this is so, can an iodine deficiency lead to damage in the developing ovum?

It is possible that iodine plays a secondary role, acting in conjunction with other factors, such as protein-calorie malnutrition. Maternal protein-calorie malnutrition during pregnancy has been postulated to be a cause of intellectual retardation in infants (35), and this has been supported by work on experimental animals (36). Other elements or trace elements may also influence the role of iodine. For example, the goiter rate in iodine deficient areas is influenced by the hardness of water supplies (9), possibly calcium interacts with iodine to cause endemic cretinism. An analogous situation occurs in sheep and cattle when a copper-molybdenum imbalance during pregnancy produces an irreversible neurological disorder in the calves and lambs (37).

SUMMARY

A controlled trial using a single depot injection of iodized oil as a prophylactic for endemic cretinism is described.

In the oil injected group six cretins were found among a total of 687 children born since the trial commenced; in five of these six cretins conception had occurred prior to the injection. The control group had 31 cretins among a total 688 children, with five of the 31 pregnant prior to the trial starting.

The injection is effective in preventing the syndrome, provided it is given prior to conception. This suggests that the irreversible neurological damage characteristic of the endemic cretin occurs prior to birth, possibly during the first trimester of pregnancy.

The mode of action of iodine in preventing the syndrome is discussed and in particular the view currently held, that maternal hypothyroidism is responsible for the fetal damage, is challenged.

ACKNOWLEDGEMENT

Supported by the Department of Public Health, Papua, New Guinea.

DISCUSSION BY PARTICIPANTS

FIERRO: How sure were you of the identification of these people?

PHAROAH: Very rarely were there any problems. About twenty children whose mothers came from another village have been excluded from the trial because I am not sure whether or not they have had iodine.

KOENIG: Having observed four children born to hypothyroid mothers, I looked at the literature on that subject. I found 74 women with 110 pregnancies. There were 49 normal children, 30 miscarriages or stillbirths, and 28 abnormal children. Among these 28 were six having congenital hypothyroidism. These six were two kindreds of three children each, from two families with inborn errors of metabolism. Other abnormalities among the 28 were developmental anomalies like anencephaly, spina bifida, and such things; and a single oligophrenic with no further classification. So among these 110 children there was no anomaly which was comparable to endemic cretinism. With the exception of the six patients with congenital hypothyroidism none of the children were hypothyroid (38).

ROSMAN: Regarding the question of whether malnutrition produces mental retardation, there is at least one rather convincing controlled study of Stoch and Smythe (35,39)indicating that it does. Malnourished children showed greatest impairment in weight, less in height, and least but nonetheless definite impairment in head growth and intelligence. The many malnourished children that we see at Boston City Hospital usually show the same picture, with a head circumference that tends to be at about the third percentile. In children seen at the Boston City Hospital, malnutrition is probably the most common cause of mild microcephaly and developmental retardation.

PHAROAH: Do they present with deaf-mutism, squint, and spastic diplegia?

ROSMAN: They may have an ataxic diplegia or spastic diplegia.

DELANGE: Do you have biochemical studies of thyroid function in the newborn defectives, to see if there was hypothyroidism during pregnancy?

PHAROAH: I have serum waiting to be done, but do not have the results yet.

IBBERTSON: As to hypothyroidism in the fetal environment, there is little evidence that maternal thyroxine crosses the placenta during the crucial period for nervous tissue development. The fact that the Zaire cretin does not show neurological abnormality is strong evidence against fetal hypothyroidism being important in the genesis of neurological defects.

KROC: Would a study comparing thyroid hormone, e.g., USP desiccated or thyroxine, be feasible and desirable? Throughout these sessions there has been an implication that iodized oil treatment is equivalent to what would be observed if T_4 or T_4 plus T_3 were administered. Is there evidence from a controlled study to support that? What about any extrathyroidal effects of iodine in development of the nervous system?

IBBERTSON: In iodine-deficient areas where iodine supplementation has been given, previously low serum thyroxine levels rise to normal, making it difficult to distinguish between the effects of thyroid hormone and elemental iodine per se.

BUTTFIELD: More important is that iodine supplements drop the TSH level down to normal, so I think you can equate the two.

PRETELL: I will show this afternoon that 48 hours after one gives iodine, T_4 increases.

STANBURY; When you give iodine to the African cretins with their damaged thyroids do their PBI's go back to normal?

DELANGE: We do not know.

ERMANS: Considering the fact that the hypothyroid cretin has a very small thyroid iodine pool, we are afraid that the administration of large amounts of iodine to these patients would block the organification by a Wolff-Chaikoff effect. This could lead to an aggravation of their thyroid insufficiency.

PRETELL: Does this happen even if TSH is high?

ERMANS: No.

BUTTFIELD: Would this not be a temporary effect? If one gives thyroxine for two or three months, then the iodized oil ought to be effective, because the subject would have a high iodine uptake.

QUERIDO: I have been considering the coincidence of hearing defect and thyroid defect in the Pendred syndrome. I wondered if it is not an enzyme defect or protein defect that is also localized in other tissues than the thyroid. If so, it could be in the placental cells. If the placenta not only transports iodide but also modifies it to an unknown compound, a defect in this mechanism could have the same effect as an insufficient supply of iodide, as is the case in endemic cretinism. This is of course highly speculative, because there are no data which indicate that the placenta metabolizes iodide.

REFERENCES

1. Marine, D. and Kimball, O.P.: Prevention of simple goiter in man. Fourth paper. Arch. Intern. Med. 25:661-672, 1920.

2. Brush, B.E. and Altland, J.K.: Goiter prevention with iodized salt: results of a thirty-year study. J. Clin. Endocrinol. Metab. 12:1380-1388, 1952.

3. Eggenberger, H. and Messerli, F.M.: Theory and results of prophylaxis of endemic goiter in Switzerland. In: Transactions of the Third International Goiter Conference, 1938. pp. 64-67.

4. Gezondheidsorganisatie, T.N.O.: De endemische Krop in Nederland, 1959.

5. McGullagh, S.F.: The Huon Peninsula endemic: I. the effectiveness of an intramuscular depot of iodized oil in the control of endemic goitre. Med. J. Aust. 1:769-777, 1963.

6. Buttfield, I.H., Black, M.L., Hoffmann, M.J., Mason, E.K. and Hetzel, B.S.: Correction of iodine deficiency in New Guinea natives by iodised oil injection. Lancet 2:767-769, 1965.

7. Pretell, E.A., Moncloa, F., Salinas, R., Kawano, A., Guerra-Garcia, R., Gutierrez, L., Beteta, L., Pretell, J. and Wan, M.: Prophylaxis and treatment of endemic goiter in Peru with iodized oil. J. Clin. Endocrinol. Metab. 29: 1586-1595, 1969.

8. Clements, F.W.: Naturally occuring goitrogens. Br. Med. Bull. 16:133-137, 1960.

9. Taylor, S.: Calcium as a goitrogen. J. Clin. Endocrinol. Metab. 14:1412-1422, 1954.

10. Stott, H., Bhatia, B.B., Lal, R.S. and Rai, K.C.: The distribution and cause of endemic goitre in the United Provinces. Indian J. Med. Res. 18:1059-1086, 1931.

11. McCarrison, R.: Observations on endemic goitre in the Chitral and Gilgit Valleys. Lancet 1:1110-1111, 1906.

12. Report of the Pan American Health Organization Scientific Group on Research in Endemic Goiter. Pan American Health Organization Advisory Committee of Medical Research, PAHO, Washington, 1963.

13. Wespi, H.J.: Abnahme der Taubstummheit in der Schweiz als Folge der Kropfprophylaxe mit jodiertem Kochsalz. Schweiz. Med. Wochenschr. 75:625-629, 1945.

14. Buttfield, I.H. and Hetzel, B.S.: Endemic cretinism in eastern New Guinea. Australas. Ann. Med. 18:217-221, 1969.

15. Costa, A., Cottino, F., Mortara, M. and Vogliazzo, U.: Endemic cretinism in Piedmont. Panminerva Med. 6:250-259, 1964.

16. Greenwald, I.: The history of goiter in the Inca Empire: Peru, Chile and the Argentine Republic. Its significance for the etiology of the disease. Tex. Rep. Biol. Med. 15: 874-889, 1957.

17. Koenig, M.P. and Veraguth, P.: Studies of thyroid function in endemic cretins. In: Advances in Thyroid Research (R. Pitt-Rivers, ed.), Pergamon Press, Oxford, 1961. pp. 294-300.

18. Norris, H.: Notice of a remarkable disease analogous to cretinism existing in a small village in the west of England. Med. Times 17:257-258, 1847-48.

19. Fagge, C.H.: Sporadic cretinism occurring in England. Medico-chir. Trans. 54:155-170, 1871.

20. Trotter, W.R.: The association of deafness with thyroid dysfunction. Br. Med. Bull. 16:92-98, 1960.

21. Pharoah, P.O.D., Buttfield, I.H., and Hetzel, B.S.: Neurological damage to the fetus resulting from severe iodine deficiency during pregnancy. Lancet 1:308-310, 1971.

22. McCarrison, R.: Observations on endemic cretinism in the Chitral and Gilgit Valleys. Lancet 2:1275-1280, 1908.

23. McCullagh, S.F.: The Huon Peninsula endemic: IV. Endemic goitre and congenital defect. Med. J. Aust. 1:884-890, 1963.

24. Stanbury, J.B.: Endemic Goiter. In: Clinical Endocrinology II (Cassidy and E.B. Astwood, eds.), New York, Grune & Stratton, 1968. pp. 195-209.

25. Querido, A.: Endemic cretinism: a search for a tenable definition. In: Endemic Goiter. Report of the meeting of the PAHO Scientific Group on Research in Endemic Goiter held in Mexico, 1968. (J.B. Stanbury, ed.), Scientific Publication No. 193, Washington, 1969. pp. 85-89.

26. Adams, D.D., Kennedy, T.H., Choufoer, J.C., Querido, A.: Endemic goiter in western New Guinea. III. Thyroid-stimulating activity of serum from severely iodine-deficient people. J. Clin. Endocrinol. Metab. 28:685-692, 1968.

27. Raman, G. and Beierwaltes, W.H.: Correlation of goiter, deafmutism and mental retardation with serum thyroid hormone levels in non-cretinous inhabitants of a severe endemic goiter area in India. J. Clin. Endocrinol. Metab. 19: 228-233, 1959.

28. Choufoer, J.C., Van Rhijn, M., Kassenaar, A.A.H. and Querido, A.: Endemic goiter in western New Guinea: iodine metabolism in goitrous and nongoitrous subjects. J. Clin. Endocrinol. Metab 23:1203-1217, 1963.

29. Hodges, R.E., Hamilton, H.E., and Keettel, W.C.: Pregnancy in Myxedema. A.M.A. Arch. Int. Med. 90:863-868, 1952.

30. Lister, L.M. and Ashe, J.R.: Pregnancy and myxedema. Report of a case. Obstet. Gynecol. 6:436-441, 1955.

31. Choufoer, J.C., Van Rhijn, M. and Querido, A.: Endemic goiter in western New Guinea. II. Clinical picture, incidence and pathogenesis of endemic cretinism. J. Clin. Endocrinol. Metab. 25: 385-402, 1965.

32. Chapman, E.M., Corner, G.W., Robinson, D. and Evans, R.D.: The collection of radioactive iodine by the human fetal thyroid. J. Clin. Endocrinol. Metab. 8:717-720, 1948.

33. Costa, A., Cottino, F., Dellepiane, M., Ferraris, G.M., Lenart, L., Magro, G., Patrito, G., Zoppetti, G.: Thyroid function and thyrotropin activity in mother and fetus. In: Current Topics in Thyroid Research (C. Cassano and M. Andreoli, eds), Academic Press, New York, 1965. pp. 738-748.

34. Brown-Grant, K.: Extrathyroidal iodide concentrating mechanisms. Physiol. Rev. 41:189-213, 1961.

35. Stoch, M.B. and Smythe, P.M.: Does undernutrition during infancy inhibit brain growth and subsequent intellectual development? Arch. Dis. Child. 38:546-552, 1963.

36. Winick, M., Fish, I. and Rosso, P.: Cellular recovery in rat tissues after a brief period of neonatal malnutrition. J. Nutr. 95:623-626, 1968.

37. Underwood, E.J.: The mineral nutrition of livestock. Published by arrangement with the Food and Agriculture Organization of the United Nations by Commonwealth Agricultural Bureau, 1966. pp. 120-146.

38. Koenig, M.P.: Die kongenitale Hypothyreose und der endemische Kretinismus. Springer, Berlin, 1968.

39. Stoch, M.B. and Smythe, P.M.: The effect of undernutrition during infancy on subsequent brain growth and intellectual development. S. Afr. Med. J. 41:1027-1030, 1967.

APPENDIX

GROUP I: ABNORMALITIES OF HEARING AND/OR SPEECH, ABNORMALITIES OF MOTOR DEVELOPMENT AND SQUINT

Oil

Case 1. Mother approximately 32 weeks pregnant at time of oil injection. Female infant, last seen when aged four years eight months, is deaf and mute, mentally defective, has an upper motor neuron lesion involving arms and legs with extensor plantars responses and is unable to sit unsupported.

Case 2. Mother injected October 6, 1966. Female infant born August, 1967 and died October, 1970. At age three years eight months was unable to sit or crawl, the limbs being hypotonic. The child was deaf and mute and had an internal strabismus.

Case 3. Male born January, 1967. Mother approximately 26 weeks pregnant when injected with oil. Walking delayed until three years of age. Last examined aged four years four months; the gait is abnormal and mother states the child is not talking but claims the child can hear. Clinically he does not appear to hear a tuning fork, he is probably partially deaf. There is an intermittent squinting of either eye.

Saline

Case 1. Male born November 4, 1967. Is deaf, mute and has a transient inward and upward squinting of either eye. Commenced walking sometime after three years four months of age. Gait is abnormal, the plantar responses are extensor and 4 or 5 beats of ankle clonus can be elicited.

Case 2. Female born January 30, 1969. At age two years 11 months has a severe head lag when pulled to the sitting position and is unable to sit unsupported. She is deaf and mute and severely mentally defective. The tendon reflexes in the arms and legs are pathologically brisk and there is an internal strabismus.

Case 3. Female born September 26, 1968. At age two years eight months is unable to sit unsupported, is deaf and mute, has a severe strabismus involving both eyes and extensor plantar responses.

Case 4. Male born June 13, 1969. At age two years five months is unable to sit, has a severe squint, is grossly mentally retarded and is a deaf-mute. The tendon reflexes in both arms and legs are exessively brisk and the plantar reflex is extensor.

Case 5. Male born February 5, 1968. Unable to sit up until over two years of age and when last examined aged three years nine months was unable to walk; is a mentally retarded deaf-mute and has a transient squinting of either eye.

Case 6. Male born March 24, 1970. At 12 months was unable to sit and there was considerable head lag when pulled from lying supine to the sitting position. At 18 months the child can sit but has a very rounded back. He shows a squint and has no speech. The parents state the child is deaf.

Case 7. Male born September 18, 1969. Was unable to sit at age 14 months but had attained this milestone by age 19 months. At age two years two months is unable to stand or walk and has extensor plantar responses; the child is deaf, mute and has an intermittent strabismus.

Case 8. Male born November 15, 1967. A severely affected mentally defective, squinting deaf-mute who is unable to walk at four years of age.

Case 9. Male born September 14, 1968. At one year seven months was unable to sit upright. When last seen age three years, he was almost able to walk. The mother states that speech is not normal though at least partial hearing is present as he can hear a finger snap. There is an inward squinting of the left eye.

Case 10. Male born December, 1966, mother approximately 30 weeks pregnant at time of saline injection. The child was first seen age three years four months when walking was established though the gait was unsteady and wide-based with flexed knees and hips. At four years 11 months he is mute though partial hearing at least is present and there is an internal strabismus of the left eye.

Case 11. Male born April 10, 1968. A deaf-mute with a squint and spasticity of the legs, pathologically brisk knee and ankle jerks and extensor plantar responses. At three years eight months of age he is still unable to sit unsupported.

Case 12. Male born March 19, 1967. Mother was approximately 16 weeks pregnant at time of saline injection. The child started sitting sometime after three years of age and walking commenced between the ages of four years and four years nine months. The gait is grossly abnormal; there is a severe strabismus and he is a deaf-mute.

Case 13. Male born December, 1967. At age three years six months is just able to sit unaided but cannot stand or walk. He is deaf-mute and has a strabismus.

Case 14. Male born May 28, 1968. Died aged two years two months. Last examined when aged one year 11 months; he was deaf and had no speech; was only able to stand if supported and had an internal strabismus.

Case 15. Male born February, 1967, died aged three years nine months. A severely affected child who was unable to sit aged three; was deaf and mute and had a squint. Mother was approximately 24 weeks pregnant at time of saline injection.

Case 16. Male born October, 1968. Sitting not attained until over 13 months of age and walking at about two years, though the gait at this time was very unsteady. He has a pronounced squint of the left eye. The parents state he hears if they call in a loud voice but that speech is not normal.

Case 17. Male born April 29, 1970. Is as yet unable to sit upright or crawl aged 18 months; has marked transient squinting of either eye and does not hear a finger snap.

Case 18. Female born January, 1970. Was unable to sit until after 15 months of age and when last examined aged one year 10 months was unable to stand or walk. She has a transient squinting of either eye, is not yet talking and does not hear a finger snap.

GROUP II: ABNORMALITIES OF HEARING AND/OR SPEECH AND MOTOR DEVELOPMENT

Oil

Case 1. Female born December 13, 1966. Mother approximately 30 weeks pregnant at time of oil injection. Sitting was delayed until after three years of age and walking until about four years. The gait at four years nine months is abnormal, and the child is deaf and mute.

Case 2. Male born November 7, 1966. Mother approximately 34 weeks pregnant at time of oil injection. A mentally defective child who at four years 10 months has spasticity of the lower limbs with pathologically brisk reflexes and extensor plantar responses and is unable to walk or stand. He is also deaf-mute.

Case 3. Female born May 4, 1967, died aged three years seven months. At the time of death was yet unable to sit and was a deaf-mute. Mother was approximately 13 weeks pregnant at time of oil injection.

Saline

Case 1. Male born March 13, 1968. Began sitting at about one year eleven months and walking at three years. Gait is very unsteady and spastic. Is also deaf-mute.

Case 2. Male born November 16, 1968. Is mute but at least partial hearing is present. Began sitting at one year three months and walking at two years five months but gait is abnormal.

Case 3. Male born July, 1967. Commenced walking when aged three years nine months but gait is unsteady and spastic and knee and ankle jerks are pathologically brisk. Is also deaf and mute.

Case 4. Male born December 9, 1968. Is deaf and mute. Sitting commenced sometime after the age of two. The left ankle and knee are fixed due to scarring from a burn which partly accounts for the inability to walk, nevertheless the tendon reflexes in the right leg are pathologically brisk.

Case 5. Female born April, 1967. Mother approximately 10 weeks pregnant when injected with saline. Child first seen when aged two years seven months when walking was established but gait appeared abnormal; the tendon reflexes excessively brisk and the plantar responses are extensor. She is mute and conveys requests to her mother by means of signs though she does not appear to be deaf.

Case 6. Male born October, 1969. Sitting not achieved until after 13 months. Last examined aged two years one month. He is unable to stand or walk and when sitting there is a marked kyphosis of the back. He has no speech and there is at least a partial hearing loss.

Case 7. Female born November 7, 1968. Deaf and mute; sitting not achieved until after two years and is still unable to stand or walk at two years ten months.

Case 8. Female born April 15, 1969. Is mute but has at least partial hearing. Walking commenced aged three years and when last examined aged three years eight months, gait is unsteady, stiff with flexed knees and hips.

Case 9. Male born February 21, 1968. Deaf and mute. Sitting commenced aged two and walking sometime after three years of age. The gait is wide based and stiff.

Case 10. Male born November, 1966. Mother approximately 32 weeks pregnant at time of saline injection. The child was first seen when aged three. He could walk but the gait was broad based, unsteady and stamping. The mother complained of the child's inability to talk and this remains the major complaint, though hearing appears fairly normal.

Case 11. Male born February 10, 1968. Commenced walking aged about three years two months. Gait is stamping, unsteady and spastic. At the last examination when aged three years nine months, the parents state the child's speech is not normal, but claim that hearing is all right.

Case 12. Male born December 6, 1969. Last examined aged 13 months, and is unable to sit upright and legs are spastic. There is no response to a tuning fork or handclap.

Case 13. Female born February 26, 1969. Sitting commenced after the age of 14 months. When last examined aged two years 10 months, she is unable to walk and crawling is most ineffective and spastic. The mother says the child is not talking properly though she can hear and this is confirmed by the child's ability to hear a tuning fork.

GROUP III: ABNORMALITIES OF HEARING AND/OR SPEECH ONLY

Oil

Case 1. Male born January 15, 1967. Mother had oil injection when approximately 24 weeks pregnant. Parents state that the child does not talk at all although hearing is essentially normal. There has been no evidence of any motor retardation.

Case 2. Male born January 15, 1967. Mother had oil injection when approximately 24 weeks pregnant. When last examined aged four years ten months his parents state he is not talking at all but hearing is normal. He can undoubtedly hear a tuning fork.

Saline

Case 1. Male born March 5, 1967. Mother injected with saline when approximately 18 weeks pregnant. First seen when aged two years eight months; walking was established and the gait was normal. He is unable to talk and is deaf and this is confirmed by the fact that communication with the child is by signs.

Case 2. Male born March, 1967. Mother injected with saline when approximately 18 weeks pregnant. He is unable to talk and is at least partially deaf, when last examined aged four years two months.

Case 3. Male born July 21, 1967. Mute and partially deaf. Motor milestones were normal.

Case 4. Male born March 24, 1968. When last examined aged two years eight months, the parents complained that speech is not normal, though there does not appear to be any hearing loss. Commenced walking at about 23 months.

GROUP IV: MOTOR RETARDATION WITH AN ABNORMAL GAIT

Oil

Case 1. Male born December, 1966. Mother approximately 30 weeks pregnant when injected with oil. Motor milestones retarded; was unable to sit unsupported until over age one year and did not walk until nearly three years. Gait is abnormal and speech was retarded. When the child was aged three, the parents complained that speech was not normal although when last seen, aged five years, it was stated that the child's speech was normal and there is no gross hearing loss.

Saline

Case 1. Female born October 20, 1967. Did not commence walking until over three years of age. Gait is abnormal with flexed knees and hips and very unsteady so that the child tends to fall after every one or two steps. At three years six months, the child is able to sit but there is a marked kyphosis of the spine. There does not appear to be any deficit of speech or hearing.

THE RESULTS OF PROPHYLAXIS OF ENDEMIC CRETINISM WITH IODIZED OIL IN RURAL ANDEAN ECUADOR

Ignacio Ramírez, M.D.; Rodrigo Fierro-Benítez, M.D.; Eduardo Estrella, M.D.; Amador Gómez, M.D.; Carlos Jaramillo, M.D.; César Hermida, M.D.; and Fausto Moncayo, M.D.

National Polytechnic School, Department of Radioisotopes, and Central University, Faculty of Medicine, Quito, Ecuador

It is widely, but not universally, accepted that endemic cretinism is closely related to endemic goiter and that it is the result of severe iodine deficit in fetal life, which can produce hypothyroidism in utero and therefore failure of the brain to develop normally (1,2,3,4,5).

There can be little doubt that thyroid hormones play a significant role in the development of nervous tissues (6,7,8). In the human and rat the brain fails to develop normally when thyroxine is deficient. This effect may be regarded as specific and directly mediated or secondary to such factors as the development of the cranial cavity or the influence of metabolites, themselves the products of the activity of thyroid hormone elsewhere in the body, on the growth of the brain. It has been suggested that thyroid hormone is more important to protein synthesis (cell size) in early life than later (9). Early in uterine life the fetus is entirely dependent upon a maternal supply of thyroid hormone. When iodine deficiency is severe the maternal thyroid may retain a larger fraction of the available iodine, and then iodine deficiency may exert a most significant effect on the fetus at a time when the central nervous system is developing most rapidly. In endemic goiter areas thyroid deficiency arising because of severe iodine deprivation during a relatively limited critical period of life may explain the etiology of cretinism, deaf-mutism, mental deficiency and other serious neurological defects which are the sequelae of endemic goiter.

The problem of goiter and cretinism has been the subject of clinical and epidemiological study in the highlands of Ecuador. The control and prevention of this condition was started in March 1966 by the use of iodized oil to correct iodine deficiency and thus to test the effectiveness of iodized oil administration in preventing endemic goiter and endemic cretinism.

Two isolated villages of the Ecuadorean Andes were selected for this program. The inhabitants of Tocachi were given iodized oil, whereas those of La Esperanza served as a control population.

The aim of this work has been to study the effectiveness of iodized oil on neuromotor maturation in children born during correction of iodine deficiency. Early results indicate that iodine prophylaxis in women of childbearing age may prevent the development of neuro-motor deficiency.

SUBJECTS AND METHODS

All children born in Tocachi and La Esperanza villages after March, 1966, the time when the Tocachi inhabitants were given iodized oil, were studied chronologically at the following periods of time: 0-15 days, 4-6 weeks, 3-4 months, 6 months, 9-10 months, 12-14 months, 18 months, 24 months, 30 months, 36 months, 42 months, 54 months and 60 months (a few cases). These children were born to mothers who were carefully followed during pregnancy. All children were delivered at home; between 60 and 70 percent of deliveries were assisted by a physician. The delivery date was given by the Deliveries Office at each village for those children who were not born under our care. In an attempt to study effectiveness of iodine correction in early fetal life we excluded those children born in Tocachi whose mothers were in the sixth, seventh, eighth and ninth months of pregnancy at the time of iodization.

Information on family background, age of parents, thyroid examination, the existence of abnormalities and on constitutional patterns was collected from each of the family members. Particular attention was given to the prenatal period when studying the personal background of each child. Any abnormalities occurring during pregnancy, infection, gynecological and obstetrical problems, and whether or not the mother was or was not iodized, were recorded. Delivery type, condition of the newborn's breathing, and early progress were also registered. Usually the first examination took place at the child's home. Subsequent examinations were done at the village dispensary.

During each evaluation, anthropometric growth, neuromotor maturation, and dental and skeletal development were assessed. A general clinical examination was done with emphasis on pathology, nutritional status, and thyroid function.

Head circumference was used as a measure of brain growth in each period of time studied.

Neuromotor evaluation was recorded on each infant during the longitudinal study. This assessment is described in a previous report (10) and is based on that outlined by the Gesell Scales (11, 12, 13) and the studies of Gareiso, et al.(14). Our categories included visual, auditory, social and language development, as well as motor and intellectual development and evolution of reflex activity. The Gesell Scale is not an intelligence scale. It is intended as a screening instrument to note whether the development of a particular child is within the normal range. Recently we have used the Stanford-Binet Intelligence Scale to measure intellectual capabilities. The results of this aspect of the study are presented elsewhere.

RESULTS

This report is concerned only with the problem of neuromotor maturation. Two hundred and seventeen children (108 males and 109 females) were born in Tocachi from March 1966 to August 1971; 10.13 percent died, and twelve were excluded because they received iodine correction after the fifth month of fetal life. In the same period 447 were born in the control population of La Esperanza (226 males and 221 females); 10.51 percent died.

Since this was a longitudinal study in which the same individuals were followed in several periods of time, in total we conducted 1408 observations on Tocachi children, and 2371 on those from La Esperanza.

HEAD CIRCUMFERENCE

The results of head circumference measurement in children from Tocachi and La Esperanza are shown by superimposed curves. The graph (Fig. 1) was prepared from the calculated grand means of both sexes at the following ages: birth, one, three, six, nine, 12, 18, and 24 months, and at yearly intervals through age 6 yr. At all ages the head circumference was generally similar in both populations, as illustrated in Table 1. However, it is interesting to note that averages in Tocachi are slightly larger than in La Esperanza after the sixth month. The mean increment in head circumference in Tocachi children was not significantly different

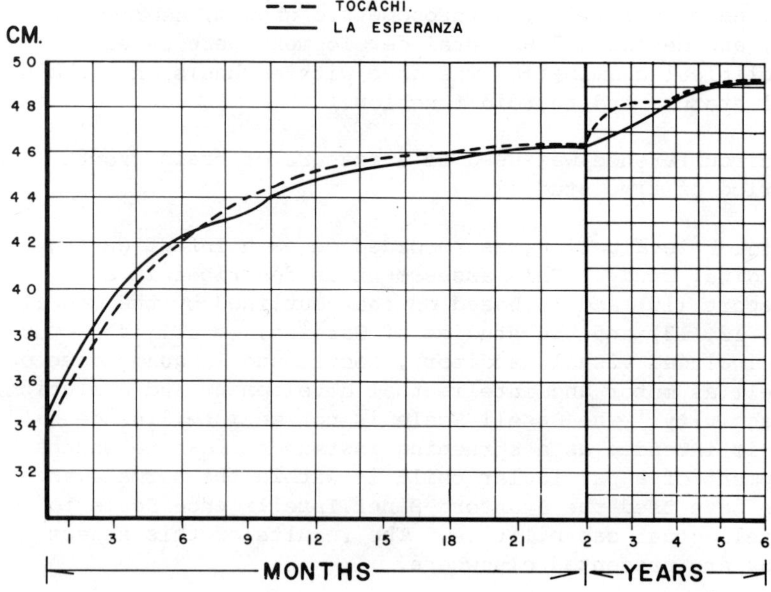

Fig. 1. Head circumference mean value of both sexes Tocachi and La Esperanza: birth, 1-3-6-9-12-18 and 24 mo.; and yearly intervals through age 6 yr.

Table 1. Head circumference, mean value for Tochachi and La Esperanza children at the time of each survey period

Age in Months	*Tocachi (cm)*	*La Esperanza (cm)*
Birth	34.2	34.3
1	36.4	36.5
3	39.2	39.6
6	42.1	42.0
9	43.8	43.2
12	44.8	44.5
18	45.8	45.6
24	46.5	46.4
36	48.1	47.2
42	48.2	48.1
48	48.3	48.6
60	49.1	49.1

from that of Esperanza children, as shown in Table 2.

Table 2. Mean increment in head circumference for Tocachi and La Esperanza children from birth to six years of age

Age	Tocachi (cm)	La Esperanza (cm)
Birth - 3 mo.	5.0	5.3
3 mo. - 6 mo.	2.9	2.4
6 mo. - 1 hr.	2.7	2.5
1 yr. - 2 yr.	1.7	1.9
2 yr. - 3 yr.	1.7	.8
3 yr. - 4 yr.	.1	1.4
4 yr. - 6 yr.	.8	.5

NEUROMOTOR MATURATION

The graphs in Figure 2-4 were prepared from the calculated grand means of total development quotient (DQ), motor development, and social-linguistic development of each sex and the sum of both sexes at all periods of time studied. At almost all ages the averages in the neuromotor characteristics in both males and females from Tocachi, were slightly better than those in La Esperanza.

There was a fall-off in averages around 18 and 24 mo. of age. This could be interpreted in the light of the poor environment in which the children develop, with increased pathology and undernutrition.

The total DQs obtained at all periods studied were grouped together in each population. A distribution of total DQs is presented in Table 3. DQs between 90-100 (normal average) in Tocachi were recorded in 67.9 percent of the examinations, while in La Esperanza they were 56.1 percent. DQs between 80-89 were 19.5 percent in Tocachi and 25.9 percent in La Esperanza. DQs between 70-79 were 7.3 percent in Tocachi and were 10.5 percent in La Esperanza. DQs below 50-69, which are considered to be deficient in terms of neuromotor maturation, were 4.9 percent in Tocachi, while in La Esperanza they were 7.2 percent. This means that in both populations neuromotor maturation deficiency was present. However, DQs between 0-19 (severe retardation) in Tocachi were not present at all, while in La Esperanza they were found in 0.2 percent of the examinations.

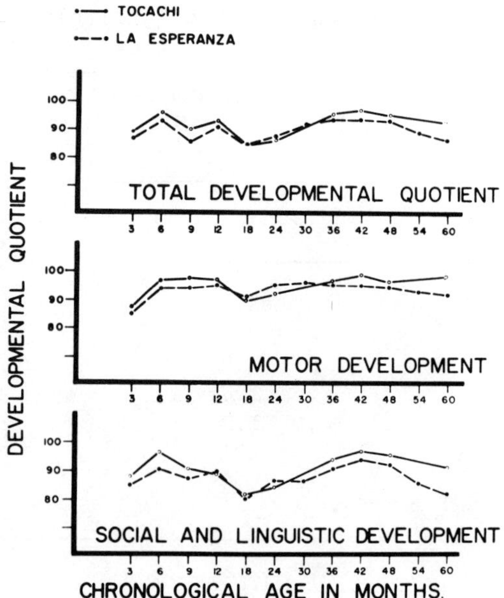

Fig. 2. The median Developmental Quotient curves of the total and individual main neuromotor maturation characteristics, for boys.

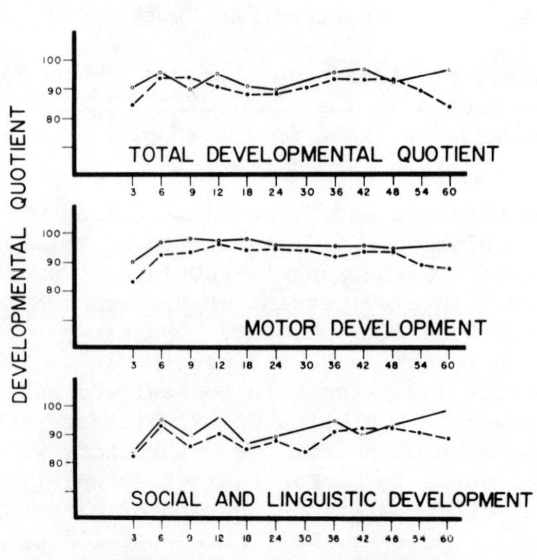

Fig. 3. The median Developmental Quotient curves of the total and individual main neuromotor maturation characteristics, for girls.

Table 3. Distribution of composite DQs of all observations

DQ	TOCACHI No.	TOCACHI Percent	LA ESPERANZA No.	LA ESPERANZA Percent
Normal				
90-100	957	67.9	1332	56.1
Low Average				
80-89	275	19.5	616	25.9
70-79	104	7.3	249	10.5
Defective				
50-69	67	4.7	146	6.1
20-49	4	.2	22	.9
0-19	0	.0	6	.2

When the observations are displayed graphically, the curve for Tocachi tended to be skewed toward the normal range in relation to the La Esperanza curve (Fig. 5).

A percentage of children in both villages had behavioural retardation as tested by manipulative tasks, perceptual, linguistic and gross motor tasks (Table 4). From these results it seems that the social and language functions are the most affected areas of neuromotor maturation in those children. When considering the grand means of all ages together we found that clearly the Tocachi children are less affected than their counterparts from La Esperanza.

The differences in frequency of the main neuromotor characteristics found in the same population can be explained by the fact that defective children presented the behavioural aspects studied with different degrees of deficit and in various combinations. This occurs in both populations, and is in full agreement with what is found in adult defectives.

Six instances of severe mental and neuromotor deficiency have appeared in La Esperanza, while there has been no new case in Tocachi. These were affected in all the neuromotor areas tested (Figs. 6, 7, 8).

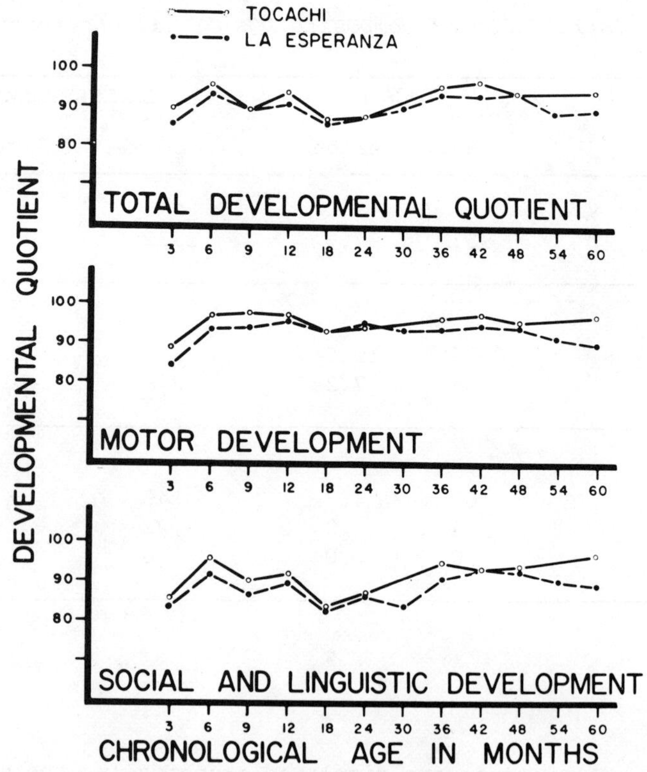

Fig. 4. The median Developmental Quotient curves of the total and individual main neuromotor maturation characteristics, for children of both sexes.

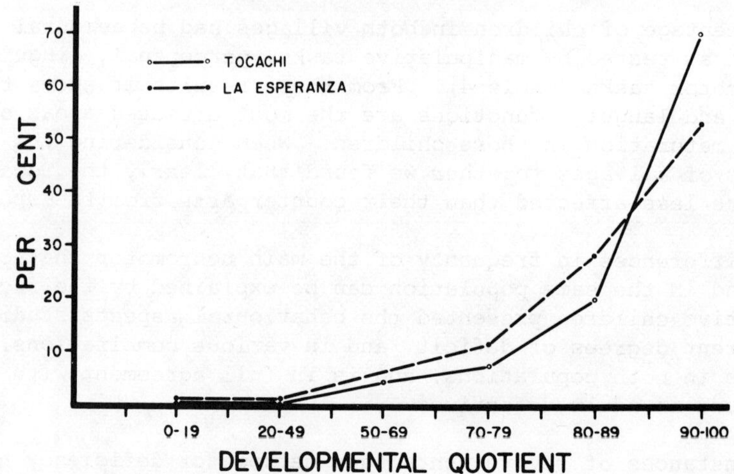

Fig. 5. Distribution of total DQ, obtained at all periods studied and grouped together in each population.

Table 4. Percentage incidence of defectives in both villages who had a behavorial retardation as tested by main neuromotor characteristics

FUNCTION	MOTOR		SOCIAL AND LINGUISTIC		INTELLECTUAL	
VILLAGE	TOCACHI (%)	LA ESP. (%)	TOCACHI (%)	LA ESP. (%)	TOCACHI (%)	LA ESP. (%)
AGE IN MONTHS 3	0	1.9				
6	0	2.3				
9	0	1.4				
12	0	2.3	4.1	4.3	0	0
18	6.1	9.6	7.1	12.3	3.5	6
24	2.0	5.0	7.1	8.4	5.0	9
36	3.8	3.0	6.1	8.1	3.8	3
48	2.0	5.9	2.0	11.6	0	3
	13.9	31.4	26.3	44.8	12.3	24.1
Mean Value	1.7	3.9	5.3	9.0	2.5	4.8

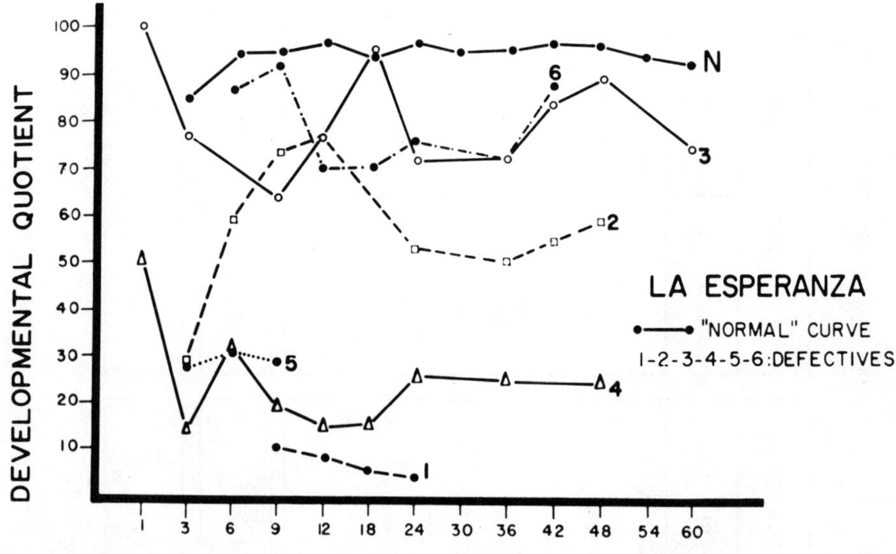

Fig. 6. Individual Motor Developmental Quotient curves of six severely retarded children born in the noniodized village, La Esperanza.

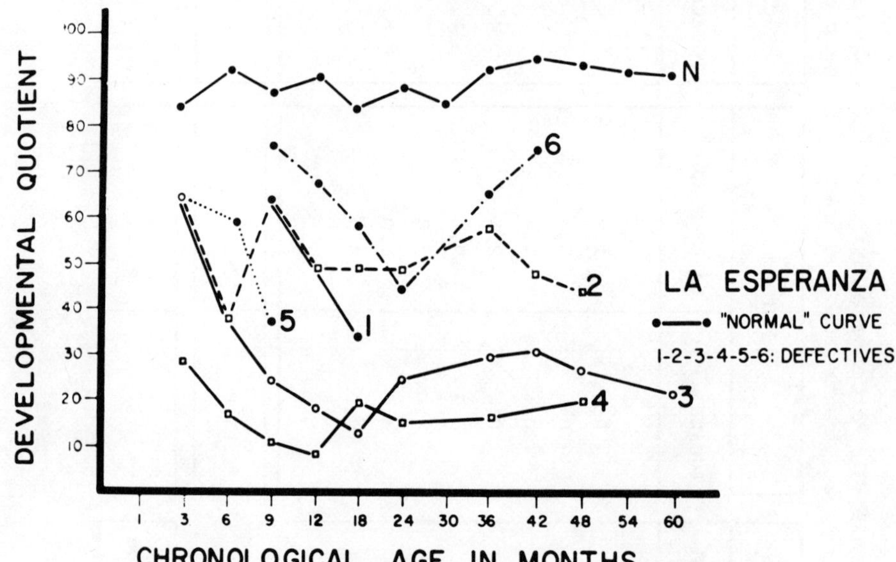

Fig. 7. Individual Social and Linguistic Developmental Quotient curves of six severely retarded children born in the noniodized village, La Esperanza.

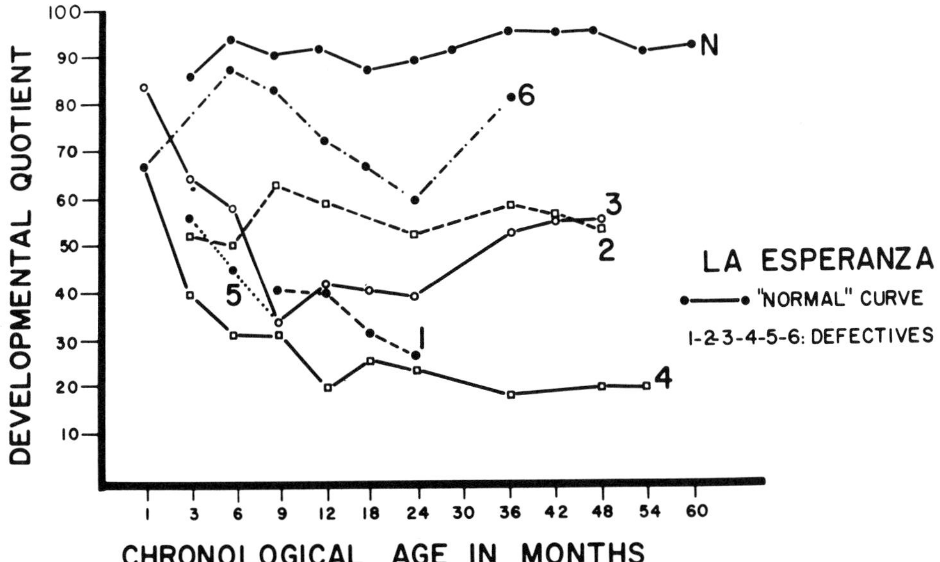

Fig. 8. Individual Total Developmental Quotient curves of six severely retarded children born in the noniodized village, La Esperanza.

SUMMARY

The results are preliminary and inconclusive and underscore the need for critical statistical analysis.

Growth and development result from an intricate pattern of genetic, nutritional, social and cultural forces which dynamically affect the child from the moment of conception.

The poor general conditions (low caloric intake, socio-economic deprivation, geographic isolation, and chronic iodine deficiency) are among the factors contributing to the prevalence of neuromotor maturation deficiency in the villages studied.

Iodine prophylaxis of the pregnant mother throughout gestation appears to be an important factor in improving the neuromotor maturation in infants and in preventing major mental retardation.

The studies on neuromotor development, when considered as a whole, suggest that there is some advance in neurological development in children of Tocachi who were protected by iodine prophylaxis as compared with children of La Esperanza who were not so protected.

ACKNOWLEDGMENTS

Appreciation is expressed to Dr. John B. Stanbury and to Dr. P. Dodge, for their contributions in this study.

DISCUSSION BY PARTICIPANTS

PHAROAH: Why did you choose the time of five months of gestation?

FIERRO: Five months was quite arbitrary. Early fetal life is the critical period in terms of nervous system formation.

BECKERS: If we admit that iodine prevents cretinism and if we admit that the fetus uses its own thyroid hormone, I think we should try to compare groups receiving iodine before the development of the fetal thyroid gland with those receiving it after.

FIERRO: You are right. We used this classification because we would not have had enough children otherwise. We will have definitive data when we have enough children whose mothers were injected during the thirteen first weeks of pregnancy or before conception.

DEGROOT: I think that in our present state of ignorance it is perfectly all right for Dr. Fierro to split his groups at five months. It is not obvious that thyroxine is even necessary during the first month of pregnancy. It is also immaterial whether or not the fetal gland is producing it because there is also the mother's thyroid to think about.

MOSIER: A great deal of brain maturation occurs after five months of fetal age. Myelination of the tracts is still incomplete at birth, and organization of the cortex, at least in the cerebellum, is still proceeding. It is possibly in the later stages that hypothyroidism makes some of its great inroads.

BALÁZS: In experimental animals, at least, thyroid function is not too important during the early part of gestation. For example, rats and rabbits can be made hypothyroid early in fetal life without apparent adverse effects visible at birth, and the effects later in life do not seem to be more severe than those caused by postnatal thyroid deficiency, which has a profound influence on brain development. It is possible that there are species differences with respect to the time in ontogenesis when thyroid function becomes essential for the development of the CNS. However, even in man the differentiation of nerve cells continues well into the postnatal period, and it seems that thyroid hormones are necessary for the normal maturation of neurons. We do not know this 'critical period' in man and thus any experimental grouping is acceptable if it is clearly defined and the studies are well done.

ROSMAN: I think there is an important difference between the rat and man. The human thyroid is functioning during the first trimester of pregnancy and myelinization continues in certain tracts well beyond birth, in some tracts into the third decade of life or longer. By contrast, the rat thyroid begins to function on the 16th or 17th day of a 21-day gestation. It is believed that most neurological development in the rat has been completed by 24 days after birth. It appears that thyroid function would be a more critical determinant in man in the first third of pregnancy, but in the rat in the last third of pregnancy.

DEGROOT: But the rat neonatal development is equivalent to human fetal development. If you add the time it takes the neonatal rat to get to the same stage of nervous development that humans have at birth, the sequence may be very similar.

ROSMAN: I think the fact that your patients showed greater impairment of social and linguistic skills than other skills is an artifact. The Stanford-Binet is a highly verbal test and consequently this population of children would be expected to show greater impairment in language skills. Secondly, social skills are likely to be less well developed if the families tested were of generally lower intelligence.

FIERRO: You are right. We were only using these tests for comparison, nothing more.

PRETELL: Our series showed the same greater deterioration of language and social adaptation.

Do you think that the Stanford-Binet tests are more important than the Gesell tests? Your Gesell tests did not show a significant difference between the two groups.

FIERRO: I do not think the Stanford-Binet tests are more important, but the Gesell also showed differences. To date we do not know how statistically significant they were.

REFERENCES

1. Eayrs, J.T.: Developmental relationships between brain and thyroid. In: Endocinology and Human Behaviour (R.P. Michael, ed.). Oxford University Press, London, 1968. pp. 317-39.

2. Blizzard, R.M.: Differentiation, morphogenesis, and growth with emphasis on the role of pituitary growth hormone. In: Human Growth (D.B. Cheek, ed.). Lea and Febiger, Philadelphia, 1968. pp. 41-57.

3. Querido, A.: Endemic cretinism: A search for a tenable definition. In: Endemic Goiter. Report of the meeting of the PAHO Scientific Group on Research in Endemic Goiter held in Mexico, 1968. (J.B. Stanbury, ed.), Scientific Publication No. 193, Washington, 1969. pp. 85-90.

4. Stanbury, J.B.: Endemic Goiter. J. Clin. Endocrinol. Metab. 2:195, 1968.

5. Fierro-Benítez, R.; Peñafiel, W.; DeGroot, L. and Ramírez, I.: Endemic goiter and endemic cretinism in the Andean Region. New Engl. J. Med. 280:296, 1969.

6. Eayrs, J.T.: Age as a factor determining the severity and reversibility of the effects of thyroid deprivation in the rat. J. Endocrinol.22:409-419.

7. Hamburgh, M. and Vicari, E.: Effect of thyroid hormone on nervous system maturation. Anat. Rec.127:302, 1957.

8. Bradley, P.B.; Eayrs, J.T.; Glass and Heath, R.W.: The maturation and metabolic consequences of neonatal thyroidectomy upon the recruiting response in the rat. Electroenceph. Clin. Neurophysiol. 13:308-313.

9. Eayrs, J.T.: The possible significance of neuropil for the mediation of cortical function. In: Regional Neuro-Chemistry (S. S.Kety, and J. Elkes, eds.). Pergamon Press, New York, 1961. p. 423.

10. Ramírez, I.; Fierro-Benítez, R.; Estrella, E.; Jaramillo, C.; Díaz, C. and Urresta, J.: Iodized oil in the prevention of endemic goiter and associated defects in the Andean Region of Ecuador: II. Effects on neuromotor development and somatic growth in children before two years. In: Endemic Goiter. Report of the meeting of the PAHO Scientific Group on Research in Endemic Goiter held in Mexico, 1968. (J.B. Stanbury, ed.). Scientific Publication No. 193, Washington, 1969.

11. Gesell, A.: Children from One Year to Four Years. Paidos, Buenos Aires, 1967.

12. Gesell, A. and Amatruda, C.S.: The Education of Children in Modern Culture. Nova, Buenos Aires, 1965.

13. Gesell, A. and Amatruda, C.S.: Diagnostico del Desarrollo Normal y Anormal del Niño. Paidos, Buenos Aires, 1967.

14. Gareiso, A. and Escardo, F.: Neuropediatrics. El Ateneo, Buenos Aires, 1956.

EFFECT OF IODINE CORRECTION EARLY IN FETAL LIFE ON INTELLIGENCE QUOTIENT. A PRELIMINARY REPORT

Rodrigo Fierro-Benítez, Ignacio Ramírez, and José Suárez

National Polytechnic School, Department of Radioisótopes, and Central University, Faculty of Medicine, Quito, Equador

In some areas in which goiter is endemic there is a high prevalence of mental deficiency without any other stigma of cretinism (1-6). When surveying the populations of Tocachi and La Esperanza in highland Ecuador in which goiter is endemic we were impressed by the high prevalence of mental deficiency in the general population. This generalized mental deficiency was independent of the typical cases of cretinism. We believe that several factors such as protein-caloric malnutrition and chronic iodine deficiency may contribute toward producing this mental deficit. All of these factors exist in the populations studied.

With these facts in mind we were interested in studying the effect of the correction of iodine deficiency on this endemic mental deficiency. The present study is concerned with this problem, and although the results are preliminary and inconclusive, they underscore the need for critical analysis of this question.

CLINICAL MATERIAL AND METHODS

The studies reported here cover a period of five years since a program of goiter prevention was begun in two rural Ecuadorean villages. Iodized poppyseed oil was given intramuscularly to women of child-bearing age in March 1966 in a village of Andean Ecuador, Tocachi, where endemic goiter is severe and cretinism commonplace. In December 1968 the fertile women were reinjected and some infants born in Tocachi since 1966 received iodine by intramuscular administration. A nearby village, La Esperanza, which is in all respects similar,has served as a control.

Study design and ongoing observations of the iodine therapy program have been described previously (7-12).

A large number of children have been born in the two villages. The "normal" children, those older than 40 months of age, were tested in both populations. The severely mentally retarded children from the control village were excluded.

Among the children born in Tocachi some had received iodine since the earliest stages of embryogenesis, during lactation, and directly by intramuscular administration. Other children only received iodine correction during the last three months of gestation, during lactation, and directly by intramuscular administration. Thus, we can classify the children who were born in Tocachi since March 1966 until October 1967 (older than 40 months at the time of study) in two main groups:

Group I: Children who received iodine during the last period of fetal life, during lactation and directly by intramuscular administration.

Group II: Children who received iodine early in intrauterine life, during lactation, and directly by intramuscular administration.

In the control village, La Esperanza, we studied a group of children with the same chronological ages as the group of Tocachi children.

The nutritional status of each child was evaluated by anthropometric measurements. Since the weight-height ratio is the best mean of evaluating nutrition we measured height and weight, as well as head circumference.

The Stanford-Binet Scale (13), as modified by us, was used to measure intellectual capacity. The modifications of the scale were in picture recognition and vocabulary, which have local characteristics. With the Stanford-Binet test it is possible to determine mental age, basal age, and most importantly, the intelligence quotient of the child.

Statistical analysis of the results was done using Experimental Design Theory (14). We have used a single factor model.

$$X_{ij} = u + T_j + C_{ij}$$

where:

u = mean

T_j = treatment effect $j = 1, 2$

C_{ij} = experimental error

RESULTS

A total of 150 children were tested, 67 in the treated population (Tocachi) and 83 in the control village (La Esperanza). Twenty six of the Tocachi children were in Group I and 41 in Group II. The corresponding numbers of children in La Esperanza were 33 and 50. There was some variation in the proportion of boys and girls in each group, but it was not greatly different. The mean chronological age of the children in Group I was 65 months. That of Group II was 40 months.

The children of both the Tocachi and La Esperanza groups had the same anthropometric characteristics. Almost all of the children presented undernutrition, but this was equal for all the groups in both villages. Thus we can dismiss nutrition as a factor for differences in intellectual function between comparable groups.

The mean value of the IQ scores in Tocachi Group I was 67.0; in Tocachi Group II it was 80.1 and in the La Esperanza groups 70.1.

From the statistical analysis of IQ of Tocachi Group II versus La Esperanza (Table 1), $F_{calculated}$ was greater than F_{table} and this was highly significant. Therefore, we rejected the null hypothesis that there exists no difference between Group II and the group of La Esperanza. Thus the children of Group II in Tocachi presented a statistically significantly higher IQ than the children in the group from La Esperanza.

From the statistical analysis of Group II versus Group I, both of Tocachi, we had:

$$F_{1,63} = \frac{2667.69}{142.61} = 18.70 \text{ (Table 2)}$$

Because $F_{calculated} > F_{table}$, this is highly significant, which means that there also exists a difference between Groups I and II from Tocachi.

Table 1. Statistical analysis of Tocachi Group II vs. La Esperanza, using the Experimental Design Theory. The model we have used is a single factor.

ANALYSIS OF VARIANCE

SOURCE OF VARIATION	D.F.	SUM OF SQUARES	MEAN SQUARE (variance)
T_j	K - 1 2 - 1 = 1	2774.63	2774.63
(error)	N - K 122 - 2 = 120	17228.65	143.57
TOTALS	N - 1 122 - 1 = 121	20103.28	

$$F_{1,120} = \frac{2774.63}{143.57} = 19.32 \quad (F_{calculated} > F_{table})$$

The IQ difference between Tocachi Group I and La Esperanza lacks significance.

Children who had an IQ below 70 were considered to be mentally deficient. From this point, we have found that in Tocachi and La Esperanza there is a significant prevalence of mental deficiency (Table 3). However, in Group II in Tocachi only 20.6 percent had IQ scores in the mentally deficient range, while in Group I in Tocachi 49 percent of the scores were in this range, and in La Esperanza 49.4 percent of the scores were in this range.

Table 2. Statistical analysis of Tocachi Group II vs Tocachi Group I, using the Experimental Design Theory. The model we have used is a single factor.

ANALYSIS OF VARIANCE

SOURCE OF VARIATION	D.F.	SUM OF SQUARES	MEAN SQUARE (variance)
Between Treatments (T_j)	K - 1 2 - 1 = 1	2667.69	2667.69
Within treatments (error)	N - K 65 - 2 = 63	8984.92	142.61
TOTALS	N - 1 65 - 1 = 64	11652.61	

When the distributions of IQ scores in each group are plotted they tend to be skewed in the direction of mental deficiency. However, the curve of Tocachi Group II has a tendency toward normality and there is an obvious reduction in the incidence of mental deficiency in relation to La Esperanza.

When the IQ distribution in the two groups of Tocachi was plotted, we observed that mental deficiency was present in both groups and that their curves remained far below the Stanford-Binet standard curve. However, we observed a reduction of the mental deficiency in Group II in relation to Group I. Forty-nine percent of the IQs in Group I were below 70 while only 20.6 percent of those in Group II were below 70. This reflects a reduction of mental deficiency of 25.5 percent in Group II with respect to Group I. This is statistically highly significant. In addition, there were fewer frankly retarded persons (IQ below 50) in Group II (2.6 percent than in Group I (6.7 percent).

Table 3. Percentage Distribution of Composite IQs (Stanford-Binet Scale). A total of 150 children were tested, the mean chronological age of children in Group I was 65 months. That of Group II was 40 months. The group of children from La Esperanza had the same chronological ages as the groups of Tocachi children.

IQ	STANFORD-BINET		TOCACHI I		TOCACHI II		LA ESPERANZA	CLASSIFICATION
100 - 109	23.5		0.0		2.6		1.1	NORMAL OR AVERAGE
90 - 99	23.0		0.0		23.1		2.8	
80 - 89	14.5		15.4		30.8		10.2	LOW AVERAGE
70 - 79	5.6		34.6		23.1		30.7	
60 - 69	2.6		23.1		15.4		28.4	
50 - 59	0.4	3.2	19.2	49.0	2.6	20.6	16.5	DEFECTIVE
40 - 49	0.2		6.7		2.6		4.5	

SUMMARY

Nutritional deficiency, socio-economic deprivation, geographic and biological isolation, and chronic iodine deficiency are among the factors contributing to the high prevalence of mental deficiency in children considered to be "normal" in the villages studied.

Iodine correction after the fifth month of intrauterine life appears to have little or no prophylactic effect in terms of preventing mental retardation.

Iodine correction early in the intrauterine life appears to be an important factor that contributes to improving the intellectual capacities of the child.

ACKNOWLEDGEMENTS

The authors are indebted to Dr. John B. Stanbury for his assistance in this study.

We wish to thank Mr. René Ortíz for his help in the statistical analysis of the data.

REFERENCES

1. Querido. A.; Endemic cretinism: A search for a tenable definition. In: Endemic Goiter. Report of the meeting of the PAHO Scientific Group on Endemic Goiter held in Mexico, 1968 (J.B. Stanbury, ed.). PAHO Scientific Publication No. 193, Washington, 1969. pp. 85-90.

2. Querido, A.: Epidemiology of cretinism. In: Endemic Cretinism. Monogr. Series No. 2 (B.S. Hetzel and P.O.D. Pharoah, eds.). Inst. Human Biology, Papua, New Guinea, 1971. pp.9-18.

3. Eugster, J.: Zur Erblichkeitsfrage des endemischen Kretinismus. Untersuchungen an 204 Kretinen und deren Blutverwendten. J. Arch. Julius Klaus-Stift. 13:383, 1938.

4. Stanbury, J.B.: The patterns of endemic cretinism. In: Endemic Cretinism, Monogr. Series. No. 2 (B.S. Hetzel and P.O.D. Pharoah, eds.). Inst. Human Biology, Papua, New Guinea, 1971. pp. 19-31.

5. Fierro-Benítez, R.; Stanbury, J.B.; Querido, A.; DeGroot, L.J.; Alban, R.; and Córdova, J.: Endemic Cretinism in the Andean region of Ecuador. J. Clin. Endocrinol. and Metab. 30:228, 1970.

6. Kelly, F.C. and Snedden, W.W. In: Endemic Goitre. World Health Organization, Geneva, 1960. p. 27.

7. Fierro-Benítez, R.; Ramírez, I.; Estrella, E.; Jaramillo, C.; Díaz, C. and Urresta, J.: Iodized oil in the prevention of endemic goiter and associated defects in the Andean region of Ecuador: I. Program design, effects on goiter prevalence, thyroid function, and iodine excretion. In: Endemic Goiter. Report of the meeting of the PAHO Scientific Group on Endemic Goiter held in Mexico, 1968 (J.B. Stanbury, ed.). PAHO Scientific Publication No. 193, Washington, 1969. p. 306.

8. Ramírez, I.; Fierro-Benítez, R.; Estrella, E.; Jaramillo, C.; Díaz, C. and Urresta, J.: Iodized oil in the prevention of endemic goiter and associated defects in the Andean region of Ecuador: II. Effects on neuromotor development and somatic growth in children before two years. In: Endemic Goiter. Report of the meeting of the PAHO Scientific Group on Endemic Goiter held in Mexico, 1968 (J.B. Stanbury, ed.). PAHO Scientific Publication No. 193, Washington, 1969. pp. 341-359.

9. Fierro-Benítez, R.; Ramírez, I.; Estrella, E.; Querido, A. and Stanbury, J.B.: The effect of goiter prophylaxis with iodized oil in the prevention of endemic cretinism. Proceedings of the Sixth International Thyroid Conference, Vienna, 1970. p. 7.

10. Fierro-Benítez, R. and Ramírez, I.: Measurements of 131-I-labelled triiodothyronine uptake by a resin as a means of diagnosing Iodine-Basedow produced by intramuscular administration of iodized oil in an area of endemic goiter. In: In Vitro Procedures with Radioisotopes in Medicine. International Atomic Energy Agency, Vienna, 1970. p. 287.

11. Dodge, P.R.; Palkes, H.; Fierro-Benítez, R. and Ramírez, I.: Effect on intelligence of iodine in oil administered to young Andean children. A preliminary report. In: Endemic Goiter. Report of the meeting of the PAHO Scientific Group on Endemic Goiter held in Mexico, 1968 (J.B. Stanbury, ed.). PAHO Scientific Publication No. 193, Washington, 1969. pp. 360-372.

12. Israel, H.; Fierro-Benítez, R.; and Garcés, J.: Iodine therapy for endemic goiter and its effects upon skeletal development of the child. In: Endemic Goiter. Report of the meeting of the PAHO Scientific Group on Endemic Goiter held in Mexico, 1968 (J.B. Stanbury, ed.). PAHO Scientific Publication No. 193, Washington, 1969. pp. 360-372.

13. Teruman, L.M. and Merrill, M.A.: *Stanford-Binet Intelligence Scale*. Riverside, Boston, 1962.

14. Hicks, Charles, R.: *Fundamental Concepts in the Design of Experiments*. Holt, Rinehart and Winston, New York, 1964. pp. 21-28.

PROPHYLAXIS OF ENDEMIC GOITER WITH IODIZED OIL IN RURAL PERU

Eduardo A. Pretell, Tobías Torres, Víctor Zenteno, and Miguel Cornejo*

Instituto de Investigaciones de la Altura (Laboratorio de Endocrinología), Universidad Peruana Cayetano Heredia, Lima, Peru

Three Andean villages at altitudes of 3,100 to 3,500 meters above sea level were studied in order to determine the prophylactic effect of iodized oil administration on endemic goiter and cretinism (1). At the time of the study the population in these villages was approximately 4,000, with an annual growth rate of about three percent. In a group of 3,000 subjects examined in a house-to-house survey, the visible goiter rate, as defined in an accompanying paper (2), was 55 percent. However, when the occurrence of palpable goiter was considered as well, the incidence of goiter rose to 83 percent. Fifty percent of the children in the 0-5 yr age group were goitrous and of these, 20 percent demonstrated visible goiter. Goiter prevalence increased with age, as did nodularity. An example of this is shown in Fig. 1. In some families every member was found with goiter as illustrated in Fig. 2. Goiter was also found among the domestic animals. The percentage of defective persons in the three villages ranged from 1.0 to 3.6 percent. Although these villages are accessible by automobile, they are still quite remote and isolated.

Measurement of iodine excretion in these three villages averaged 17 µg per 24 hr, and the radioactive iodine uptake averaged approximately 75 percent. The mean value of the total serum iodine was 5.5 µg per 100 ml and the total thyroxine

**With the collaboration of Artidoro Cáceres, Frida Fernández, and Raquel Fürgang

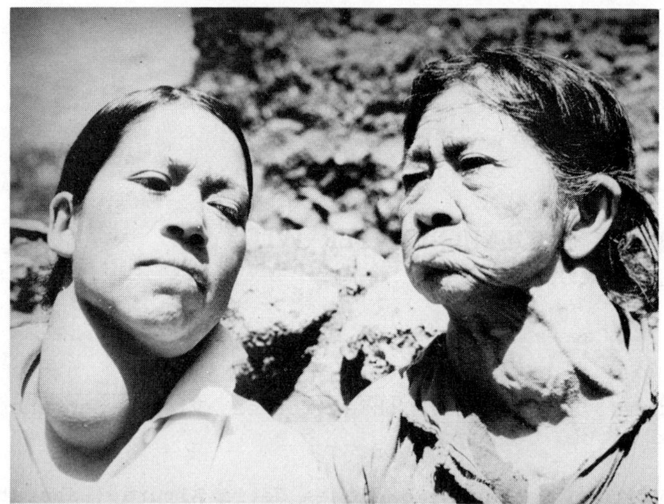

Fig. 1. Huge nodular goiters are more prominent among adults as shown in this 74 yr old mother and her 39 yr old daughter from the endemic area of Tapo.

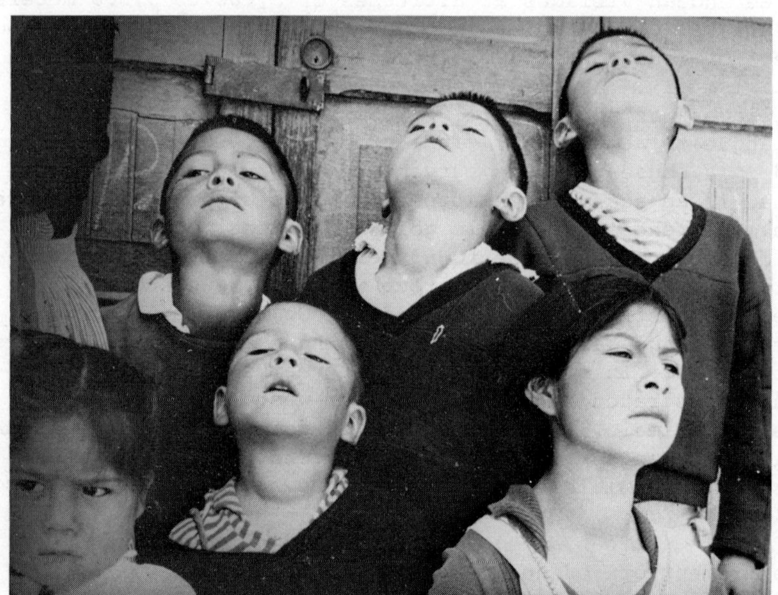

Fig. 2. Clinical appearance of a group of four brothers and two sisters all of whom have diffuse goiters of Grade I and II. The boy on the top right and the girl below were six and seven years old respectively. The other four children were below five. A six month old baby sister who does not appear in the picture was not goitrous as yet.

was 4.1 μg per 100 ml measured as iodine, with a range of 1.7 to 6.4 μg per 100 ml. As a result, many persons were below the accepted normal range for a population without endemic goiter; however, these patients had no clinical evidence of hypothyroidism.

In October, 1966, 1,700 persons from these villages were injected either with iodized oil or placebo, and were reinjected three years later along with a new group of persons injected for the first time. The program design is described elsewhere (1,2).

In order to control carefully the progress of women in the child-bearing age and to follow as many pregnancies throughout gestation as possible from both the iodized and placebo groups, a full-time physician was appointed to rotate continuously among the villages. Newborn infants were recorded at the time of delivery.

This report is particularly concerned with the evaluation of these children who were born into the program and now have been followed up to five years after injection of their mothers. The marked effects of thyroid hormone deficiency during intrauterine and early post-natal life, resulting in physical growth and mental retardation, have already been demonstrated in human beings (3-6) and in animals (7-9). Though hypothyroidism has been reported among children (10) and developmental delay is well known in cretins from iodide-deficient endemic goiter areas, as yet it is not well established that the deficiency of iodine alone is the only cause, or whether any developmental delay actually occurs in non-cretin children. We hope, therefore, at this time to provide additional information on the role of iodine deficiency in early development as well as the effect of iodine supplementation in mothers-to-be.

The negative effect of chronic iodine deficiency on maternal thyroid hormone synthesis, but not necessarily on the fetus, is described in an accompanying paper (II).

SUBJECTS AND METHODS

A total of 456 newborn children was registered, of whom approximately 44 percent belonged to the placebo or iodine-deficient (Group D) and the other 56 percent to the iodized group (Group I). Of these, 84 percent have been covered by comprehensive follow-up evaluations which included the following:

1. *Physical examination*, including the assessment of goiter.

2. *A full anthropometric series* including body weight, stature or supine length, sitting height or crown-rump length, head and chest circumferences, as well as upper arm circumferences, triceps,

subscapular and waist skinfold thickness and biacromial and bi-ilicristal diameters in order to characterize the nutritional status of the subject. The measurements were made according to recommendations given by WHO (12). A Lange caliper was used for the skinfold measurements.

3. *Radiology studies* made from birth through several different ages in order to demonstrate bone maturation according to standard methods. The examination included a PA x-ray of the left hand and wrist using a Bucky field-portable x-ray unit at a tube to film distance of 91.5cm. The bone age was then calculated according to the patterns of Greulich and Pyle (13).

4. *Motor and neuropsychological appraisal* in 60 percent of these children utilizing the Gesell test (14). In some cases, a more critical neuropsychological development was measured by the Stanford-Binet (15) and the Brunet-Lézine (16) tests. The Stanford-Binet evaluation was employed in the two to four yr-old group only and the Brunet-Lézine in those under two yr of age. In a few children older than two yr, but with a marked mental retardation, the Brunet-Lézine test was employed. Audiometry, voice, buccofacial praxis, articulation praxis and verbal expression and comprehension were tested by methods adapted to our environment by Dr. Cáceres' team (17). The more critical studies were done only in the village of Huasahuasi.

5. *Electroencephalographic studies* made with an eight channel Nikon Kode portable unit on 15 subjects in each group between the ages of two and four yr. These studies were carried out under sleeping conditions after Seconal administration (.025-.075 gm) in most of them.

6. *Urinary excretion of iodide (UEI)* measured in a sampling of the overall newborn population, between the ages of two and 4 1/2 yr according to methods previously described (1).

The above studies were mainly cross-sectional. On some occasions, semi-longitudinal evaluations were carried out. All investigators were unaware of the injection status of the subjects throughout the determination of the above parameters. Grouping of results according to protocol injection of the mothers occurred only after the qualification of the studies was concluded.

RESULTS AND COMMENTS

At the time of birth there was no difference in the children of placebo or iodized-oil injected mothers, although there did appear to be a slight tendency for weight to be higher in the iodized group. Head circumference and Apgar scores were in the normal range in both groups. Placental weights were lower than in usual standards, but they were not different from those expected in any population at 3,500 meters above sea level (18). Mean values of the data recorded at birth are included in Table 1.

Table 1. Data at birth of children born to iodized and placebo mothers

	Weight (gm)	Length (cm)	Cephalic Circumference (cm)	Apgar	Placental wt. (gm)
PLACEBO	2981 ± 69*	44.7 ± 3.2	33.9 ± 0.3	9.0 ± 0.2	488 ± 50
IODIDE	3197 ± 181	49.4 ± 0.3	34.2 ± 1.2	7.9 ± 0.7	413 ± 157
P VALUE	ns	ns	ns	ns	ns

*Mean ± SE

Birth rate was slightly higher in the iodized group than in the placebo one. Two hundred fifty-four births were registered among 390 fertile-aged women in the former while in the latter there were 202 births among 402 fertile-aged women. Infant death rate, on the other hand, although significantly higher when compared to well-developed countries, was similar to other rural areas in Peru (19), with no significant difference between iodized and placebo groups - i.e. approximately 11 percent in the former and 12 percent in the latter during the first two years of life.

No congenital goiter was found in either group. The data obtained in regard to height and weight were similar in both placebo and iodized groups in both sexes as shown in Figs. 3 and 4. These factors beyond 12 months of age are in the third percentile for North American standards (20), but when compared to another population in Peru (21) not involved with endemic goiter, the figures are comparable. Thus, these changes appear to be characteristic of the rural Peruvian population rather than of the endemic area alone. A slow and prolonged growth pattern has been demonstrated in high altitude Peruvian natives (22). However, there appeared to be little difference between the iodine and placebo groups as both attained nearly the same stature year by year. The iodine group tended to show slightly higher growth rate values, but there was considerable overlap (Table 2). Post-natally there was an observable tendency for weight to increase more than height, which might suggest that there is no severe malnutrition among these children. Additional support for this theory was provided by the skinfold and upper arm circumference measurements as shown in Table 3. While both groups

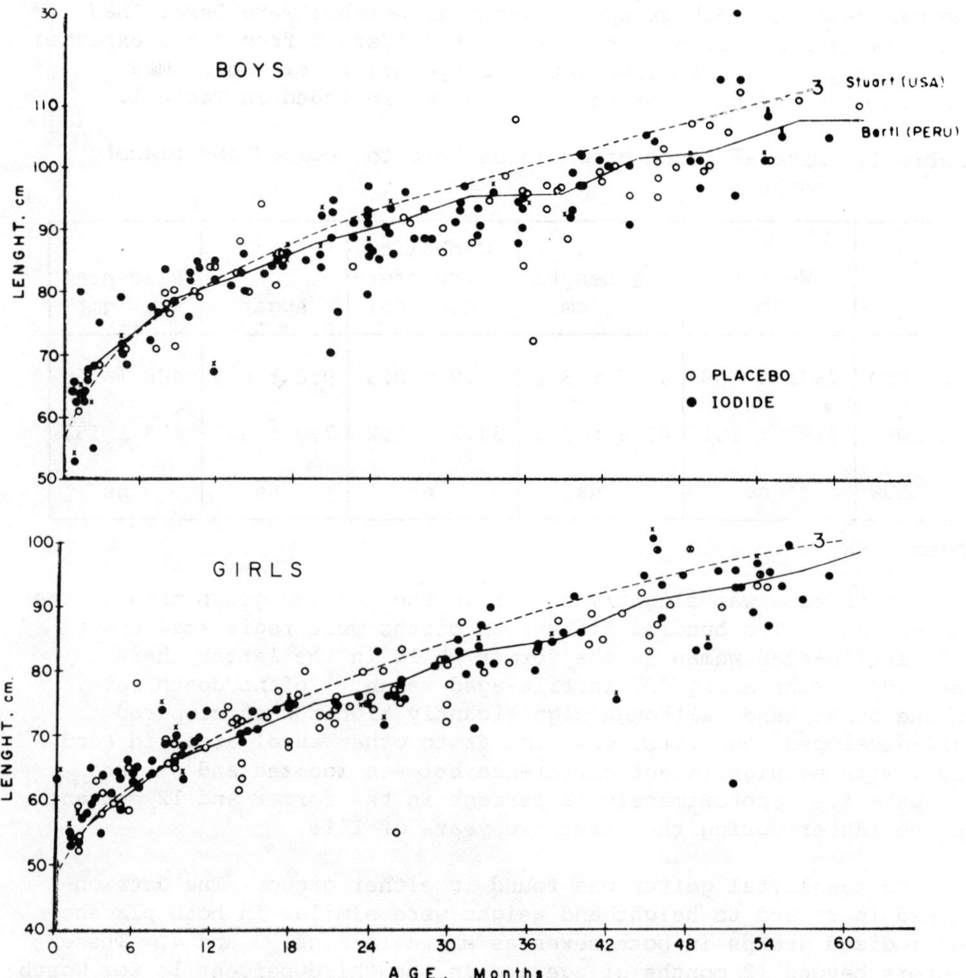

Fig. 3. Stature and supine length of a cross-sectional sample of 0-5 yr old children, as compared to North American patterns and to another non-goitrous rural population in Peru.

appeared to have nearly the same upper arm circumference, the sums of skinfolds were slightly, but not significantly, greater in the placebo group. Although it seems unlikely that this finding may reflect a slow thyroid function in the iodine-deficient group, this possibility has not been ruled out. In any event, whatever the factors responsible for the slightly greater fat deposition of the placebo group, they did not appear to be reflected in taller statures. Moreover, in both groups there was a drop in the skinfold values from birth through 12-18 months of age.

Birth x-rays disclosed no evidence of intrauterine hypothyroidism as indicated by the appearance of ossification (23). In only two subjects was there any indication of retardation in bone maturation and this was not definite. It is interesting to

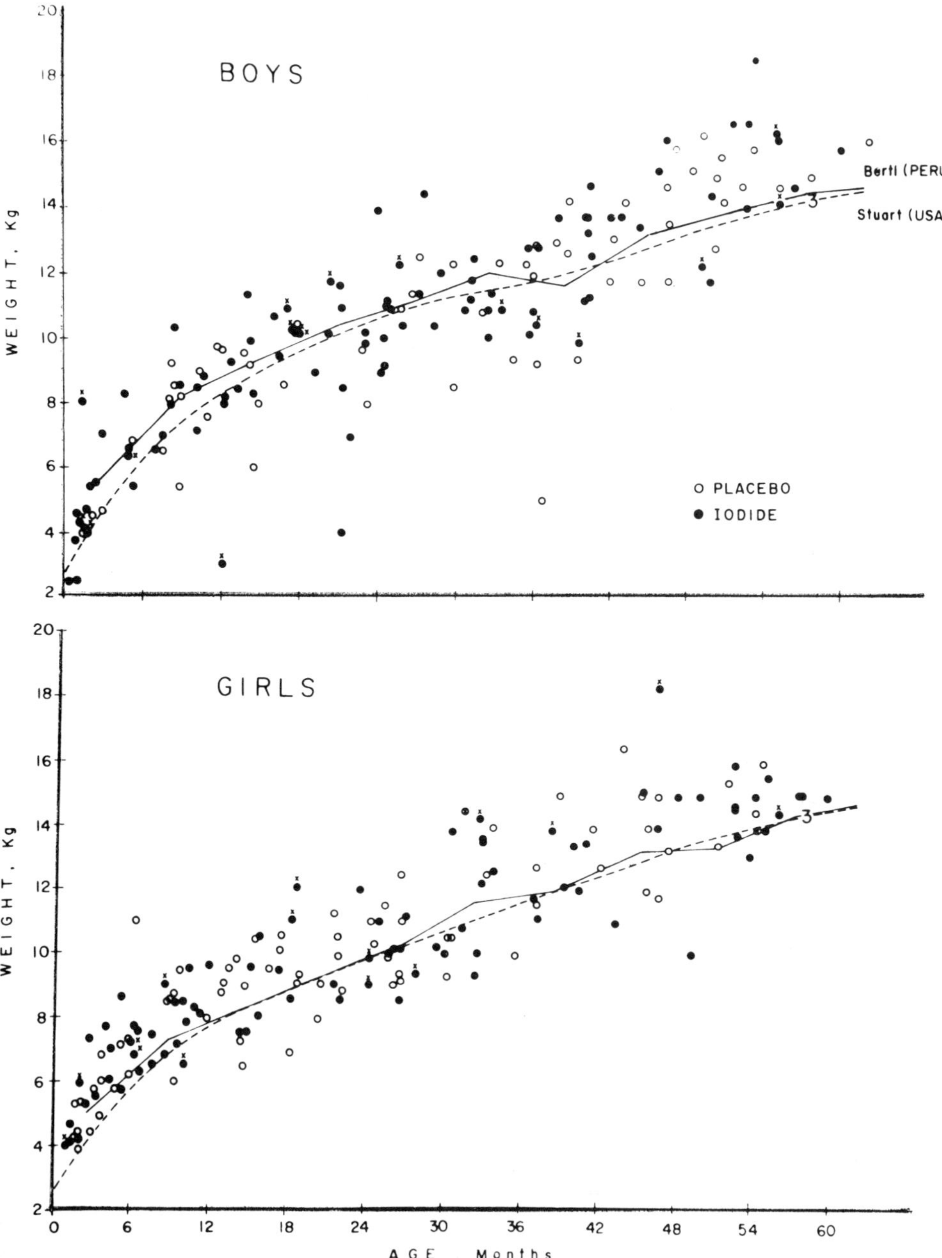

Fig. 4. Weights of the same cross-sectional sample as described in Fig. 3.

Table 2. Growth Rate (cm/month) in children born to iodide deficient (placebo) and iodide treated (iodide) mothers

Age Months	0-6	6-12	12-24	24-36
PLACEBO	2.52	1.58	0.85	0.55
IODIDE	3.16	1.75	0.83	0.84

Table 3. Skinfold thickness (mm) and upper arm circumference (cm) of children born to iodide-deficient (P) and iodide-treated (I) mothers

Age	Group	N	Triceps	Scapula	Waist	Sum of Skinfolds	Upper Arm Circumference
2 - 6 months	P	17	7.4	5.9	5.8	19.1	13.1
	I	28	6.5	5.1	4.5	16.1	12.6
6 -12 months	P	15	7.9	5.6	5.5	19.0	14.4
	I	15	6.6	4.5	4.4	15.5	13.8
1 - 2 years	P	19	7.8	4.2	4.0	16.0	14.0
	I	21	7.0	3.9	3.4	14.3	14.1
2 - 4 years	P	44	8.3	4.1	3.7	16.1	14.8
	I	23	7.9	3.8	3.8	15.5	14.8
4 - 5 years	P	14	8.0	4.1	3.9	16.0	15.0
	I	21	7.5	3.6	3.8	14.9	15.5

note that post-natal bone maturation continued quite normally until the 12th to 18th month, when there was evidence of some slowing down which resulted in a 12 months' lag with respect to chronological age through the third year and a lag of up to 25 months through the fifth year. However, there was no difference between the iodized and the non-iodized group (Fig. 5). It is possible that this bone retardation is related to weaning and weaning diarrhea, as well as to other significant factors

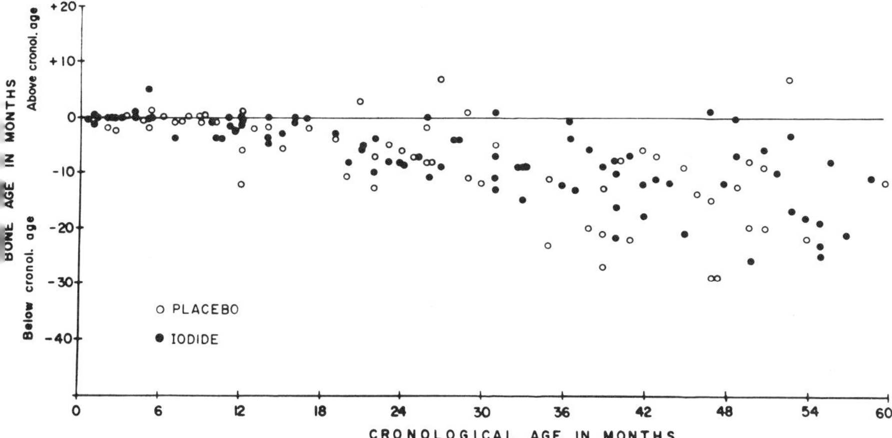

Fig. 5. Bone age maturation as compared to chronological age. A progressive "delay" is apparent beyond the 12th-18th months of age in both groups.

in rural areas of developing countries. The possibility that this bone delay, when coupled with nutritional factors, may be a genetic characteristic of our populations, has not been ruled out. If true, comparison to North American standards would be inappropriate. Our results are consistent with similar findings reported by Baker *et al.* (24) in other non-endemic areas in the highlands of Peru as well as with those reported by Israel *et al.* (25) in children from endemic goiter areas of Ecuador.

The motor and neuropsychological results which we have obtained applying the Gesell tests to about 70 percent of the newborn population from both iodized and placebo groups are shown in Fig. 6. An interesting pattern was observed: both groups appeared to follow the normal curves until approximately 18 months, at which time they began to fall below normal developmental patterns. There were 20 to 30 percent of the subjects who scored below 90 during the first 12 months, but this percentage did not differ between the two groups. Scores were more affected by linguistic defects than by inadequate motor or social skills.

The Stanford Binet and Brúnet-Lezine assessments were carried out in 49 subjects in the placebo group and 43 in the iodized oil group. For the purpose of statistical analysis, however, exclusion has been made of those children born to mothers

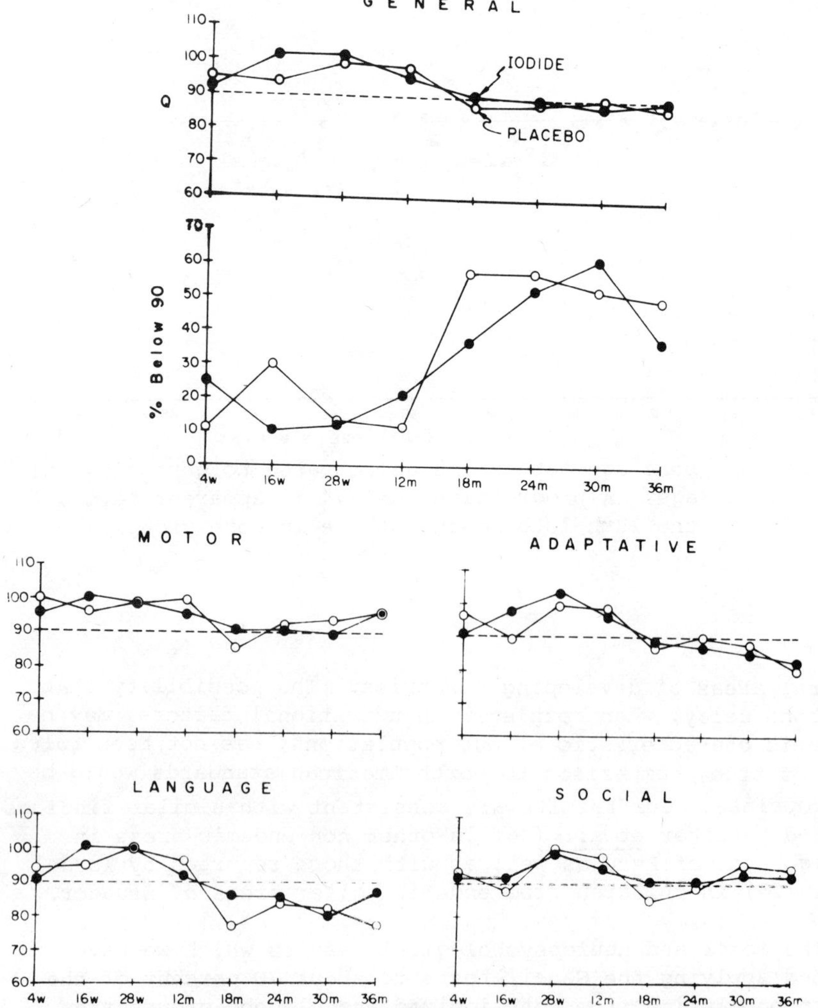

Fig. 6. Developmental quotients assessed by Gesell tests.

injected while already pregnant. Therefore, the results illustrated in Table 4 and Fig. 7 apply only to those children of mothers who received iodized oil or placebo prior to conception. While differences in the mean IQ scores shown in Fig. 7 were not significant between the two groups, there was a tendency for higher results in the iodized group regardless of the age interval. Moreover, Table 4 demonstrates that while only 15 percent of those in the placebo group obtained IQ scores of 90 or over, 26 percent were in the 80-90 "dull" range and 59 percent were in the below normal category. In the iodized group 34 percent demonstrated

Table 4. Percent distribution of iodine-deficient (D) and iodine-supplemented (I) children according to their IQ scores

	AGE, Months						TOTAL	
	3-12		13-24		25-58			
	D(10)	I(8)	D(11)	I(12)	D(25)	I(15)	D(46)	I(35)
Normal	20	50	0	25	20	33	15	34
Dull	30	37	18	17	28	27	26	26
Borderline	40	12	9	25	28	27	26	23
Mental Deficiency	10	0	73	33	24	13	33	17
Language Deficiency	10	0	64	42	72	73	58	46
Hearing Deficiency	0	0	11	0	14	0	11	0

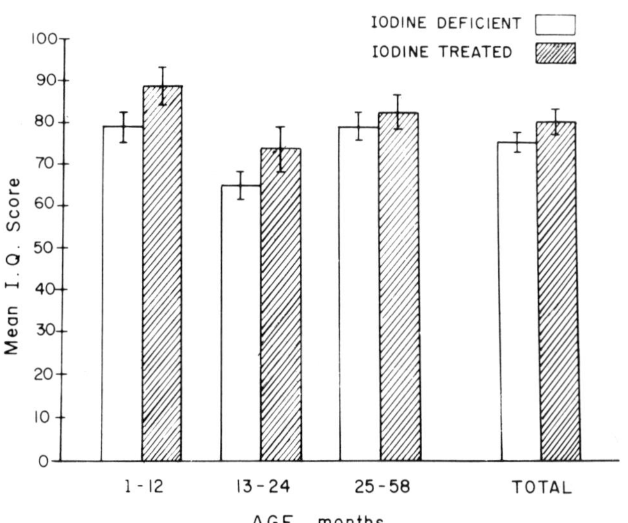

Fig. 7. Comparison of intellectual status in terms of intelligence quotients (IQ) between children born to iodine-deficient and iodine-treated mothers.

an IQ higher than 90 with 26 percent also in the borderline area, but only 40 percent in the below-normal category. Language and hearing deficiency was also more frequent among the placebo children, and 11 percent of these showed some hearing impairment but not deafness.

Electroencephalographic studies were done on a sample of Huasahuasi children. Those children born to mothers injected after conception were excluded from the results, leaving 12 in the iodine-deficient group and nine in the iodized group. All but one EEG showed normal traces. The abnormal one was in the iodine-deficient group and showed disorganized background activity with bursts of theta and delta activity and scattered low waves, which is suggestive of mildly diffuse, disorganized activity. The small number of observations prevented drawing firm conclusions from this study.

The urinary excretion of iodide in a sample of 32 children born to iodine-deficient mothers demonstrated a mean value of 27 μg per 24 hr. In 11 children with an age span of 24 to 57 months born to iodized mothers UEI values ranged from seven in the older children to 107 in the younger ones with a mean value of 42 μg per 24 hr. It would seem from these data, that iodized mothers are capable of supplementing their offspring with adequate amounts of iodide through placental transfer and through lactation after birth for periods of up to 24 months.

Unfortunately, the results of this study still do not permit us to arrive at definite conclusions about the benefit of iodide supplementation on the physical and neuropsychological development of children born to mothers previously injected with iodized oil as compared to children born to iodine-deficient mothers. A comparable delay in development was similarly observed in both groups and was also found to be true in a separate parallel study (26). Although a more critical neuropsychological evaluation showed a tendency for higher IQ mean values in the iodized group, on an individual basis there was no significant relationship between physical growth and intelligence status. This latter observation is consistent with those made in children even more mentally retarded (27). Recent information from New Guinea (28) and Ecuador (29) on the prevention of easily detectable neurological damage amongst children born to iodized mothers is strong evidence in favor of the important role played by iodine deficiency in the pathogenesis of cretinism. However, the drop in the percentage of defectives seen in Ecuador in their control group from the original 10 percent found in the overall population before starting the iodized oil program to only two percent in the population born over a five yr period, while the iodine deficiency remained the same, supports the assumption that this deficiency is not the only cause of cretinism, but rather is a permissive factor. Medical care and possibly an improvement in the socio-economic conditions introduced in this area might have been contributing to these changes. There is also a general consensus as to the underlying role of heredity in the pathogenesis of defects associated with endemic goiter as demonstrated by the variability in the percent of cretinism amongst villagers suffering the same degree of iodine deprivation (30). Heredity possibly accounts for the occurrence of few defectives, since the base-line prevalence of defectives in our series ranges from 1.0 to 3.6 percent, which is significantly lower than the 10 percent observed in Ecuador. It is also possible that, although no obvious cretins have been detected in our series, the IQ difference between iodized and control groups observed in Huasahuasi village, where the prevalence of defectives was the lowest, might become more significant in the other villages where the higher prevalence is possibly due to a genetic trait.

We have examined one patient recently from the iodized group who is now nearly two yr of age, but is unable to walk and is markedly retarded. She demonstrates hypertelorism, her Stanford-Binet score was 71, and her bone age was retarded to five months. She is clearly retarded in comparison with her sibs. We intend to investigate the cause of this retardation. A single case of Down's syndrome has also been observed in the iodized group as well as one well-documented patient with a 21 trisomy in her karyotype in the iodine-deficient group.

Therefore, we must conclude that if one is to judge the actual benefit of iodine supplementation alone as a means of eliminating the development of handicapped children from the world-wide endemic areas, not only must more sophistocated neuropsychological assessments (other than that used to identify cretins), more than one psychological instrument and the electroencephalogram be employed, but also, factors other than iodine deficiency must be taken into consideration. Minor mental handicaps, aside from the gross abnormalities seen in cretinism, must be recognized as well in children protected by iodine prophylactic programs.

SUMMARY

Studies in agrarian villages in highland Peru have been conducted in order to determine the effectiveness of iodized oil prophylaxis against endemic goiter and cretinism. After random injections in the population, observations have been made over a period of five years which have not yet disclosed definite differences between the control children and those born to mothers who received iodized oil prior to conception. Both groups have shown some delay in neuromotor and physical development beginning some time between the 12th and 18th months of life. Thus, our data do not enable us to conclude at present that iodized oil prophylaxis in itself is significantly beneficial in terms of neuropsychological or physical development in our population groups. The existence of a tendency for higher IQ's in the iodized group, however, cannot be ignored and needs further investigation. As both groups were under the same socio-economic and ecological circumstances, other climatic, nutritional, social and economic factors have undoubtedly played a major role which may obscure the effect of iodide administration. The importance of heredity in cretinism and mental defects also cannot be overlooked.

ACKNOWLEDGEMENT

Supported by Fondo Nacional de Salud y Bienestar Social of Peru, Contract No. 51 and U.S. Public Health Service, Grants AM 12748 and AM 10992.

DISCUSSION BY PARTICIPANTS

PRETELL: A study on nutrition in these Andean villages was carried out by the National Institute of Nutrition and showed a low intake of animal protein. Most of these people eat meat perhaps once a week. Caloric supply is about normal.

ERMANS: I think there is some danger in comparing the effects of iodized oil in a population with control patients living in the same area. In a previous study, a survey of goiter prevalence was made in a given village of Idjwi using as controls two groups of untreated subjects, the first one being a group of subjects living in the same village, and the second, subjects living in a neighboring village in which iodine prophylaxis was not introduced. After one year, the non-injected subjects living in the village treated with iodized oil showed a clear-cut regression of goiter size and prevalence. In the neighboring village no change at all occurred. This result seems to be related to recirculation of iodine in the areas in which large amounts of iodine were given. Another interesting point is the observation by a zoologist (S. O.) who is measuring the size of the thyroid glands in rats captured in the goitrous region. These glands were found to be initially enlarged, but after administration of iodized oil to the inhabitants of the village, the size of these glands was definately reduced.

IBBERTSON: I wonder if Dr. Ermans would agree that it is possible to increase body iodine stores without materially influencing the amount of iodine appearing in the urine. I agree that it is difficult to maintain a control population. In the Himalayas all the human excreta goes into a pile of leaves in the bottom of the household and once a year this is carried out in the fields and dumped. The iodine comes back in the crops and the whole population becomes iodized as a result, so that a control population in this sort of setting is useless.

PRETELL: I agree. We have been able to measure the urinary excretion of iodine in the non-treated group to 19 months after the program was started. We also noted, as will be demonstrated, a small drop in the prevalence of goiter in the non-treated population, but the uptake and the urinary excretion of iodine were the same.

REFERENCES

1. Pretell, E.A.; Moncloa, F.; Salinas, R.; Guerra-García, R.; Kawano,A.; Gutierrez, L; Pretell, J. and Wan, M.: Endemic goiter in rural Peru: Effect of iodized oil on prevalence and size of goiter and on thyroid iodine metabolism in known endemic goitrous populations. In: _Endemic Goiter_, Report of the meeting of the PAHO Scientific Group on Research in Endemic Goiter held in Mexico, 1968 (J.B. Stanbury, ed.). Scientific Publication No. 193, Washington 1969. pp. 419-437

2. Pretell, E.A.: The optimal program for prophylaxis of endemic goiter with iodized oil. In this volume.

3. Andersen, H.J.: Nongoitrous hypothyroidism. In: _Endocrine and Genetic Diseases in Childhood_ (L.I. Gardner, ed.). Saunders, Philadelphia, 1969, pp. 216-234

4. Man, E.B.; Mermann, W.M. and Cooke, R.E.: The development of children with congenital hypothyroidism: A note on early temporary replacement therapy for two goitrous infants. _J. Pediat._ 63:926-941, 1963.

5. Van Wyk, J.J.: Hypothyroidism in childhood. _Pediatrics_ 17:427-437, 1956.

6. Fisher, D.A.; Hammond, G.D. and Pickering D.E.: The hypothyroid infant and child. _Amer. J. Dis. Child._ 90:6-21, 1955.

7. Bargman, G.J. and Gardner, L.I.: Otic lesions and congenital hypothyroidism in the developing chick. _J. Clin. Invest._ 46:1828-1839, 1967.

8. Crane, J.T.; Pickering, D.E.; Van Wagenen, G. and Smith, F.S.: Growth and metabolism in normal and thyroid-ablated infant rhesus monkeys (Macaca Mulata). Amer. J. Dis. Child. 87: 708-723, 1954.

9. Lusted, L.B.; Pickering, D.E.; Fisher, D.A. and Smith, F.S.: Growth and metabolism in normal and thyroid-ablated infant rhesus monkeys (Macaca Mulata). Amer. J. Dis. Child. 86: 426-435, 1953.

10. Najjar, S.S.: Hypothyroidism in children from an endemic goiter area. J. Pediat. 64:372-380, 1964.

11. Pretell, E.A.: Role of the placenta and of plasma hormone binding in the pathogenesis of cretinism. In this volume.

12. Nutritional status of populations: A manual on anthropometric appraisal of trends. World Health Organization, Geneva, 1968.

13. Geulich, W.W. and Pyle, S.I.: Radiographic Atlas of Skeletal Development of the Hand and Wrist, Stanford University Press, 1959.

14. Gesell, A. and Amatruda, C.S.: Diagńostico del Desarrollo Normal y Anormal del Niño. Paidos, Buenos Aires, 1967.

15. Terman, L.M. and Merrill, M.A.: Medida de la Inteligencia. Espasa-Calpe, Madrid, 1970.

16. Lézine, I. and Brunet, O.: El Desarrollo psicológico de la Primera Infancia. Troknell, Madrid, 1966.

17. Cáceres-Velásques, A.: Patología del Lenguaje Verbal Expresivo. Doctoral Thesis, Universidad Peruana Cayetano Heredia, Lima, 1971.

18. Sobrevilla, L.A.: Romero, I.; Krueger, F., and Whittembury, J.: Low estrogen excretion during pregnancy at high altitude. Am. J. Obst. & Gynec. 102:828-833, 1968.

19. Mongrut-Muñoz, O.: Los servicios de salud y el desarrollo de la población en el Perú. Acta Herediana, 3:5-16, 1971.

20. Stuart, H.C. and Reed, R.B.: Longitudinal studies of child health and development. Series II. Pediatrics (Suppl.) 24:875-878, 1959.

21. Baertl, J.M.: Morales, E.; Verastegui, G. and Graham, G.: Diet supplementation for entire communities. Growth and mortality of infants and children. Amer. J. Clin. Nutr. 23:707-715, 1970.

22. Frisancho, A.R. and Baker, P.T.: Altitude and growth: A study of the patterns of physical growth of a high altitude Peruvian Quechua population. Am. J. Phys. Anthrop. 32:279-292, 1970.

23. Pretell, E.A.; Wan, M. and Palacios, P.: Fetal thyroid function in endemic goiter. In: Further Advances in Thyroid Research (K. Fellinger and R. Höfer, eds.). Medizinischen Akademie, Vienna, 1971, pp. 45-52

24. Baker, T.S.: Little, A.V. and Frisancho, A.R.: Infant growth in a high altitude population. Am. J. Phys. Anthrop. 2:248-249, 1967.

25. Israel, H.; Fierro-Benítez, R. and Garcés, J.: Skeletal and dental development in the endemic goitre and cretinism areas of Ecuador. J. Trop. Med. Hyg. 72:105-113, 1969.

26. Ramírez, I.; Fierro-Benítez, R.; Estrella, E.; Jaramillo, C.; Díaz, C. and Urresta, J.: Iodized oil in the prevention of endemic goiter and associated defects in the Andean Region of Ecuador. In: Endemic Goiter, Report of the meeting of the PAHO Scientific Group on Research in Endemic Goiter held in Mexico, 1968 (J.B. Stanbury, ed.). Scientific Publication No. 193, Washington,1969, pp. 341-359

27. Pozsonyi,J. and Lobb, H.: Growth in mentally retarded children. J. Pediat. 71:865-868, 1967.

28. Pharoah, P.O.D.; Buttfield, I.H. and Hetzel, B.S.: Neurological damage to the fetus resulting from severe iodine deficiency during pregnancy. Lancet 1:308-310, 1971.

29. Fierro-Benítez, R.; Ramírez, I.; Estrella, E.; Gomez, A.; Hermida, C.; Jaramillo, C.; Urresta, J. and Suarez, J.: Prevencion del cretinismo y otros defectos asociados al bocio endemico mediante aceite yodado. Rev. Ecuat. Med. 8: 99-115, 1970.

30. Hennessy, W.B.: Goitre prophylaxis in New Guinea with intramuscular injection of iodized oil. Med. J. Aust. 1:505-512, 1964.

THE OPTIMAL PROGRAM FOR PROPHYLAXIS OF ENDEMIC GOITER WITH IODIZED OIL

Eduardo A. Pretell

Instituto de Investigaciones de la Altura, (Laboratorio de Endocrinologia), Universidad Peruana Cayetano Heredia Lima, Peru

No one knows what the optimal dosage, size or schedule is for the prevention of endemic goiter with iodized oil. McCullagh first used iodized oil as a prophylactic in endemic goiter in 1957 in New Guinea and published his results in 1963 (1). Hennesey confirmed McCullagh's findings and demonstrated the effectiveness and safety of the method (2). More recent studies have not only supported the usefulness of iodized oil in the prevention of endemic goiter, but have also provided additional information on its fate, effective duration, and influence on goiter size and thyroid function. Thus far, many thousands of subjects in the goitrous areas of New Guinea (3), Peru (4), Zaire (5), Ecuador (6) and Argentina (7) have been treated by this method. In spite of considerable variation in study protocol and variations in dosage of iodine, with respect to age groups, ranging from 95 to 1600 mg, the results have been similar in most respects.

It is the purpose of this paper to review our experimental studies on the fate of iodized oil labeled with ^{131}I in rats, as well as our own five-year follow-up data on the use of intramuscular iodized oil (Ethiodol*) in endemic goitrous subjects, using different doses according to age. The effect of the injection on urinary excretion of iodide (UEI), thyroid function and goiter has been partially published (4,8,9), and the results up to date will be discussed. These observations have permitted us to estimate the duration of effectiveness of a single injection.

*Poppy-seed oil containing 475 mg of iodine per ml, obtained from Laboratories André Guebert (France), marketed by E. Fougera & Co., Inc., Hicksville, N.Y.

The epidemiological and ecological characteristics of the villages in Andean Peru used for the studies, as well as the baseline thyroid function tests and the severity of the iodine deficiency, have been published elsewhere (4,8).

The evaluation of goiter size has been made using the criteria given by Perez et al. (10) as modified at the First Meeting of the PAHO Scientific Group on Research in Endemic Goiter (Caracas, Venezuela, 1963) in which the O_A category refers to the absence of goiter and the O_B degree represents goiter observed only by palpation. Therefore, visible goiter (VG) only refers to Grade I through IV goiters and palpable goiter (PG) refers to all grades of goiter including O_B.

In October 1966 approximately 1700 persons from the villages studied were injected either with placebo or iodized oil. The dose ranged from 0.2 ml to 0.5 ml in infants zero to 12 months of age, 1.0 ml was administered to children below 5 yr and 2.0 ml in subjects from six to 45 yrs. In adults with nodular goiter, 0.2 ml was given to prevent the risk of the Jod-Basedow syndrome. Half the subjects in each village were injected with iodized oil and the other half were given an injection of placebo containing no iodine. Selection was random, although an attempt was made to match age groups and sex in order to achieve optimal criteria for comparing results.

Three years after the initial injection, approximately 60 percent of the same subjects were reinjected and a new group of subjects was injected for the first time. The doses used in the second injection program were 0.2 ml from 0 to 6 months of age, 0.3 ml from 6 to 12 months, 0.5 ml from 12 months to 6 yr and 1.0 ml from 6 to 45 years, according to the recommendations of the "Technical Group Meeting on Use of Iodized Oil in the Prevention of Endemic Goiter and Cretinism: (Third Meeting of PAHO Scientific Group on Research in Endemic Goiter, Puebla, Mexico, 1968). The dose of 0.2 ml for adults with nodular goiter was kept the same.

ABSORPTION, METABOLISM AND EXCRETION OF INTRAMUSCULAR INJECTED IODIZED OIL

Although the intramuscular injection of iodized oil has proven to be an effective and safe means to prevent and treat endemic goiter, little is known about its absorption from the muscle and its subsequent metabolism in the body.

It has been assumed that iodized oil once injected into the muscle may act as a reservoir from which a slow absorption may occur. However, tissues other than the thyroid, such as adipose tissue and the reticuloendothelial system, may also act as a reservoir. It is also possible that lipoprotein complexes are formed from which a rapid liberation of iodine occurs during the first three to six months, followed by a subsequent slow release over a period of years which causes a more prolonged effect on the thyroid. Buttfield, et al. published results obtained in New Guinea four and a half years after iodine injection which seem to suggest this possibility (11). In order to obtain more information concerning this aspect, biochemical studies on the bonding of iodine to oil and its subsequent degradation were studied in vitro. Iodized oil (Ethiodol) was previously labeled in our laboratory with ^{131}I (12). Chromatography disclosed that 99.3 percent of the label was bound to the oil with no change over a period of two months of observation. Ethiodol-^{131}I incubated with human serum in a dilution of 1/100 at 37°C was partially and progressively deiodinated as shown by the paper chromatographic analysis. The free iodide, which was only 0.7 percent before incubation increased to 2.9 percent at five minutes and 13.2 percent at 15 hr after incubation. At the same time the percent of radioactivity remaining at the origin of the chromatogram increased from 2.5 to 6.7 between the five minutes and 15 hours of incubation, which suggests that some binding of the label to the serum proteins or lipoproteins may have taken place (9).

During this preliminary study it was also demonstrated that iodized oil can be readily extracted from the serum or eluted from the chromatogram with ethanol or butanol. This observation should be taken into consideration when evaluating follow-up studies with BEI measurement after iodized oil administration.

The absorption and metabolism of Ethiodol-^{131}I was also studied in rats which were kept in metabolic cages for up to 23 days (9). During this time urine and feces were collected, and the rats were sacrificed at different times for measurement of the radioactive iodine in various tissues. In groups of rats kept up to 23 days, 87 percent of the radioactive iodine was retained at the site of injection, 8 percent appeared in the urine and feces and 0.2 percent was concentrated by the thyroid, the tissue accumulating the greatest quantity of radioactive iodine (Table 1).

The daily urinary excretion of ^{131}I was significantly higher during the first two days following injection and was mainly present as free iodide. We were only able to account for 95 percent of the administered radioactivity and thus there was some suspicion that other tissues might also be accumulating the iodized oil. The next most abundant site of deposition of the radiolabeled iodized oil or ^{131}I was adipose tissue (Fig. 1). The low radioactivity in the tissues, however, precluded further investigation of the chemical form in which the ^{131}I was accumulated by the tissues.

Table I. Fate of injected Ethiodol-^{131}I in rats 23 days after intramuscular administration

	Percent Dose				
N^{o}	Site of injection	Urine + Feces	Thyroid	Recovery	Other Tissues
5	86.6 ± 2.2*	8.4 ± 2.0	0.19 ± 0.018	95.1 ± 1.8	4.9

*Mean ± SE

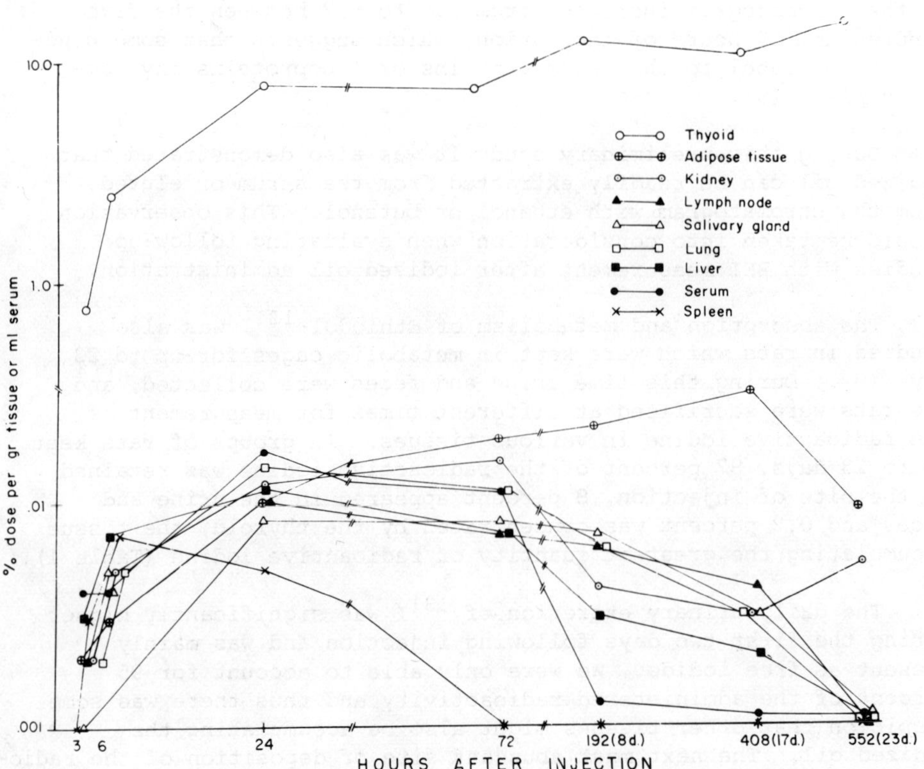

Fig. 1. Tissue accumulation of radioiodine following administration of Ethiodol-^{131}I. Each point represents the mean value from 4-5 rats.

Additional evidence of the slow absorption of the iodized oil from the intramuscular depot was given by X-ray study (Fig. 2) of a patient who had been given 1.0 ml of Ethiodol six months earlier. The opacification from the Ethiodol at the injection site is clearly observed, in contrast to Buttfield's observation of rapid absorption of the oil (3), but in accordance with more recent studies by Malamos _et al._ (13). This particular patient had nodular goiter and developed severe hyperthyroidism three months after the injection of the iodized oil. She was hospitalized for a full metabolic study which will be fully reported elsewhere (14). A large amount of non-organic iodide was accumulated by the thyroid, as was demonstrated when the patient was given KSCN (1 gr three times a day for five days) and there was a sharp increase in $UE^{127}I$ from 120 μgr/24 hr to 383 μgr and 908 μgr at the first and fifth day after KSCN was started. At

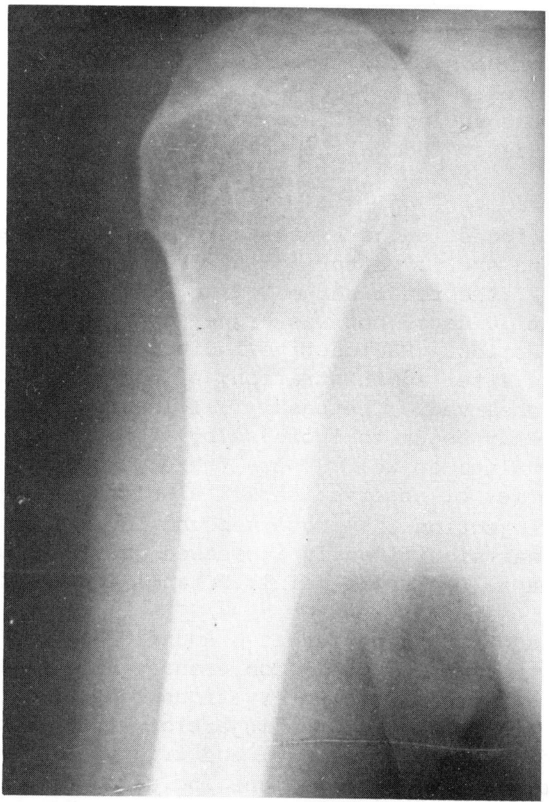

Fig. 2. X-ray from the right arm of a 45 yr old woman injected with 1.0 ml Ethiodol six months previously. Notice the opacification of the iodized oil in the upper third of the arm.

the same time the NBE^{131}I increased from .026 percent dose per liter to .084 percent dose per liter and the BII increased from 3.3 μgr per 100 ml to 4.8 μgr per 100 ml to 4.8 μgr per 100 ml at the fifth day. These results are consistent with a large accumulation of iodide in the thyroid and with results obtained by Japanese workers in subjects receiving high intakes of iodine (15).

EARLY OBSERVATIONS ON THYROID FUNCTION, SERUM COMPOUNDS AND URINARY LOSSES OF IODIDE AFTER INJECTION OF IODIDE OIL

Studies have been done on six iodine deficient subjects between 16 and 18 yr of age who received 1.0 ml of Ethiodol. Baseline studies were done before injection. Thyroid radio-iodine uptake was measured at 72 hr, 30 days, and 6 months; blood samples were taken at 48 hours, 7 and 30 days, and at 6 months for iodinated compound assays; and urine was collected daily during the first 30 days and on alternate days thereafter for urinary ^{127}I analysis. The methods used in these studies have been described elsewhere (4,8). The butanol insoluble iodine (BII), and the cholesterol and triglycerides in serum were determined in the Boston Medical Laboratory through the courtesy of Dr. J. Benotti.

The effect of injection of a huge amount of iodine as Ethiodol on the thyroid gland shortly after administration was evaluated. As shown in Table 2, the total serum iodine (TI) rose as high as 57 μg per 100 ml at 30 days, but was higher than normal within 48 hours after injection. Radioactive iodine uptake was rapidly blocked at 72 hours after administration; a drop from 73 percent to 26 percent was observed. The basal T_4-I levels were 2.3 μg per 100 ml and had already begun to increase by 48 hours along with increased free T_4 values as well. Thus, there was no evidence in this particular series of observations of a Wolff-Chaikoff effect. By 48 hours after injection the protein-bound iodine concentration of the serum was significantly increased and reached its peak at about 30 days. This was mainly butanol insoluble iodine.

These results, first reported at a Round Table on Endemic Goiter (Fifth International Thyroid Conference, Rome, Italy, June, 1970), are consistent with observations recently published by Malamos *et al.* (13). Whether the injection of Ethiodol contributed to the rise in cholesterol and triglycerides needs further investigation. The observations included in Table 2 were found in one patient.

Table 2. Thyroid radioiodine uptake and serum levels of thyroid hormones and other iodinated compounds, cholesterol and triglycerides after iodized oil injection

	Thyroid uptake %dose/24h	TI μg%	PBI μg%	BII μg%	T_4-I μg%	Free T_4 μg%	Choles-terol mg%	Triglycer-ides mg%
Basal	73 ± 6*	4.7 ± 0.4	4.6 ± 0.5	-	3.2 ± 0.2	0.91 ± .07	-	-
48 hr	-	11.1 ± 2.2	10.2 ± 2.1	3.9	4.3 ± 0.3	1.40 ± .09	136	100
72 hr	26 ± 7	-	-	-	-	-	140	110
7 days		41.2 ± 4.2	27.2 ± 3.8	23.6	6.2 ± 0.4	1.82 ± .25	-	-
30 days	15 ± 3	57.1 ± 4.9	50.1 ± 3.8	33.1	7.0 ± 0.4	2.16 ± .21	-	-
6 months	11 ± 1	13.7 ± 1.0	10.5	4.0	5.5 ± 0.3	1.86 ± .10	152	127

*Mean ± SE

De-iodination appears to take place in the muscles and probably in the blood stream as well, as we have demonstrated in in vitro studies. Thus, inorganic iodine is readily available to the thyroid, but is also actively cleared by the kidney, as shown in Fig. 3. After administration of iodized oil there was a rapid

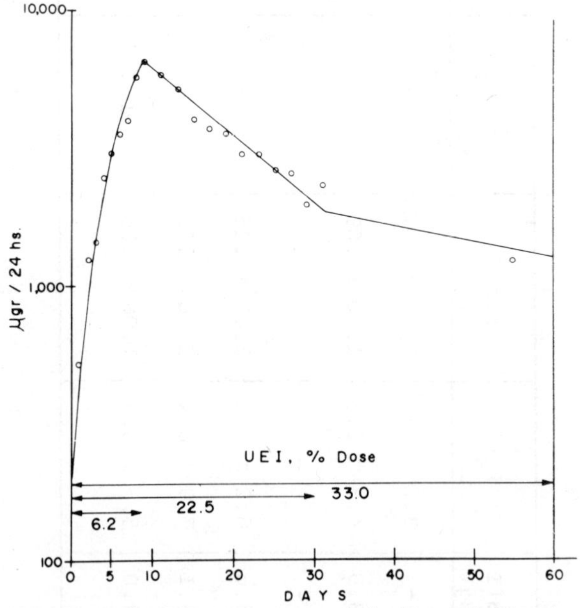

Fig. 3. Early urinary losses of iodine following the injection of 1.0 ml (475 mg I) of iodized oil.

increase in urinary excretion of stable iodine from control values of 40 µg to almost 10 mg per 24 hr. Urinary excretion of iodine accounted for approximately 22 percent and 33 percent of the administered iodine during the first 30 days and after 60 days respectively. These findings indicate that a significant amount of the injected iodine of the Ethiodol is lost in the urine during the early weeks after administration and that the long-term effect is due only to a residual fraction which is stored. A similar observation became evident during metabolic studies in rats.

Column chromatographic analysis (Bio. Rad. AG 50 W-X2, 100-200 mesh, cation exchange resin, H^+ form)* of the chemical nature of the iodine appearing in the urine indicated that during the early stages following injection, the iodine present was predominantly inorganic. This finding has also been demonstrated in the urine of rats given

*Part of the analysis were done at the Boston Medical Lab., Boston, Mass.

^{131}I labeled iodized oil (Table 3) and is in accord with data reported by Delange et al. (5).

Table 3. Chromatographic analysis of urinary iodide after iodized oil injection

COLUMN CHROMATROGRAPHY OF URINARY ^{127}I

Time	Inorganic Iodide	Organic Iodide
48 hr	0.22 (61%) µg/ml	0.14 µg/ml
7 days	4.60 (81%)	1.10
30 days	1.20 (71%)	0.48
60 days	0.56 (67%)	0.28
6 mo	0.43 (81%)	0.12

PAPER CHROMATOGRAPHY OF URINARY ^{131}I

Percent Distribution of Radioactivity

Time	Origin	Free-I	I-Tyrosines ?	I-Thyronines ?
24 hr	1.8	89.6	3.6	4.5
8 days	3.6	72.3	10.3	13.6

LONG-TERM FOLLOW UP STUDIES ON THE EFFECT OF IODIZED OIL

The UEI followed a multiple exponential decline, falling sharply at the early stages after injection, but more slowly toward the end of the study. A preliminary report from our laboratory indicated that administration of larger doses of Ethiodol would most likely result in a greater loss into the urine without there necessarily being a longer retention time in the body (4). This factor was also observed by Delange et al. (5). The different doses used in our program, according to age groups have enabled us to better document this observation. The results are shown in Fig. 4. Two age groups

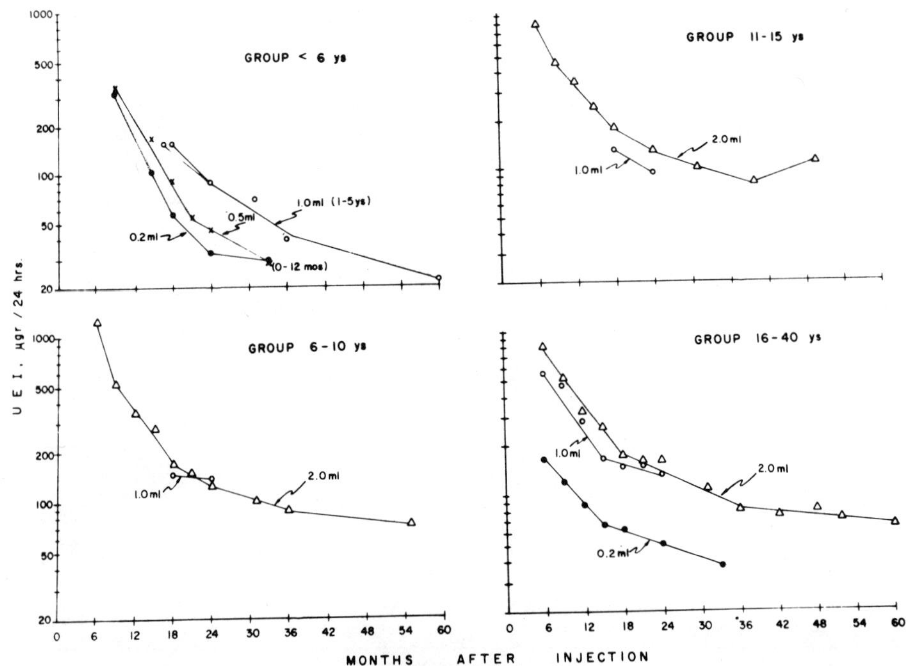

Fig. 4. Mean urinary excretion of iodide values in various age groups following the injection of different doses of iodized oil.

of subjects were studied, one less than 4 yr of age, and the other more than 16 yr of age. Both groups received 0.2 ml of Ethiodol (95 mg of iodine). The younger group excreted more iodine. A similar observation was made in another group between 6 and 10 years of age as compared to an older group of more than 16 years, who received 2.0 ml of Ethiodol (950 mg of iodine). Again, the early urinary excretion of iodine was significantly higher in the younger group than in the older one; however, after 12 months similar observations were made in both groups. When two different doses were compared within the same age group, the larger dose resulted in higher urinary excretion during the early days after administration. Therefore, no significant differences in the $UE^{127}I$ 12 to 18 months after injection were observed after administration of either 0.2 ml or 0.5 ml in children 1-12 months of age or 1.0 ml and 2.0 ml in age groups 6-10 years, 11-15 years and 16-49 years.

Longitudinal studies of the serum thyroid hormones and the thyroid radioiodine uptake are shown in Fig. 5, which clearly illustrates the prolonged effect of a single injection in maintaining normal thyroid function for as long as three and possibly four years in subjects injected with 2.0 ml. Similar observations were made in those given 1.0 ml dose. When 0.2 ml was used the T_4 level approached basal values by the 18th to 24th months and the thyroid uptake was above normal, although by the 38th month this value was still below basal values. A high plasma inorganic iodine (PII) at 13th-19th months, with low thyroid iodine clearance resulting in normal absolute iodine uptake (AIU) has been reported previously (4). Malamos et al. reported (14) higher AIU values, but those were measured at an earlier period after injection.

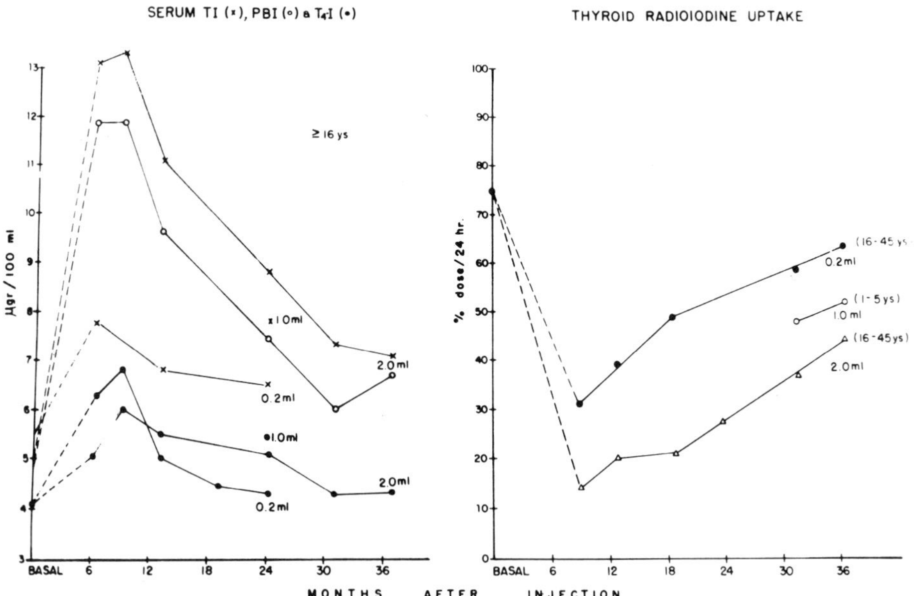

Fig. 5. The changing pattern of thyroid function after iodized oil administration. The dose and age group are indicated in the graph.

The effect of the reduction of goiter rate in the iodized group injected in 1966 is shown in Fig. 6. The 0-5 group is graphed separately from the other age groups since its basal goiter prevalence was significantly different and the size of doses used were smaller. Maximum effect was practically achieved by the 18th-24th month. The VG rate fell 80 percent in the groups of subjects older than six years and 78 percent in children below five years during the 38 months of observation. The PG rate decreased to a lesser extent because goiter of the O_B degree did not disappear in all of them. At 32 months (Fig. 7), 86 percent of the subjects had shown a "positive" response to the injection. Within this group 61 percent of the subjects had shown a complete disappearance of goiter and 26 percent showed a partial shrinkage in size of goiter. While in the former group most of the goiters were of the diffuse type and O_B and I degree, in the latter group the percent of nodular goiters and goiters of large size had been more prominent. There were

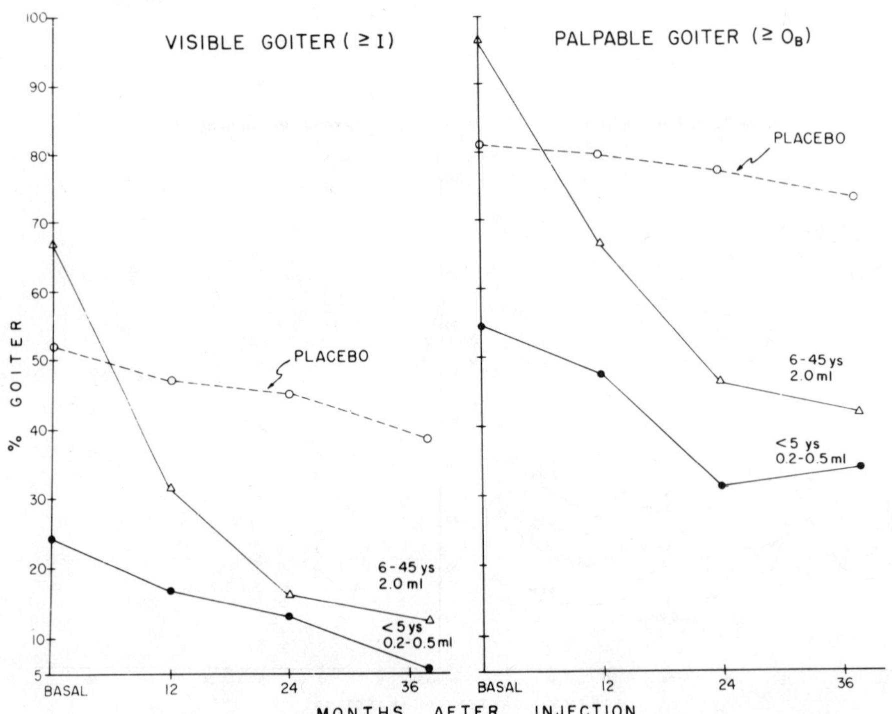

Fig. 6. Effect of iodized oil on the prevalence of goiter. The group of children below 5 yr has been plotted separately and those adults with large nodular goiters injected with 0.2 ml have been excluded from the remainder of the adults injected because of the reduced duration of effect of iodized oil treatment.

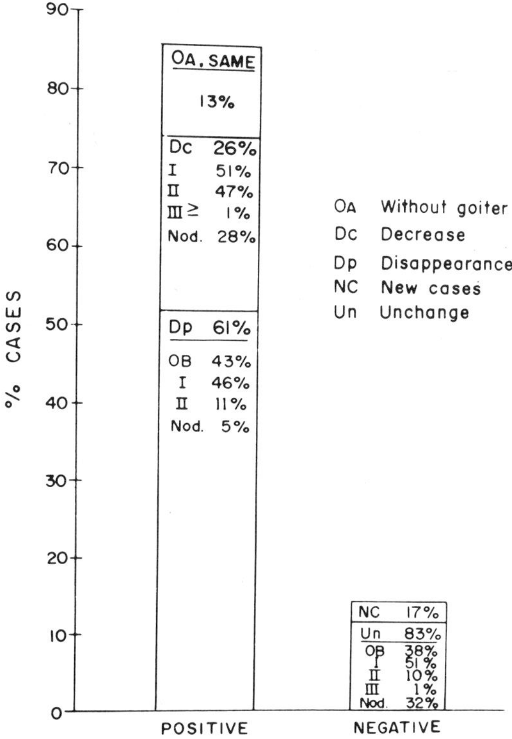

Fig. 7. Glandular response to iodized oil. This evaluation has been made on an individual basis comparing the size of goiter at the 32nd month as to the reduction in the size observed through the 24th month follow-up.

subjects accounting for about 14 percent of the total injected group, who showed no change at all in goiter, with an actual slight increase or even appearance of goiter in some cases (9). This observation may be due partially to ascertainment, while goiters may have become more evident because of the disappearance of soft hyperplastic tissue which enabled nodules previously undetected to become apparent. Nevertheless, it is somewhat disturbing that there is a residual group of patients who appear not to respond to iodide. This suggests the possibility of an auxiliary goitrogenic factor. Gaitan in Cali, Colombia, has demonstrated a geographic clustering of patients who appear not to respond to iodide administration and who were concentrated in an area which received its water from a particular well which he demonstrated contained a possible goitrogenic factor (16). Thyroid function tests and UEI were not different in the subjects with "negative" responses when compared to those who responded favorably to the treatment. It is worth noting that over the period of observation there was a slight drop in the prevalence of goiter in the placebo group. This may have been related to an aging factor (8) or to possible contamination of the ground with urinary iodine. This phenomenon has been observed by others (5) when a placebo group was maintained in the same area with the iodized group, but not observed in Ecuador, where the groups were in two separate villages (6).

RELATIONSHIP BETWEEN DOSE OF IODIZED OIL AND EFFECTIVE DURATION

Our data enabled us to make an estimate of the maximal duration of a given dose of iodized oil necessary to maintain a minimal urinary excretion of 50 μg per 24 hr above basal values (Table 4).

Table 4. Relationship between dose of Ethiodol and effective duration to maintain a UEI of 50 μg per 24 hr above basal values

Age Group	Dose ml	Predicted months [Ref. (8)]	Actual Months
	0.2	13.0	17.0
< 5 years	0.5	19.5	19.5
	1.0	24.0	28.0
	0.2	13.0	14.5
>16 years	1.0	24.0	?
	2.0	29.0	42.0

Calculations indicate that 2.0 ml to an adult patient should fulfill these criteria for approximately 42-48 months, while 0.2 ml should last approximately 15 months. Although our follow-up studies with a dose of 1.0 ml in this group are still too recent to draw conclusions, the present trend of the UEI curve leads us to assume that a similar result will be observed as that with a 2.0 ml dose. In infants 0-12 months of age there seems to be no wide difference between doses ranging from 0.2 to 0.5 ml. The effective duration time is 17 to 20 months. In children 1-5 years of age, a 1.0 ml dose lasts approximately 28 months.

In the age groups 6-10 years and 11-15 years, both 1.0 ml and 2.0 ml doses do not appear to last longer than in the adult group, probably because of the higher early waste of iodine in the urine. The actual values closely agree in most instances with the predicted values obtained from the empirical formula which was derived from our first observations (8).

The first indication of insufficient iodine is a decrease in urinary excretion of iodine below normal values. Although an inverse correlation exists between the quantity of UEI and the radioactive iodine uptake, as was demonstrated by Stanbury _et al._ (17), it is only later when the UEI has approached values below 50 µg per 24 hr above basal values (Fig. 4) that the radioiodine uptake returns to values above normal (Fig. 5). The difference, however, does not seem to be greater than six months. Thus, uptake over 50 percent in the adult group occurs by the 20th month for 0.2 ml dose and between 42-46 months for 2.0 ml dose. Serum thyroxine level trends (Fig. 5) are also consistent with the above calculations. A second increase of the palpable goiter rate in children below five is observed after the 24th month and this may occur after 42-46 months in the other groups. Therefore, it seems reasonable to conclude from these data that the optimal dosage should be 0.5 ml of Ethiodol for infants 0-12 months of age every two yr, 1.0 in children 1-10 yr every 30 months, and in subjects 11-48 yr 1.0 ml every 36 months or 2.0 ml every 48 months, with restriction of administration to those persons older than 45 yr or those adult subjects with nodular goiter who are more likely to suffer the side effect of thyrotoxicosis. However, we conclude that an exception should be made in the case of women of childbearing age with nodular goiter, since protection of the newborn against iodine deficiency is a prime objective.

SIDE EFFECTS

Side effects were negligible in our series. Local temporary painful induration was seen occasionally and there has been a single case among 2025 subjects treated of well-documented hyperthyroidism which developed three months after injection. In Ecuador, Fierro also reported three cases of Jod-Basedow in a series similar to ours (6). However, Watanabe _et al._ (7) in Argentina have two cases among 95 subjects injected. In any case, the occurrence of Jod-Basedow has only been demonstrated in adults with large nodular goiters. The epidemic thyrotoxicosis seen in Tasmania following iodization of bread (19) is definitely more significant than the one observed after iodized oil. The fact that most of the Tasmanian subjects were 50 yr or older, while in our series none was injected beyond 45 years of age, could be an explanation for this difference.

We do not believe, as stated before (4), that reducing the dose of iodized oil to 0.2 ml in aged subjects with large nodular goiter will prevent the risk of Jod-Basedow in those who are susceptible, since PII necessarily rises above normal even with this dose. The only absolutely safe measure would seem to be to avoid injection in adults beyond 45 years and in those with large nodular goiter. However, in view of the actual occurrence of thyrotoxicosis we feel that this absolute measure should not always be applied, particularly in the women of childbearing age as discussed before.

Lack of congenital goiter in children born in iodized oil treated women indicates the safety of the method in pregnant women.

SUMMARY

This paper presents the optimal scheme for iodized oil injection as a means of prevention and treatment of endemic goiter. The fate of the iodine after injection, its binding, absorption, metabolism, and excretion were studied with the aim of determining which dosage provides maximum protection for the longest period of time in the various age groups with a minimum of initial wastage and a reduction in side effects.

Available data suggest that over a wide dose range differences in duration and effectiveness may be trivial, since a larger dose is rapidly degraded initially both in the muscle sites and in the plasma, but more slowly thereafter in order to supply the long-term needs of the subject.

Exhaustion of stores after iodized oil administration is indicated initially by a fall below normal values in the daily urinary excretion of iodide and only later by other evidence of iodide deficiency, such as a rising radioiodine uptake.

Iodized oil is effective in reducing goiter size and incidence, but even many months after administration there is still a residual group of subjects who have goiter and a few who have developed enlarged thyroids in spite of administration of iodized oil. The reason for this last occurrence is not clear.

It seems reasonable to conclude that a safe schedule for reinjection would be 20-24 months in infants injected with 0.2 to 0.5 ml Ethiodol and in adults given 0.2 ml and 30 months in children injected with 1.0 ml. In the subjects injected either with 1.0 or 2.0 ml dose the reinjection should take place after 36 or 48 respectively.

DISCUSSION BY PARTICIPANTS

QUERIDO: I remember Dr. Pharoah's saying Saturday morning that he thought at this moment iodized oil could last ten years. I just wonder what made him say so.

PHAROAH: Blood samples have been drawn from pregnant women approximately four to five years after an iodized oil injection and serum T_4 analysis performed. Many of these women, since receiving the iodized oil, have had one infant and were again pregnant and, therefore, their iodine demands may be considered to be greater than that of the rest of the population. Yet the serum T_4 in this group compared to the control saline group showed considerably higher values. Hence my claim that a 4 ml iodized oil injection is effective for at least five years and may even be sufficient for 10 years.

DELANGE: I would like to comment on Pretell's paper. From our experience in Zaire, we completely agree on all the points he mentioned. An important one is that after a long time there is no difference in thyroid function according to the initial dose of iodized oil given. This result seems to confirm that the dosage proposed by the Pan American Health Organization in 1968 is valid. Dr. Thilly has also collected information concerning the point which Dr. Pharoah has pointed out. Dr. Thilly has followed during five years a population of Idjwi injected with the same doses of iodized oil that Dr. Pretell just mentioned. The results of that study are summarized on Fig. A. The prevalence of goiter, which was 47 percent before the treatment, decreased sharply after one year, remained the same two years and a half later, and began to be slightly increased again at five years. The same evolution is observed for the thyroidal uptake. With regard to the thyroidal exchangeable iodine pool the values were extremely low before the treatment, near normal after one year of treatment, and then began to decrease. The trend for serum thyroxine is similar to that observed by Pretell: the normal level observed one year after the treatment did not undergo any significant modifications during the following four years of observation.

In spite of this normal thyroxine level, we suggest that one must consider a reinjection after five years. The slight increase in goiter prevalence and uptake and the reduction in exchangeable iodine reserves support this point of view.

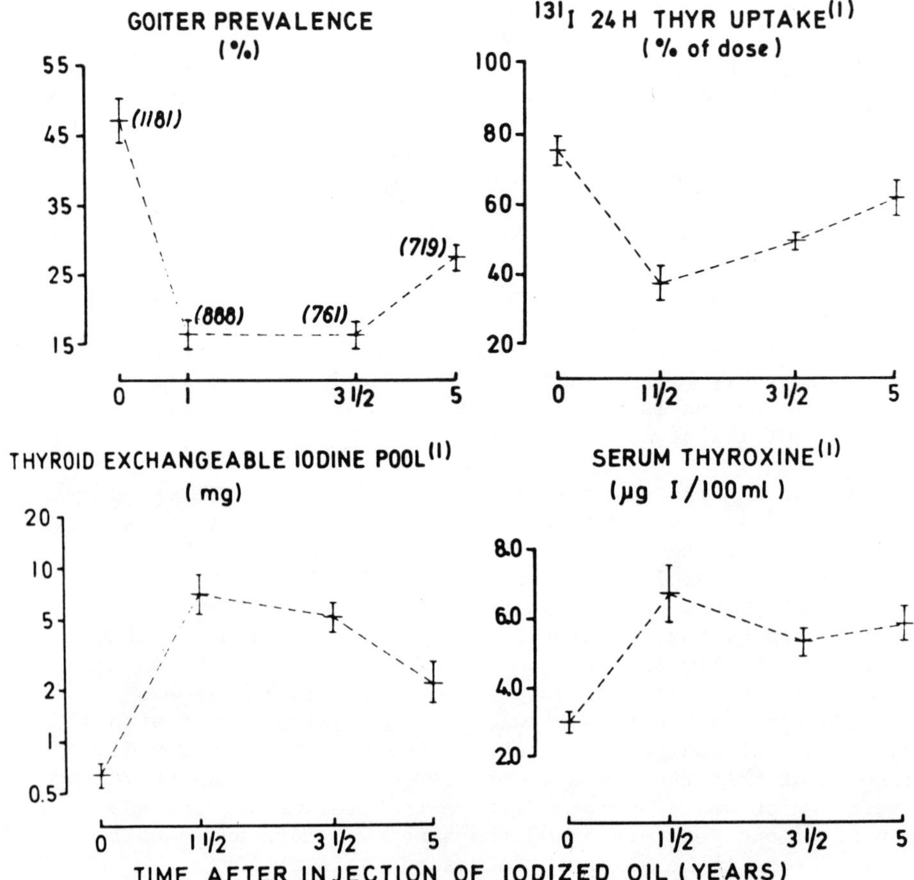

Fig. A. Comparison of goiter prevalence and various parameters of thyroid function in untreated subjects and in groups of patients treated by iodized oil at various intervals of time before the determinations [Results presented as mean ± SEM, number of subjects under brackets]. (1) Number of subjects for time 0, 1 1/2, 3 1/2, and 5 are respectively 14, 7, 16, 10.

KOENIG: I was amazed at this 20 percent goiter not disappearing. I have reported that we have 23 percent goiter in our medical students. I gave this figure to J. Crooks of Dundee, who said that this is approximately the figure he gets in Iceland, in a population which has a very high iodine input. I gather from all this that this 20 percent is the "physiological" incidence of goiter.

STANBURY: I don't think we can let that figure of 20 percent go as the minimum physiological level. Matovinovic has been examining near Ann Arbor, in Appalachia, Savannah, Georgia, and in Texas recently. His figures have been running around four or five percent in Savannah and as high as about 12 percent in Tecumseh, Michigan. But even these are small goiters, just above the level of detectability. I think the minimal value that one can obtain is pretty small - not 20 percent.

PARIS: Dr. Pretell, did you observe a high incidence of goiter in the children born to mothers treated with iodized oil, that is, large goiters like those reported in offspring of asthmatic women given iodides during gestation?

PRETELL: In the early data we published on this, we made the point that no goiter had been seen. We have been careful in looking for such defects. One might expect it because of the high concentration of inorganic iodine.

DELANGE: Does this population eat lima beans? I ask because lima beans contain large quantities of cyanogenic glucosides which could act as a goitrogen. This could perhaps contribute to the severity of the goiter endemic and also the remaining prevalence of goiter despite adequate iodine prophylaxis.

PRETELL: They eat them occasionally. Mostly they eat corn and potatoes. We are going to try to do some genetic studies in this group in an attempt to identify other factors.

DEGROOT: The effect of iodine in causing fetal goiter probably involves administration of a few hundred ml potassium iodide per day. Even though you have given massive amounts of iodinated oil the free iodine available is reduced to a reasonable level after 10-15 days. Perhaps that is why they do not get fetal goiter.

PRETELL: Besides that, we have demonstrated by column and paper chromatography that a large part of the iodine is organic during the first period after injection.

COSTA: Does any iodine remain encysted in the muscle?

PRETELL: No.

PITTMAN: Not all the iodine that appears in urine is necessarily iodide. Dr. George Dailey studied twelve patients in Birmingham that had myelograms. One seemed to get a better estimate of iodide using salivary instead of urinary iodine.

ACKNOWLEDGEMENT

Supported by Fondo National de Salud y Bienestar Social of Peru, Contract No. 51, U.S. Public Health Service Grants AM 12748 and AM 10992, and Pan American Health Organization (HP-A-Peru-4201).

The author wishes to thank Dr. John B. Stanbury for his encouragement and continued support in this study. We also wish to acknowledge our co-workers Dr. F. Moncloa and Dr. R. Guerra-García from Instituto de Investigaciones de la Altura and Dr. R. Salinas from Instituto Nacional de Nutricion, for their contribution to this study, as well as to Dr. P. Palacios, Dr. L. Tello, Dr. T. Torres, Dr. A. Kawano, Dr. L. Gutierrez, Dr. L. Beteta and Dr. V. Zenteno for their participation in the field work, to Dr. Benotti for the laboratory analysis and to Miss M. Wan for her technical assistance.

REFERENCES

1. McCullagh, S.F.: The Huon Peninsula endemic: I. The effectiveness of an intramuscular depot of iodized oil in the control of endemic goiter. Med. J. Aust. 1:769-777, 1963.

2. Hennessy, W.B.: Goitre prophylaxis in New Guinea with intramuscular injections of iodized oil. Med. J. Aust. 1:505-512, 1964.

3. Buttfield, I.H. and Hetzel, B.S.: Endemic goiter in New Guinea and the prophylactic program with iodinated poppyseed oil. In: Endemic Goiter. Report of the meeting of the PAHO Scientific Group on Research in Endemic Goiter held in Mexico, 1968 (J.B. Stanbury, ed.). Scientific Publication 193, Washington, 1969. pp. 132-145.

4. Pretell, E.A.; Moncloa, F.; Salinas, R.; Kawano, A.; Guerra-García, R.; Guiterrez, L; Beteta, L.; Pretell, Jr. and Wan, M.: Prophylaxis and treatment of endemic goiter in Peru with iodized oil. J. Clin. Endocrinol. Metab. 29:1586-1949, 1969.

5. Delange,F.; Thilly, C.; Pourbaix, P. and Ermans, A.M.: Treatment of Idjwi Island endemic goiter by iodized oil. In: Endemic Goiter. Report of the meeting of the PAHO Scientific Group on Research in Endemic Goiter held in Mexico, 1968 (J.B. Stanbury, ed.). Scientific Publication 193, Washington, 1969. pp. 118-131.

6. Fierro-Benítez, R.; Ramírez, I.; Estrella, E.; Jaramillo, C.; Díaz, C. and Urresta, J.: Iodized oil in the prevention of endemic goiter and associated defects in the Andean region of Ecuador. In: Endemic Goiter. Report of the meeting of the PAHO Scientific Group on Research in Endemic Goiter held in Mexico, 1968 (J.B.Stanbury, ed.). Scientific Publication 193, Washington, 1969. pp. 306-321.

7. Watanabe, T.; Degrossi, O.J.; Santillan, C.; El Tamer, E.; Sotorres, A.; Altschuler, N. and Forcher, H.: Profilaxis del bocio endemíco utilizando aceite yodado. Rev. Argent. Endocrinol. Metab. 17:83-89, 1971.

8. Pretell, E.A.; Moncloa, F.; Salinas, R.; Guerra-García, R.; Kwano, A.; Guiterrez, L; Pretell, J. and Wan, M.: Endemic goiter in rural Peru: Effect of iodized oil on prevalence and size of goiter and on thyroid iodine metabolism in known endemic goitrous populations. In: Endemic Goiter. Report of the meeting of the PAHO Scientific Group on Research in Endemic Goiter held in Mexico, 1968 (J.B.Stanbury, ed.). Scientific Publication 193, Washington, 1969. pp. 419-437.

9. Pretell, E.A.: El uso del aceite yodado en el tratamiento y profilaxis del bocio endemíco. Respuesta glandular y aspectos del metabolismo del yodo. In: Simposios, Second Bolivarian Congress of Endocrinology (R. Calderon,; E. Kesseru and F. Moncloa, eds.). Litografica del Peru S.A., Lima 1970, pp. 60-68.

10. Perez, C.; Scrimshaw, N.S. and Munõz, J.A.: Technique of endemic goitre surveys. In: Endemic Goitre. Geneva, WHO, 1960. pp.369-384.

11. Buttfield, I.H. and Hetzel, B.S.: Endemic goiter in Eastern New Guinea with special reference to the use of iodized oil in prophylaxis and treatment. Bull. W.H.O., 36:243-262, 1967.

12. Albani, H. and Mitta, A.E.A.: Preparacíon de Lipiodol UF-I. Comisión Nacional de Energia Atomica. Buenos Aires, 1968.

13. Malmos, B.; Koutras, D.A.; Mantos, J.; Chiotak, L; Sfontouris, J.; Papadopoulos, S.N.; Rigopoulos, G.A.; Pharmakiotis, A.D. and Vlassis, G.: Endemic goiter in Greece: Effects of iodized oil injection. Metabolism 19:569-580, 1970.

14. Pretell, E.A.; Tello, L; Salem, L.E. and Wan, M.: Sindrome de Jod-Basedow: Estudios cinéticos del metabolismo del yodo. Abstract. IV Peruvian Congress of Endocrinology, Trujillo, Peru, April 29-May 2, 1971. p. 29.

15. Nagatki, S.; Shizume, K. and Nakao, K.: Thyroid function in chronic excess iodide ingestion: Comparison of thyroid AIU and degradation of thyroxine in euthyroid Japanese subjects. J. Clin. Endocrinol. Metab. 27:638-647, 1967.

16. Gaitan, E.; Wahner, H.W.; Correa, P.; Bernal, R.; Jubiz, W.; Gaitan, J.E. and Llanos, G.: Endemic goiter in the Cauca Valley: I. Results and limitations of twelve years of iodine prophylaxis. J. Clin. Endocrinol. Metab. 28:1730-1740, 1968.

17. Stanbury, J.B.; Brownell, G.L.; Riggs, D.S.; Perinetti, H.; Itoiz, J. and Del Castillo, E.B. Endemic Goiter, the adaptation of man to iodine deficiency. Harvard University Press, Cambridge, 1954.

18. Stewart, J.C.; Vidor, G.I.; Buttfield, I.H. and Hetzel, B.S.: Epidemic thyrotoxicosis in northern Tasmania: Studies of clinical features and iodine nutrition. Aust. N.Z.J. Med. 3:203-211, 1971.

SECTION 4
CRETINISM AND HEARING

EMBRYOGENESIS OF THE EAR AND ITS CENTRAL PROJECTION

A. Costa

Mauriziano Hospital

Turin, Italy

The induction of the ear begins as a part of the primary organization occurring during gastrulation, and continues through later stages. Paired mesodermal inductor regions are localized in the primary organizer of the early gastrula. The beginning of the second period of induction is characterized by the approximation of the presumptive ear ectoderm to the adjacent neural fold.

DEVELOPMENT OF THE INTERNAL EAR

Ectodermic thickening, the otic placode, appears on the side of the developing rhombencaphalon in embryos of about seven mesodermal segments (Fig.1); in later somites proliferation of the surrounding mesoderm elevates the ectoderm around the placode, so that the latter appears as the otic pit. By the 30 somite stage, the otic pit becomes separated from the surface to form the otic vesicle or otocyst. The otocyst is related anteromedially to the acoustic-facial portion of the neural crest, which represents the primordium of the acoustic-facial ganglion (Fig.2). The geniculate ganglion of the facial nerve soon separates, leaving the primordium of the acoustic ganglion, the cells of which remain throughout life in the bipolar condition. Soon a hollow diverticulum appears from the medial aspect of the otocyst, and becomes elongated to form the endolymphatic sac.

The otocyst is first constricted into an upper vestibular pouch and a lower cochlear pouch. From the former, three

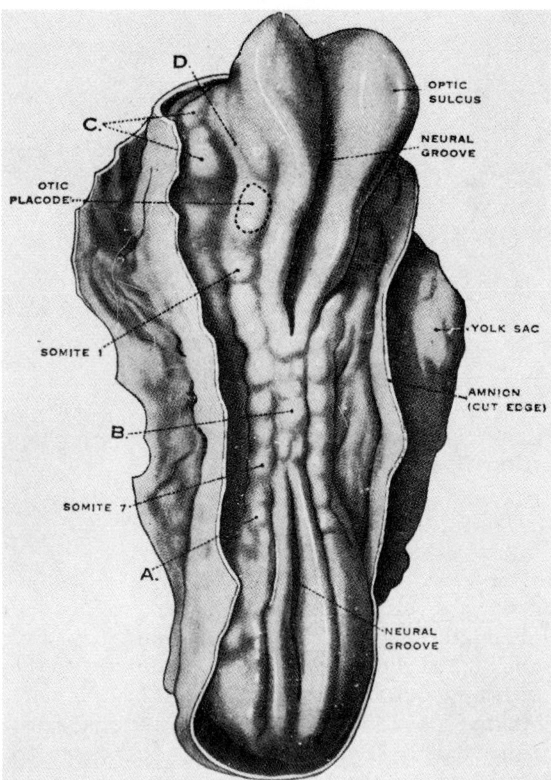

Figure 1. The dorsal aspect of a model of a seven-somite human embryo on about the 22nd day (7).

flattened hollow plates, at right angles to each other, become elevated to form the primordia of the superior, posterior and lateral semicular canals. The lower part of the vestibular pouch, into which the semicircular canals open, becomes the utricle. The cochlear pouch soon becomes divided into an upper portion, the saccule, and a lower portion which elongates rapidly and becomes curved to form the cochlea. The communication between the saccule and the cochlea successively narrows to form the ductus reuniens (Fig.3). The communication between the saccule and the utricle becomes constricted to form the utriculosaccular duct.

The otocyst is initially lined with a single layer of epithelium, but thickened epithelial areas arise later, in relation to the ingrowth of nerve fibers, and are situated in the saccule (saccular macula), the utricle (utricular macula), the dilated ampulla of each of the semicircular canals (ampullary maculae), and along the whole length of one side of the cochlear

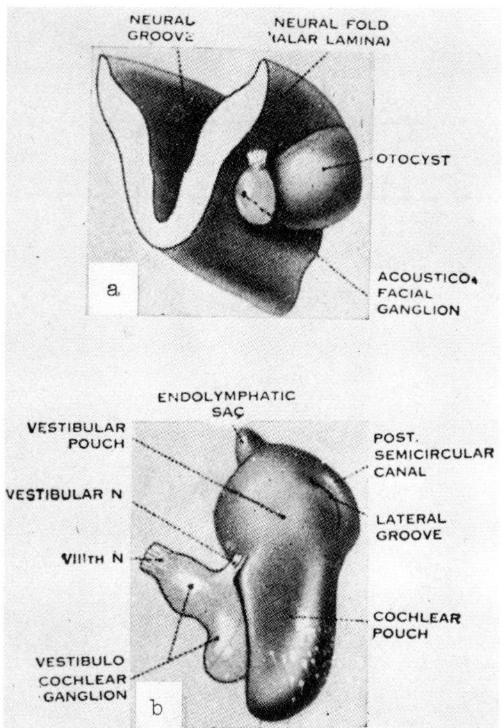

Figure 2. a. The otocyst is related to the acoustic-facial portion of the neural crest (7).

b. A hollow diverticulum appears from the medial aspect of the otocyst and becomes elongated to form the endolymphatic sac (7).

ducts (cristae acusticae). Each of these specialized areas receives a sensory nerve from the vestibular or cochlear division of the acoustic nerve (Fig.4).

All these essential parts of the membranous labyrinth are defined by the end of the second month. Virtually no malformation of the inner ear is known: it seems to be imcompatible with life. The thickened primordium of the spiral organ, which is adjacent to the scala tympani, differentiates into the organ of Corti. The maculae of the saccule, utricle and the semicircular ducts become the sensory equilibration organs (Fig. 5).

DEVELOPMENT OF THE MIDDLE EAR AND OF THE EXTERNAL EAR

The external auditory meatus derives in part from the first ectodermal cleft. Its area in contact with the endoderm of the

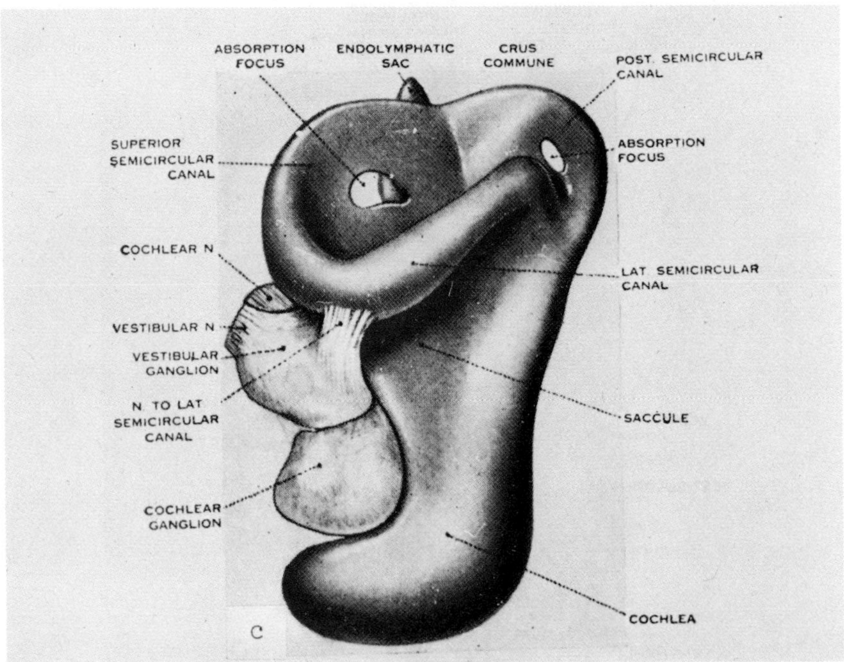

Figure 3. The otocyst is constricted into an upper vestibular pouch and a lower cochlear pouch (7).

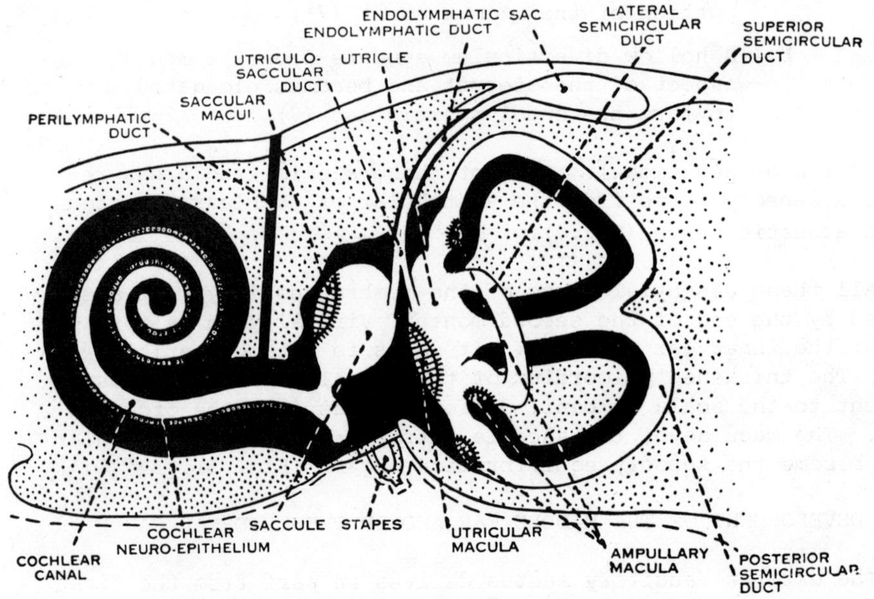

Figure 4. The otocyst with thickened epithelial areas in relation to the ingrowth of nerve fibres (7).

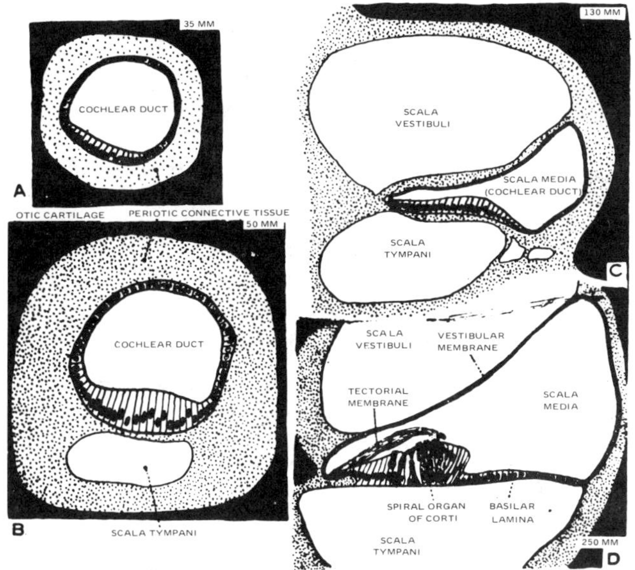

Figure 5. Histogenesis of the internal ear in fetuses of 35 (a), 50 (b), 130 (c) and 250 (d) mm (7).

tubotympanic recess, which is formed chiefly from the first endodermal pharyngeal pouch, becomes the tympanic membrane, the mesoderm being interposed between the two epithelial layers (Fig. 6). The rudiments of the incus and malleus are formed from the dorsal cartilage of the first visceral arch (Meckel's cartilage). The stapes is formed from the upper end of the second arch cartilage (Reichert's cartilage). The development of the muscles of the middle ear parallels that of its various structures with which they are in contact.

The external ear arises from a number of ectodermal hillocks which surround the opening of the ectodermal cleft (Fig.7).

THE VESTIBULAR NERVE

The cells of the vestibular ganglion (Scarpa's ganglion) are constantly acetylcholinesterase-positive during fetal development. The dendrites of these neurons have sensory endings in the hair cells on the maculae of the semicircular ducts, the utricle and the saccule. Their neuraxes reach the brain stem in front of the cochlear root. Soon after their entrance into the medulla oblongata the great majority of the vestibular root fibers bifurcate into two branches, one ascending, the other descending. From the former, fibers pass directly into the cerebellum and reach the medullary center and many parts of the cerebellar cortex.

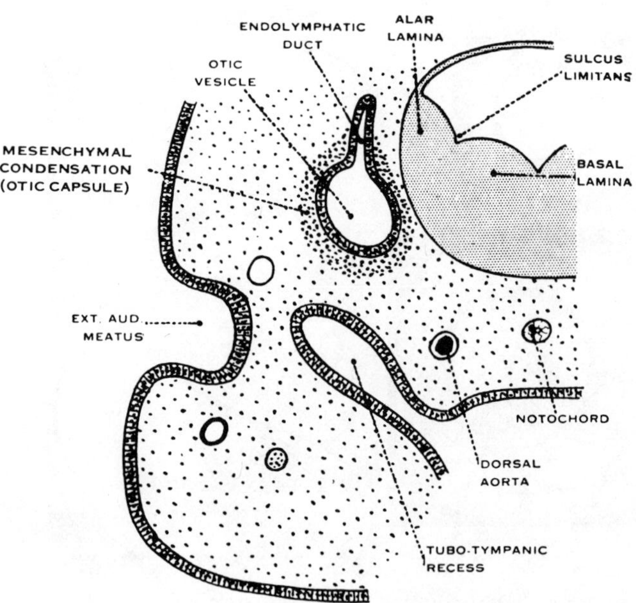

Figure 6. Early stage in the development of the external auditory meatus and of the tubotympanic recess (7).

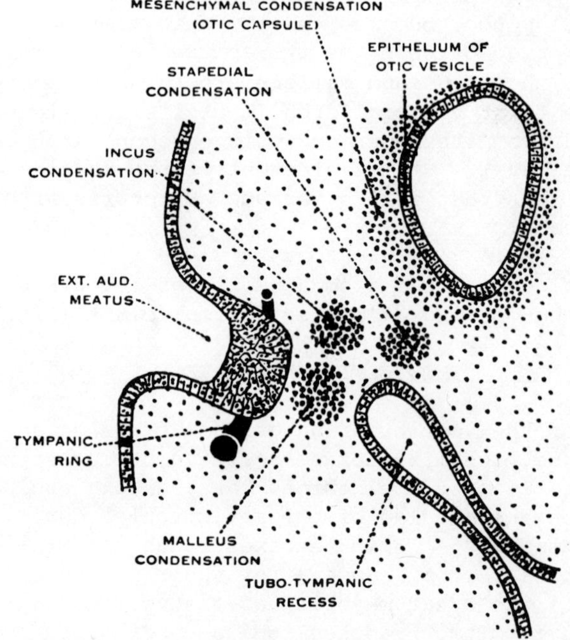

Figure 7. A drawing of a stage later than shown in Fig.6 in the development of the tubotympanic recess and associated structures (7).

The vestibular root fibers generally end in the vestibular nuclei, which in mammals are:

a. clusters of cells among the intramedullary vestibular fibers,

b. the medial or Schwalbe's nucleus,

c. The superior or Bechterew's nucleus,

d. the lateral or Deiter's nucleus, and its caudal continuation,

e. the descending or spinal vestibular nucleus,

f. the accessory or external cuneate or Burdach's nucleus.

The neurons of these nuclei have a cell body of stellate shape, with long dendrites which may extend into adjacent nuclei, or even into certain fiber paths of the vestibular system. Deiter's nucleus gives rise to the descending vestibulospinal system which extends throughout nearly all the spinal cord, and constitutes a path conducting impulses for the changes in position of the body and the maintenance of equilibrium. The lateral vestibulospinal tract ends at the motor neurons of the muscles of the limbs. The medial vestibular or Schwalbe's nucleus seems to be concerned in the fine elaboration of the eye movements. The medial longitudinal fasciculus conveys messages to the nuclei of the eye muscles and of the muscles moving the head and the neck in response to changes of position of the body.

Connections of the vestibular centers with the temporal lobe have been ascertained. Vestibular fibers seem to reach the cortex following almost the same pathway as the acoustic fibers. Fibers reaching the vestibular ganglion from the brain stem have been described by Ramon y Cajal and others.

THE COCHLEAR NERVE

The bipolar ganglion cells (Corti's ganglion) are imbedded in the petrous bone. Their dendrites go to Corti's organ, their neurons enter the medulla oblongata, lateral to the restiform body. Close to their place of entrance they come into relation with the nucleus ventralis cochlearis. Here the fibers dichotomize: the descending fibers run mainly to the dorsal cochlear nucleus, the tuberculum acusticum. Some of the root fibers seem to pass directly to the contralateral nuclei through the trapezoid body.

The acoustic pathways from the medulla oblongata to the cortex are complex: the further cell stations are:

a. the superior olivary nuclei,

b. the nucleus of the lateral lemniscus,

c. the inferior colliculus on the roof of the midbrain,

d. the medial geniculate body.

Between the cochlear nuclei and the medial geniculate body, there are at least two neurons. The snyapses may be located in any of the three cell masses mentioned. Many but not all of the fibers decussate. The most prominent of these decussations is the trapezoid body. It is the most central one and is at the level of the superior olive. Lateral to the olive, the trapezoid body and the fibers from the dorsal cochlear nucleus unite to form a compact bundle of fibers, the lateral lemniscus. This, rostral to the superior olive, forms, with the medial lemniscus, an ascending sensory system. The lateral lemniscus terminates in part in the inferior colliculus and in part in the medial geniculate nucleus of the thalamus.

The inferior colliculus is the midbrain auditory center. From this, and even more from the superior colliculus, impulses are relayed into the tectobulbar and tectospinal paths. The inferior colliculus may relay auditory impulses to the medial geniculate body by way of the brachium of the medial geniculate nucleus. It does not contribute fibers directly to the cortex. The medial geniculate nucleus is a metathalamic auditory center, a necessary relay station in the pathway to the auditory cortex. Pathways are provided from the auditory centers to the motor nuclei of the eye and neck muscles by the peduncle of the superior olive. Their functional significance relates to the reflexes of turning the eyes and head towards the sound. The superior olive seems to have connections with the facial nucleus, producing reflex movements of the ear muscles.

Auditory projection fibers to the cortex arise from the medial geniculate nucleus of the thalamus. In mammals, the cochlear root also carries vestibular fibers from the posterior ampulla and the sacculus. Hence it retains some degree of vestibular function. These vestibular fibers are already myelinated in the 23 cm human embryo, while myelin sheaths do not appear in the cochlear root fibers until the 28 cm stage. An efferent "olive-cochlear bundle" has been described. Its fibers lie along the cochlear nerve, from which they part to form the intraganglionic spiral bundle and reach hair cells of the organ of Corti. These fibers show a marked acetylcholinesterase activity, whereas the fibers deriving from the peripheral and central extensions of Corti's ganglion never show any such activity. The function of this bundle, efferent from the olive to the cochlear, in the mechanism of hearing, is still uncertain. It has to be fitted into the feed-back systems of the sensory apparatuses.

THE ACOUSTIC AREA OF THE CORTEX

The acoustic area of the cortex is situated in the superior transverse temporal gyrus. The cytoarchitectonic and myelo-architectonic fields of the temporalis region of man have been indicated by different numbers. Among these are the superior temporalis area (field 22), the parainsularis area (field 52), the anterior internal transverse temporalis area (field 41) and the posterior external temporalis area (field 42). These fields are situated along the dorsal or superior face of the first temporal convolution. The sensory auditory area of Campbell is surrounded by the auditory psychic area. Differences have been observed in the cytoarchitectonics of this area between caucasian and non-caucasian races, and it has also been shown that the spread of the auditory radiations varies markedly among Europeans. There seems to be a point-to-point correspondence between the cochlea and the acoustic area of the cortex. In man and in primates low tones are picked up near the tip of the cochlea (helicotrema) and are transmitted to the occipital end of the acoustic area, whereas high tones are picked up near the oval window and transmitted to the frontal end of this area.

Evidence is still not complete with regard to the connections of the acoustic area of the cortex. Minkowski found that, on destruction of areas 5-7-22, a large thalamic area, including the medial geniculate nucleus, the dorsolateral thalamic nucleus and the pulvinar, showed degeneration. A lesion of the middle part of the first temporal convolution and its continuation into the gyri transversi is sufficient to lead to degeneration of the whole projection tract from the medial geniculate, together with the degeneration of the cells of this nucleus. Double-sided lesions in this region cause cortical deafness in man, proof that the auditory center is located here.

On the basis of the distribution of the auditory fibers, it has been recognized that in man the posterior portion of Heschl's convolution may be concerned primarily with connections with the contralateral hemisphere. Thus, the connecting fibers run through the posterior portion of the corpus callosum. The medial and inferior temporal gyri are phylogenetically younger; they differ structurally and functionally from the rest of the region, and their function is not yet sufficiently understood. An efferent path (temporopontine path) arises in the anterior part of the second and third temporal convolutions, and in the medial temporalis area. The connections of this region with the pons, and through that with the cerebellum, provide a means of placing the cerebellar functions under the control of the cerebral cortex.

These relationships indicate that the temporal region originally served static or spatial functions, and proves the close relationship which has existed during evolution, between the vestibular and cochlear nerves. The presence of a center of hearing near a static temporopontile region suggests that the gnostic auditory sense may have been metamorphosed from the rhythmic body sense.

DEVELOPMENTAL CHRONOLOGY OF THE EAR AND THYROID

The chronological development of the ear and of the thyroid is summarized in Table I. It should be remembered that the term "embryo" has here been used for the human organism up to the end of the second month, after which the fetal period begins.

In these stages the presumptive age from conception is deduced from the length, weight, histological development and maturation of the body. The length, expressed in mm, is measured from the crown to the rump (C.R.). At the end of the third week the dorsal portion of the mesoderm has become divided by transverse furrows into a number of segments or somites, visible through the semitransparent skin (Fig. 1). At the beginning of the second month, 40-44 hollow lumps (the mesodermal somites) have been formed on each side of the notocord.

SUMMARY

The frequency of deafmutism in association with endemic goiter prompts an examination of the embryogenesis of the ear in relation to the development of function of the fetal thyroid. The earliest primordium of the ear is recognizable as the otic placode by two and a half weeks of human embryonic life. The primitive cells of the thyroid in the foregut can probably be recognized at the same time. The organ of Corti differentiates by the tenth week whereas the thyroid begins functioning only by the twelfth week. Thus by the initiation of thyroid function the ear is already well along in its differentiation and development. Ossification of the ear does not begin until about the 20th week. Already by this time colloid is recognizable in the follicles of the embryonic thyroid.

Table 1. Chronological Development of the Ear and Thyroid in the Human Embryo and Fetus

AGE	LENGTH	DEVELOPMENT OF THE EAR	DEVELOPMENT OF THE THYROID
Embryological period			
2½ weeks	1.5 mm (7 somites)	The otic placode is distinguishable; the primordium of the acoustic ganglion develops.	A thickening of the endodermal cells of the foregut represents the thyroid primordium.
4 weeks	3.5-4 mm (17-20 somites)		The endodermal thickening forms a diverticulum in the underlying mesoderm. The pharyngeal pouches become established.
end of first month	5 mm (30-40 somites)	The otic pit becomes separated from the surface to form the otocyst. The endolymphatic sac appears.	
5-6 weeks	5-10 mm		The pedicle of the diverticulum elongates; its distal part acquires a bilobate shape, and is composed of a solid mass of endodermal epithelial cells. The thyroglossal duct becomes fragmented.
6 weeks	12 mm	The middle and external ear develop.	
	14.5 mm		The fourth pharyngeal pouch fuses with the expanding lateral lobes of the median thyroid primordium.
	20 mm		Early follicles, without colloid, begin to appear. Influence of fetal TSH? Differentiation of the parafollicular cells?
Fetal period			
8 weeks	23 mm		The thyroid, parathyroid and thymus have reached their final shape.
10 weeks	40 mm	The organ of Corti differentiates	
early part of third month			Stainable colloid appears in some follicles. Uptake of radioiodine occurs.
12 weeks-end of third month.	70-100 mm		Colloid shows peripheral vacuoles. Functional activity is evident in many follicies, which concentrate radioiodine.
20 weeks	160 mm	Ossification of the ear occurs.	

ACKNOWLEDGEMENTS

Fig. 1-7 reprinted from Hamilton, Boyd and Mossman (7) by permission of the publisher.

DISCUSSION BY PARTICIPANTS

STANBURY: Isn't the important point that the ear is virtually complete before the thyroid begins to function?

COSTA: Yes.

KOENIG: If I recall correctly, the middle ear develops after the first trimester, with the pneumatization of the sinuses. According to Nager (13) the otic lesions must occur in the last two-thirds of fetal life.

REFERENCES

1. Arey, L.B.: Developmental Anatomy; A Textbook and Laboratory Manual of Embryology. 7th. ed. Saunders, Philadelphia, 1965.

2. Ariëns Kappers, C.U.; Huber, G.C. and Crosby, E.C.: The Comparative Anatomy of the Nervous System of Vertebrates, Including Man. Hafner, New York, 1960.

3. Bairati, A.: Trattato di anatomia umana. Minerva Med. 1961.

4. Balázs, R.: Biochemical effects of thyroid hormones in the developing brain. In: Cellular Aspects of Neural Growth and Differentiation (D.C. Pease, ed.). Berkeley, Univ. California Press, 1971. UCLA Forum Med. Sci. 14:273-311, 1971.

5. Boyd, J.D.: Development of the human thyroid gland. In: The Thyroid Gland (R. Pitt-Rivers and W.R. Trotter, eds.). Butterworths, London, 1964.

6. Campenhout, E. van.: Le development du nerf auditif. Acta Otorhinolaryngol. Belg. 11:283-287, 1969.

7. Hamilton, W.J.; Boyd, J.D. and Mossman, H.W.: Human Embryology; Prenatal Development of Form and Function. W. Heffer, Cambridge, 1962.

8. Debain, J.J.: Enciclopédie Medico Chirurgicale-Oto-rhino-laringologie. 20190 C IC, C 30, 1954.

9. Candiollo, L. and Levi, A.C.: Studies on the morphogenesis of the middle ear muscles in man. Arch. Klin. Exp. Ohren. Nasen. Kehlkopfheilkd. 195:55-67, 1969.

10. Rossi, G.: L'acetylcholinesterase au cours du development de l'oreille interne du cobaye. Acta Otolaryngol. Suppl. 170, 1961.

11. Schindler, O.; Demichelis, G.; Ferrero, G.; Busca, G.P. and Gallizia, G.: Considerazioni sulla cibernetica della funzione acustica. Riv. Otoneurooftalmol. 41:709-716, 1966.

12. Yntema, C.L.: Ear and nose. In: Analysis of Development (B.H. Willier, P.A. Weis and V. Hamburger, eds.). W.B. Saunders, Philadelphia, 1955. pp. 415-429.

13. Nager, F.R.: Die Beziehungen des endemischen Kretinismus zum Getororgan. In: Handbuch der HNO-Heilkunde (A.Denker and A. Kahler, eds.). Vol. 6. Springer, Berlin, 1926. pp. 617-635.

EXPERIMENTAL PRODUCTION OF OTIC LESIONS WITH ANTITHYROID DRUGS

Gerald J. Bargman and Lytt I. Gardner

Genetic and Endocrine Unit, Department of Pediatrics
State University of New York, Upstate Medical Center
Syracuse, New York

Deafness is a classic but not universal finding in endemic cretinism. Trotter (1) has reviewed the forms of thyroid disease that have been observed in association with hearing deficits. We report here the results of an experiment designed to study the effects of propylthiouracil in producing goitrous hypothyroidism on the middle and inner ear hearing structures (including the auditory nerve and its central projection) in developing chick embryos.

METHODS AND MATERIALS

Following techniques reported by Romanoff and Laufer (2), fertile chick eggs were injected with two mg of propylthiouracil (PTU) into their albumin on the tenth incubation day. L-Thyroxine (one to 100 μg in divided doses of five μg) was also inoculated in the same manner, either simultaneously with PTU or on subsequent days up to and including the 17th incubation day. Control inocula included sterile saline and sterile water. All embryos were incubated at 99.5°F (37.8°C) with the humidity maintained at 60 to 65 percent. Each egg was turned frequently and candled twice per day. Dead embryos were discarded, whereas the survivors were allowed to continue incubation until hatch time. After hatching, specimens were studied for obvious gross defects. The thyroid glands, middle and inner ear hearing mechanisms, as well as the auditory nerve and brain stem were then dissected and studied microscopically using hematoxylin and eosin stain (3) or silver impregnation (4). The latter technique was that of Cajal and DeCastro as described by Levi-Montalcini (4). No decalcification methods were employed.

RESULTS

The embryos injected with PTU, compared to control embryos, had a higher mortality rate and required a longer incubation period before hatching occurred. Gross observation of newly hatched chicks who had been injected with sterile water or sterile saline showed no remarkable physical differences when compared to uninjected specimens. However, chicks who survived exposure to PTU as embryos exhibited the following consistent physical changes when compared to the control specimens: shorter crown-rump length, reduced wet weight, and omphalocele with incomplete resorption of the yolk sac (Fig. 1). Death occurred within

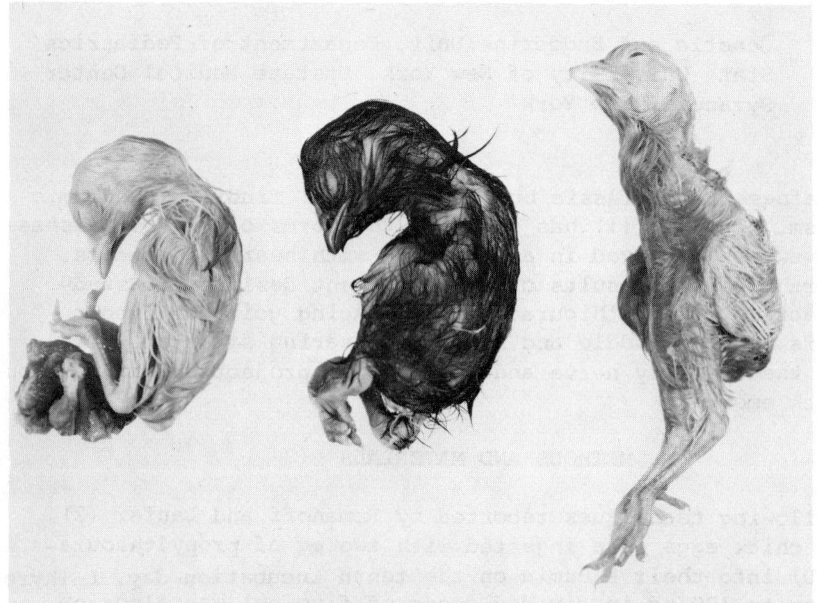

Fig. 1. The bird on the left was fixed immediately after hatching, and illustrates the reduced size and umbilical hernia (incomplete absorption of the yolk sac) consistently found in chicks exposed to propylthiouracil on the 10th incubation day. The middle chick received 65 μg of l-thyroxine simultaneously with 2 mg of PTU. It exhibits no obvious gross anomalies when compared to a saline treated specimen (right).

five days unless exogenous thyroid hormone therapy was initiated 24 to 48 hr after hatching. The thyroid glands of these chicks were found to be markedly enlarged with prominent vascularization (Fig. 2,3).

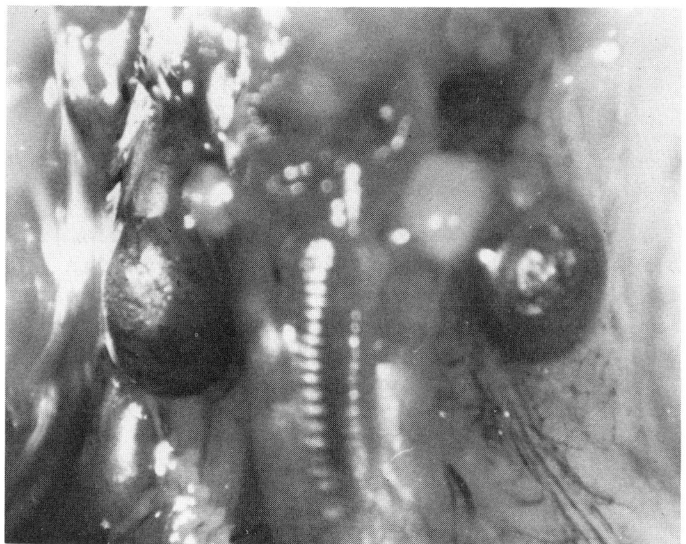

Fig. 2. The marked enlargement and prominent vascularization of the thyroid glands in chicks injected with 2 mg PTU is demonstrated. The laminated structure in the midline of the photo is trachea (x 2.5).

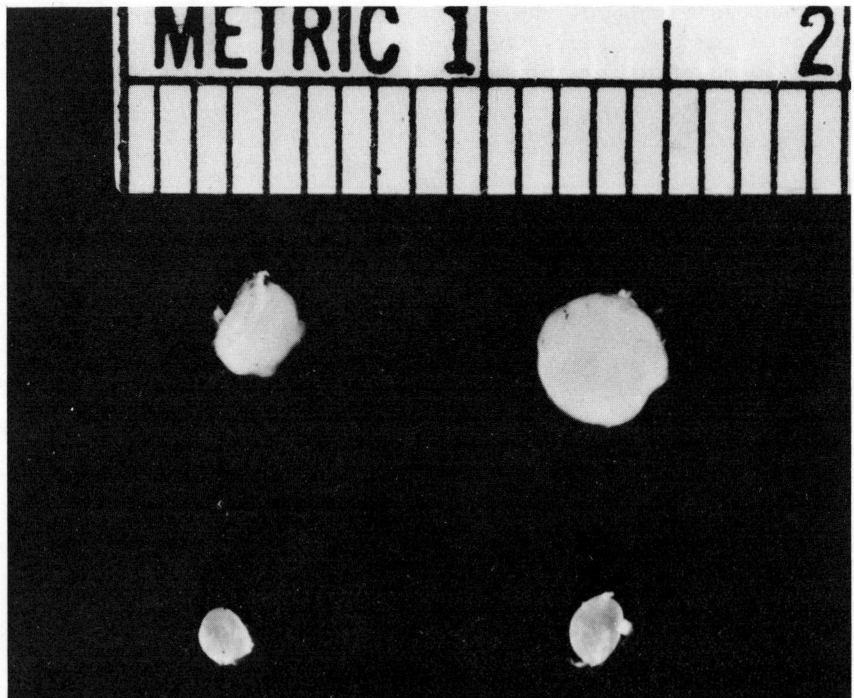

Fig. 3. This photograph compares the intact, formalin fixed thyroid glands from a hatched chick treated with PTU as an embryo (top) and from a control (bottom). The glands from the chick exposed to PTU are not only hypertrophic but also opaque because of increased cellularity.

Histologically, these thyroid glands revealed acinar cell hypertrophy and, unlike the work reported by Ritter and Lawrence (5), distinct colloid vesicles were not detectable (Figs. 4,5).

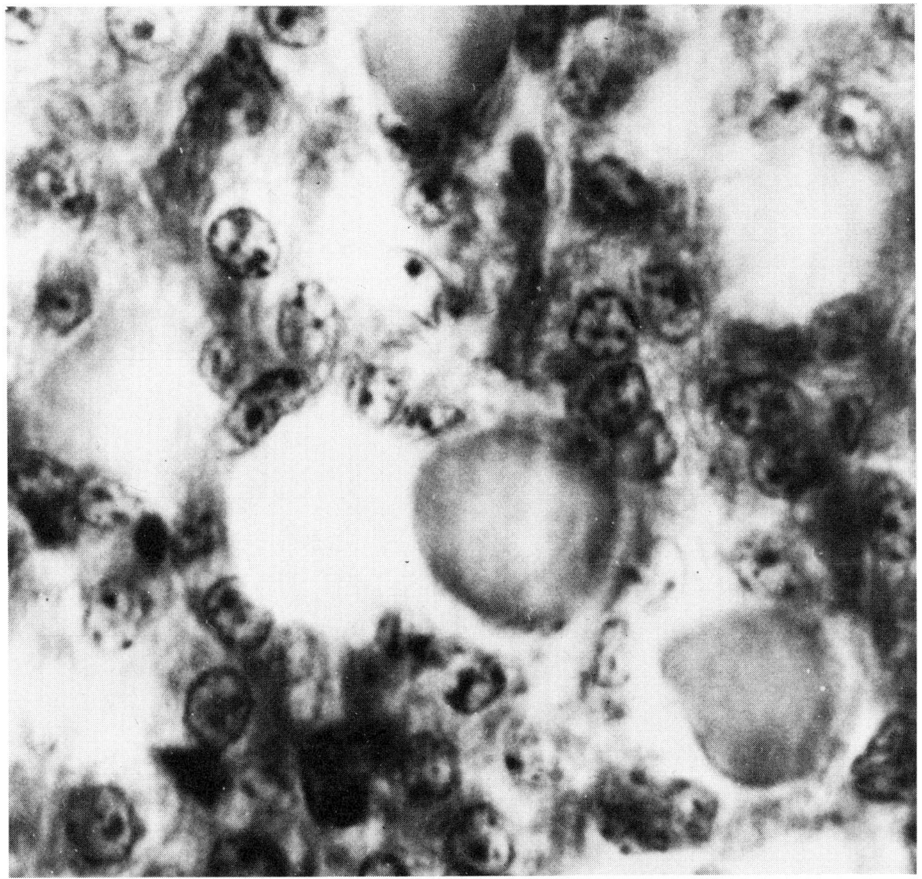

Fig. 4. A 10 micron section of a control thyroid gland is represented above. Note the distinct acinar cell-lined follicles containing colloid (H&E x 1000).

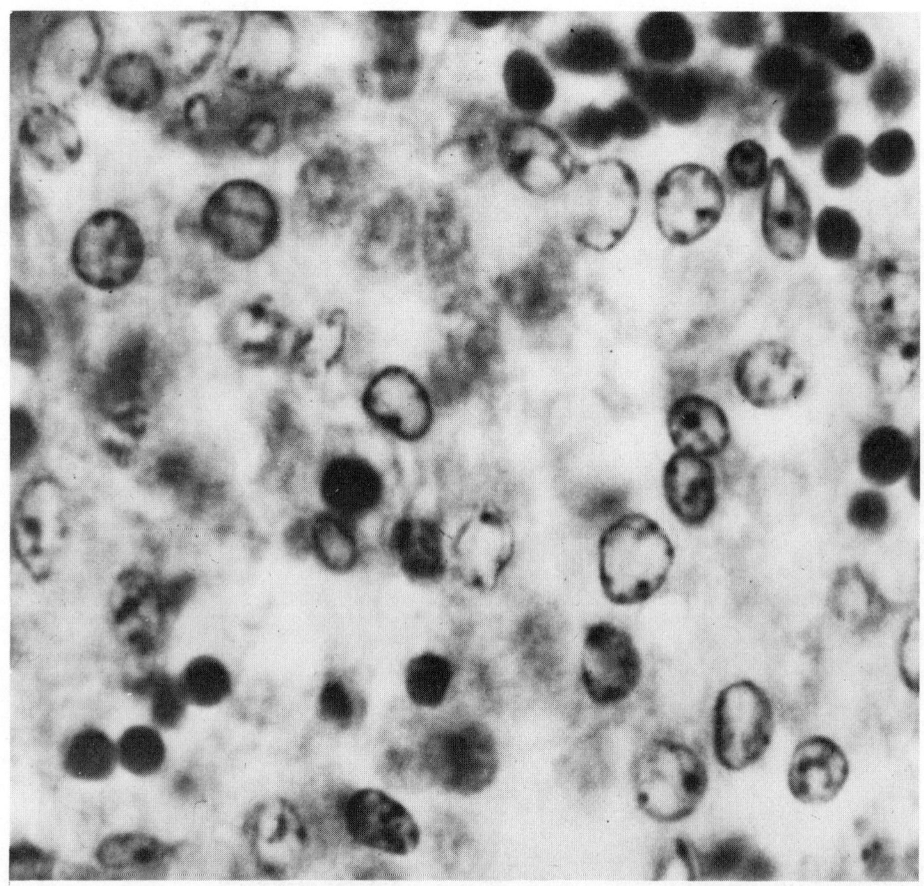

Fig. 5. This 10 micron section is representative of an entire thyroid gland from a PTU treated specimen. Well circumscribed acinar-lined follicles and colloid are not distinguishable. The scattered darkly stained cells are erythrocytes, demonstrating increased vascularity of the gland (H&E stain x 1000).

Our microscopic findings are consistent with chemically induced hypothyroidism in the chick as described by Mitskevitch (6). Histological examination of the middle and inner ears from PTU-treated chick embyros revealed alterations confined to the sensory hair cells of the cochlea in the area of the macula lagenae (Figs. 6,7).

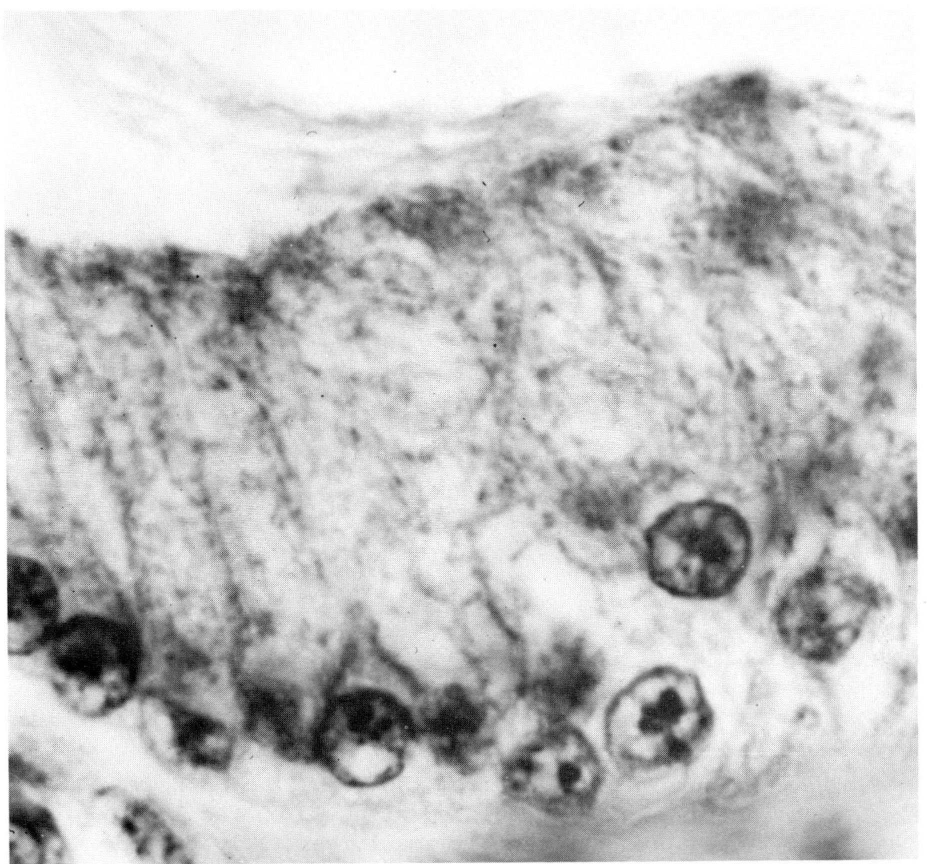

Fig. 6. Sensory hair cells from the area of the cochlear maculae lagenae of control chicks show distinct nuclei at their base and intracellular material (H&E stain x 1470).

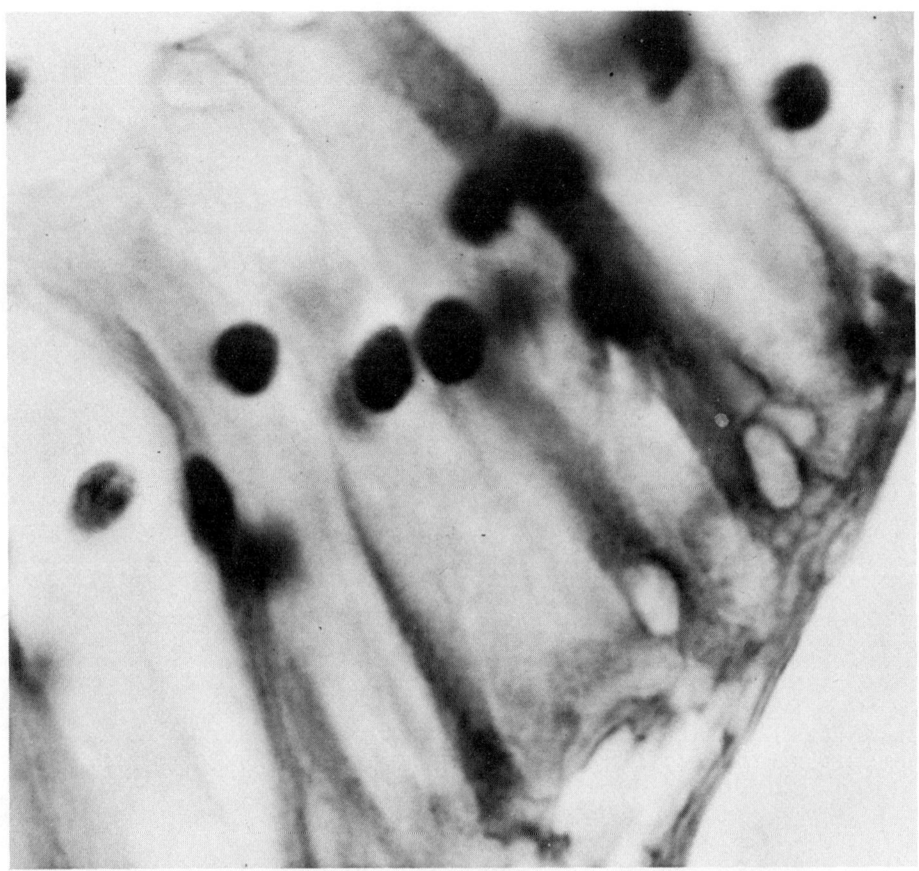

Fig. 7. Sensory hair cells from the cochlea of a newly hatched chick inoculated with PTU on the 10th incubation day exhibit small, centrally placed nuclei and obliteration of intracellular material (H&E stain x 1470).

The cytoplasm of these cells was composed mainly of a semi-opaque, glossy, weakly acidophilic material with a loss or obliteration of intracellular granularity. The nuclei of these cells were found to be relatively small and more centrally located within the individual cells. Chicks showing these cochlear changes also exhibited histologic alterations in the spiral ganglion of the cochlea. The bipolar nerve cells of the ganglion were smaller and relatively widely separated by the accumulation of an intercellular substance resembling, on silver impregnation, the material composing the abnormal cytoplasm of the affected sensory hair cells. Nuclear boundaries and chromatin material within these nerve cells were difficult to identify (Figs. 8, 9).

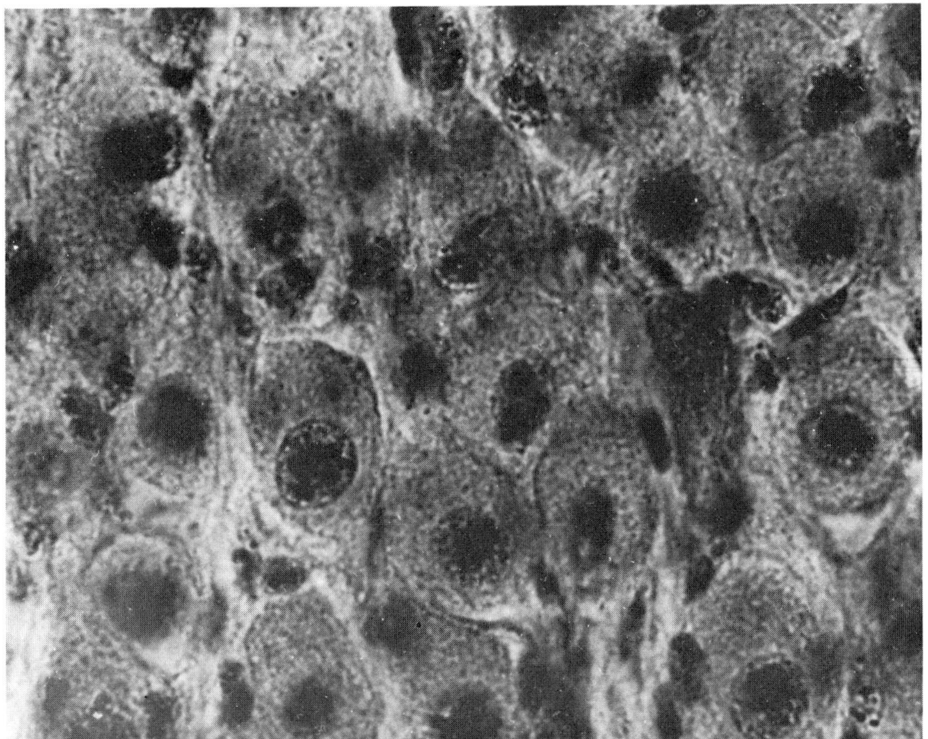

Fig. 8. Cells from the spiral ganglion of the cochlea of a saline-treated specimen are illustrated above. Distinct nuclei and rather coarse dark-staining cytoplasmic granules are present. Note how closely "packed" the individual cells are (Silver impregnation x 1000).

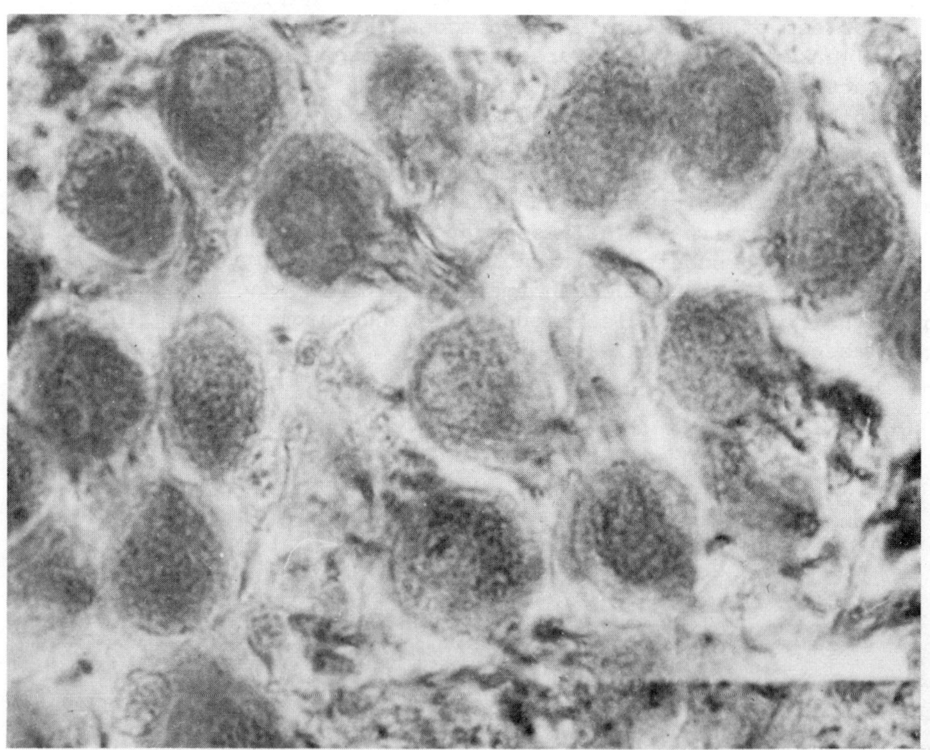

Fig. 9. The spiral ganglion of the cochlea from chicks exposed to PTU as embryos reveals cells lacking distinct nuclei and dark-staining cytoplasmic granularity. The intercellular space is very obvious (Silver impregnation x 1000).

No consistent histological abnormalities in the axons of the cochlear nerve and their associated nuclear centers in the medulla oblongata were found in hypothyroid specimens. Except for evidence of delayed calcification, no pathological changes were found in the structures (columella) of the middle ear. The type of morphologic abnormality of the chick Organ of Corti described by Ritter and Lawrence (5) was not found.

If 50 to 75 μg of l-thyroxine was given simultaneously with, or as long as 120 hours after, the PTU injection on the tenth incubation day, the mortality rate was increased, but survivors generally hatched earlier than with PTU alone. The characteristic thyroid lesions and abnormal histological findings of the sensory hair cells in the cochlea and its ganglion were not detected when l-thyroxine was given with PTU as described above (Figs. 10,11,12).

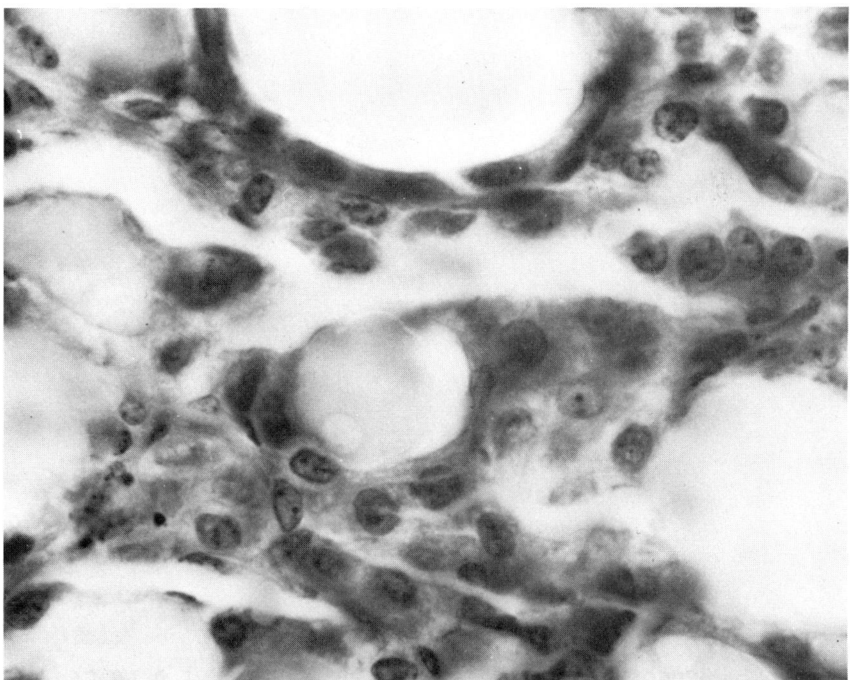

Fig. 10. Distinct acinar-lined follicles containing colloid can be seen in this 10 micron section of thyroid obtained from a chick who received PTU (2 mg) and l-thyroxin (55 μg) on the 12th incubation day (H&E x 1025).

In accordance with the work of Stoll *et al.* (7), we found that l-thyroxine appears to be a very toxic agent, at least when inoculated by itself into the albumin of 10 to 17 day developing chick embryos.

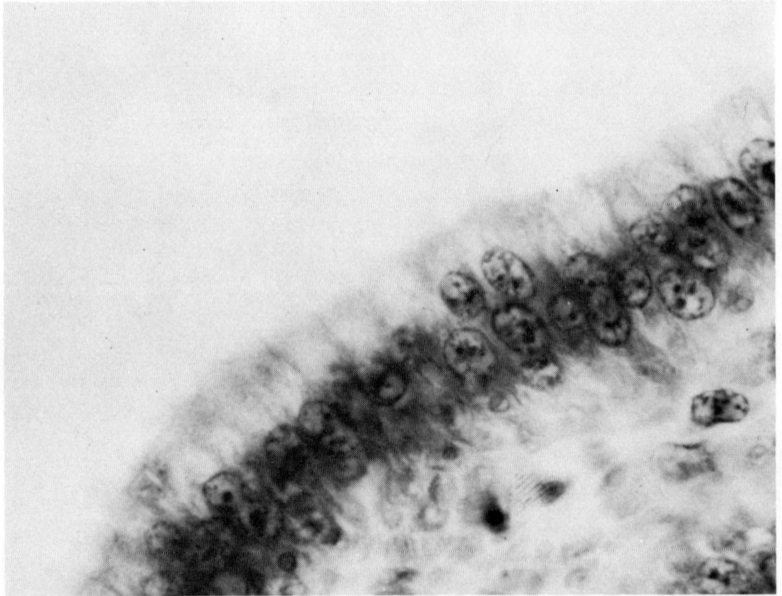

Fig. 11. Sensory hair cells from the cochlea of a chick treated with PTU (2 mg on 10th incubation day) and l-thyroxine (60 μg on 12th incubation day) are presented above. Distinct basilar nuclei and cytoplasmic granulations are present. Note the hair-like projections from the top border of these cells (H&E x 1025).

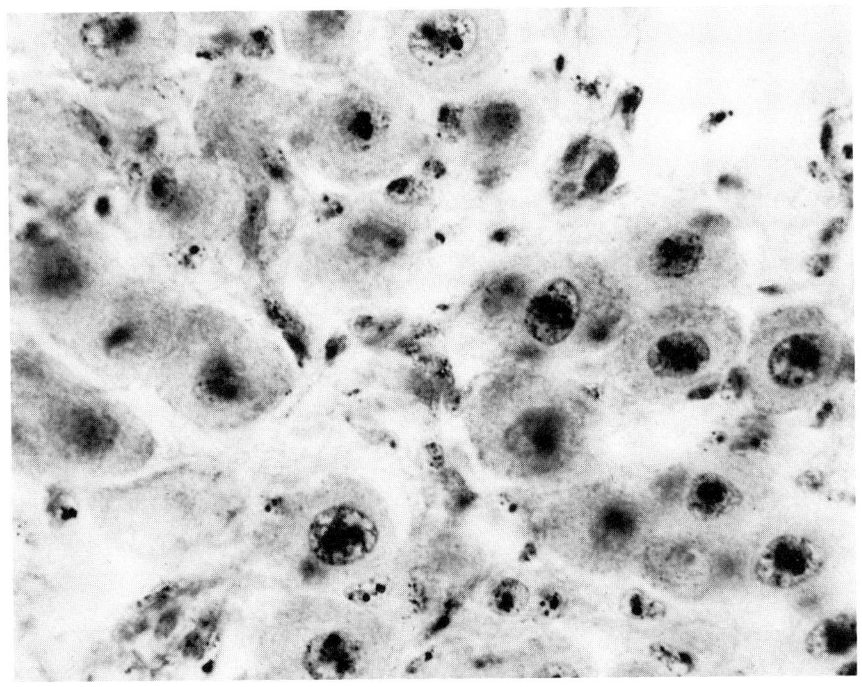

Fig. 12. Cells in the spiral ganglion of the cochlea from a chick injected with PTU (2 mg on 10th incubation day) and l-thyroxine (60 μg on 12th incubation day) reveal well-demarcated nuclei with dark staining chromatin material. Dark cytoplasmic granulations are also present. The intercellular space in this photomicrograph has been exaggerated by technical artifact (Silver impregnation x 1025).

DISCUSSION

A brief review of the embryology seems in order. On the second incubation day the thyroid glands of the chick embryo begin as a single midline ventral outpouching from the primordial pharyngeal wall, at the level of the first and second branchial pouches. This outgrowth subsequently differentiates into two separate structures, each migrating laterally to its eventual position at the base of the neck (8). These paired but unattached embryonic glands begin to elaborate thyroxine after approximately 9.75 days of incubation (9). Histologically the chick thyroid resembles the thyroid gland of man (8,10).

The chicken cochlea is derived from a ventral outgrowth of the otocyst starting at about six days of incubation. Growth and differentiation of this structure continues until about 11.75 incubation days when its degree of anatomical maturation is essentially the same as that of the adult. Neuroepithelium confined to the ventral otocyst grows and subdivides into all the necessary sensory tissue including the auditory nerve and its branches. The development of this nervous tissue is concomitant with differentiation of the structures derived from the otocyst (11). The chicken cochlea differs morphologically from that of man in several respects. It is a membranous, 5 mm long, slightly concave, finger-like tube, within a similar shaped bony shell. This membranous tube contains a central channel (scala media) that ends blindly in a region called the maculae lagenae (Fig. 7). Endolymph from the membranous labyrinth fills the entire scala media while above and below it are perilymph-containing cavities known as the scala vestibuli and scala tympani, respectively. The floor of the scala media is referred to as the basement membrane, while its roof is known as the tegmental membrane or tegmentum vasculosum. Covering the basement membrane are columnar cells which, in the area of the maculae lagenae, have differentiated into sensory hair cells. This specific area of neuro-epithelium is called the acoustic papilla. Lying above, and in close apposition to the cells of the acoustic papilla, are a group of transverse fibers (tectorial membrane) supported at one end by the basement membrane and its columnar cells. The other end of these fibers is anchored to a small cartilaginous shelf jutting into the scala media. Post-ganglionic afferent and efferent fibers from the spiral ganglion of the cochlea penetrate this cartilaginous shelf and ramify among the sensory hair cells (acoustic papilla) just beneath it. The combination of basilar membrane, accessory supporting cells, sensory hair cells, tectorial membrane and nerve fibers are collectively referred to as the Organ of Corti. The spiral ganglion of the cochlea, containing the bipolar nerve cells, lies just medial to the bony cochlea. Afferent fibers from this ganglion pass through the cochlear branch of the auditory nerve into the main trunk and then into the specific nuclei within the medulla oblongata. These medullary centers include the ventral cochlear nucleus, nucleus laminaris, nucleus angularis, and nucleus magnocellularis. In our study auditory nerve tracts were not traced beyond these nuclei.

As alluded to previously, our findings are different than those obtained in the work reported by Ritter and Lawrence (5). They observed that injection of 2 mg of propylthiouracil into the albumin of four to nine day old chick embryos produced lesions in the Organ of Corti characterized by "toothlike sensory hair cells" separated from supporting tissues by edema. Propylthiouracil inoculation after nine days presumably had no effect on the cochlea. Morphologic alterations of the spiral ganglion were not mentioned and subsequent thyroid hormone therapy apparently was not attempted.

De Vos (12), producing a form of acquired hypothyroidism in mice, rats and hamsters, found that a daily oral dose of propylthiouracil (0.1 percent solution) started shortly after birth and maintained for an appropriate period thereafter (6 to 21 weeks), resulted in a "slight degeneration of the spiral ganglion." This, however, was not consistently observed. He did not demonstrate whether the pathological changes in the spiral ganglion were reversible with exogenous thyroid hormone replacement. The spiral ganglion was not re-examined after stopping the propylthiouracil regimen.

Interpretation of the data derived from our experimental model suggests that production of anatomic lesions of the cochlea and cochlear ganglion in embryonic chicks exposed to PTU, is related to chemical production of a metabolic error of the thyroid and subsequent hypothyroidism. The fact that these morphologic otic abnormalities could be prevented or possibly reversed with the appropriate dose and temporal scheduling of thyroxine therapy serves to strengthen this concept. If the cochlear mechanism were directly affected by propylthiouracil one would not expect thyroxine to have any protective or preventive effect.

SUMMARY

Post-hatch examination of chicks which, as embryos, were exposed to 2 mg of intraalbumin propylthiouracil (PTU) on their tenth day of incubation, revealed the following consistent alterations when compared to controls: increased mortality, delayed hatching, reduced weight and crown-to-rump length, incomplete yolk sac absorption and death within five days unless exogenous thyroid hormone was provided in the first 24 to 48 hr after hatching. Specific morphologic alterations were observed in their thyroid glands as well as in the sensory hair cells and spiral ganglion of the cochlea. Data are presented indicating that if 50 to 75 μg of l-thyroxine is given simultaneously with, or as long as 120 hr after the PTU injection on the tenth incubation day, one cannot detect the gross defects, marked thyroid lesions or abnormal histology in the cells of the cochlea and its ganglion. A relationship between embryonic thyroid gland function and histological otic lesions in the chick embryo is suggested.

ACKNOWLEDGEMENTS

This study was supported by grants T1-AM-5277 and AM-02504, National Institute of Arthritis and Metabolic Diseases, National Institutes of Health, U.S. Public Health Service.

Acknowledgement is made to the American Society for Clinical Investigation for permission to reproduce material from our study in the *Journal of Clinical Investigation.*

DISCUSSION BY PARTICIPANTS

GARDNER: Based on the foregoing experimental findings and on information appearing elsewhere in this volume, I would like to suggest the following concerning the connection between deafness and the thyroid. As a working hypothesis I propose that the deafness associated with endemic cretinism and with certain genetically determined goitrous states is somehow related to *thyroid, hyperplasia or dysplasia per se*. Several lines of observation suggest this:

1. In sporadic, athyreotic non-goitrous cretinism such as we see in Europe and North America deafness is not a complication, yet these infants have very low levels of thyroxine and are severely hypothyroid.

2. In the endemic cretinism of Idjwi Island in the Congo reported by Dr. DeLange *et al*. the patients had a much lower incidence of goiter than the general population and appeared to have thyroid destruction. Deafness was essentially unknown in this group.

3. In areas of endemic cretinism in other parts of the world where the syndrome is characterized by thyroid hyperplaxia, deafness is a common associated defect.

4. Certain patients with genetically determined biochemical errors of the thyroid with thyroid hyperplasia not infrequently show deafness as an associated finding.

I therefore suggest the possibility that thyroid hyperplasia in itself, whether caused by iodide deficiency, by an inborn metabolic error, or by a metabolic error produced by propylthiouracil may be responsible for pathological changes in the tissues involved in hearing. One could postulate an as yet unknown ototoxic factor elaborated by the hyperplastic or dysplastic thyroid gland.

PHAROAH: The goiter rate among cretins is no higher than in the normal population for the same age group, so by and large they do not have thyroid hyperplasia.

STANBURY: It would seem crucial to do the experiment in which you add iodine along with thyroxine. Did you do that?

GARDNER: No.

MOSIER: It has been reported that the thyroid gland in the newborn is hypoplastic (13). Is there any incidence of deaf-mutism in mongoloids?

FIERRO: There have been many reports of newborns with goiters when the mothers have been receiving PTU for hyperthyroidism. Do you know any evidence of cretinism or damage to the auditory system in these children?

KOENIG: I have gone through the literature on mothers getting PTU. I found 187 pregnancies in women taking antithyroid drugs, either carbamizole or PTU. There were 15 abnormal children, with three hypothyroid or cretinous children, one mongoloid, and none called deaf (14).

HERSHMAN: I would like to take issue with the speculation that the hyperplastic thyroid elaborates a neurotoxic substance. There is no basis for it and there is a basis for thinking that thyroid hormone influences the development of the nervous system. The effect of the antithyroid drug is through a feedback mechanism. Thyroxine inhibits that whole process.

GARDNER: Why don't you see deafness in the athyreotic cretin?

STANBURY: I do not think they are very hypothyroid *in utero*. You can get some delay, as we will discuss later in relation to iodine deficiency, but not great delay. They probably have enough thyroid *in utero* to take care of their otic development.

The Pendred syndrome is another problem which is completely baffling. DeGroot's patients who are deaf and insensitive to thyroid hormone have a defect which, I would assume, goes back to the earliest embryonic life. That is why they are deaf.

BALAZS: It is justifiable to propose a hypothesis when it can be tested experimentally, as in the case of Dr. Gardner's studies. One could destroy the thyroid by other means, for example by radioactive iodine. These experiments would indicate whether or not the thyroid gland is necessary for the development of the otic lesions.

DEGROOT: Is it possible that the damage you saw on the ganglia was independent of or secondary to the damage you saw in the organ of Corti?

ROSMAN: One certainly can get secondary changes this way. The photomicrographs that Dr. Gardner presented showed nerve cell changes that were virtually identical to those seen in central chromatolysis or "axonal reaction", with homogenization of nerve cell cytoplasm that can occur with a lesion distal to the histologically altered nerve cells.

REFERENCES

1. Trotter, W.R.: The association of deafness with thyroid dysfunction. Br. Med. Bull. 16:92-98, 1960.

2. Romanoff, A.L. and Laufer, H.: The effect of injected thiourea on the development of some organs of the chick embryo. Endocrinology 59:611-619, 1956.

3. Armed Forces Institute of Pathology. Manual of Histologic and Special Staining Technics. McGraw-Hill, New York, 2nd edition, 1960.

4. Levi-Montalcini, R.: The development of the acoustico-vestibular centers in the chick embryo in the absence of the afferent root fibers and of descending fiber tracts. J. Comp. Neurol. 91:209-241, 1949.

5. Ritter, F.N. and Lawrence, M.: Reversible hearing loss in human hypothyroidism and correlated changes in the chick inner ear. Trans. Am. Laryngol. Rhinol. Otol. Soc. 270-284, 1960.

6. Mitskevich, M.S.: Glands of Internal Secretion in the Embryonic Development of Birds and Mammals, Moscow, Academy of Science of U.S.S.R., 1957. (Translated for the National Science Foundation by the Israel Program for Scientific Translations, Jerusalem, 1959).

7. Stoll, R., Coulaud, H., Faucounau, N. and Maraud, R.: Sur l'action teratogene des hormones thyroidiennes chez l'embryon de poulet. Les mecanismes morphogenetiques de la strophosomie. Arch. Anat. Microsc. Morphol. Exp. 55:59-76, 1966.

8. Romanoff, A.L.: The Avian Embryo; Structural and Functional Development. Macmillan, New York, 1960.

9. Trunnell, J.B. and Wade, P.: Factors governing the development of the chick embryo thyroid. II. Chronology of the synthesis of iodinated compounds studied by chromatographic analysis. J. Clin. Endocrinol. Metab. 15:107-117, 1955.

10. diFiore, M.S.H.: An Atlas of Human Histology. 2nd edition. Lea and Febiger, Philadelphia, 1963.

11. Lillie, F.R.: The Development of the Chick: An Introduction to Embryology. Holt, Rinehart & Winston, New York, 1908.

12. de Vos, J.A.: Deafness in hypothyroidism. J. Laryngol. Otol. 77:390-414, 1963.

13. Pennacchietti, M.: Idiotie mongolienne et hyperthyroidisme. Rev. Neurol. (Paris) 2:276-288, 1932.

14. Koenig, M.P.: Die kongenitale Hypothyreose und der endemische Kretinismus. Springer, Berlin, 1968.

THE PATHOLOGY OF THE EAR IN ENDEMIC CRETINISM

M. P. Koenig and M. Neiger

The Medical University Clinic and University

Clinic for Ear, Nose, and Throat Diseases

Bern, Switzerland

A report on the otic lesions in endemic cretinism is hampered by the fact that since the classic descriptions by Nager (1), Mayer (2) and others, all summarized in the textbook article of Denker, 1927 (3), no new investigations have been published in the literature available to the authors. An additional complication lies in the fact that the cases described in the literature were selected arbitrarily in so far as the term "endemic cretinism" or "endemic deafness" is concerned. Another difficulty must be mentioned, which is the discrepancy, repeatedly observed by different authors, between the perceptive type of deafness found clinically in almost all endemic cretins studied by audiograms and the main involvement of the middle ear described as the typical otic lesion of endemic cretinism in the anatomicopathologic studies.

H. Bircher (4) was the first, in 1883, to insist on a relation between endemic goiter (and cretinism) and deaf-mutism. Since then, the majority of investigators have recognized this relationship. Nager (5) has made an extensive review of the information accumulated until 1926. This report will summarize the facts published in this excellent article, as well as in that of Denker (3).

SELECTION OF CASES

Among the patients from whom material was available at autopsy for morphologic (macroscopic and histologic) investigations of the ear, there were three typical endemic cretins, eight individuals with deafness, oligophrenia, goiter and "some cretinous features," and four with deaf-mutism and goiter, but of normal stature and normal intelligence. One cretinous dog was studied. In his original article, Nager (1) noted that among the nine patients he had studied all were representative of "endemic degeneration," i.e., were either typical dwarfed cretins with oligophrenia, deaf-mutism, goiter and motor disabilities, or were endemic idiots with congenital deaf-mutism and goiter, or were simple congenital deaf-mutes with goiter and neither other cretinous features nor oligophrenia.

ANATOMICOPATHOLOGIC EXAMINATIONS

A summary of the clinical features and middle ear lesions described by Nager (1) appears in Table I. In view of the fact that tissue alterations occur rather quickly after death, it is important to realize that the autopsies made by Nager and the other investigators of that time were done several hours or even days after death. With these reservations, the following changes appear to characterize endemic cretinism.

The temporal bone is affected as a whole, being small and ill-shaped. The mastoid process is poorly developed and its pneumatization may be totally lacking.

The mucous membrane of the tympanic cavity is considerably thickened, particularly in its subepithelial elements, but without signs of inflammation. This connective tissue is rich in fat and, even in old individuals, contains so-called "embryonic" mucous tissue.

Because of the impressive hyperostosis, the promontorium becomes consistently enlarged and deformed (Fig. 1). As a consequence, the round and oval windows are more or less distorted, and the round window may be totally closed. A deformation of the ossicles is also observed, especially of the stapes. The stapes may be entirely fixed to the facial nerve (Fig. 2).

These changes in the middle ear seem to be most typical for endemic cretinism (and "endemic deaf-mutism"), and have not been found in any other condition. Yet, apparently not all endemic cretins examined by Nager showed these alterations, which is in accord with the well-known fact that not all cretins are deaf.

Alterations in the inner ear have not been described with such regularity or specificity. In fact, atrophy of the organ of Corti, as well as other "degenerative changes," have been described by Mayer (2). Table II summarizes the results obtained by Nager (1) in his nine observations mentioned above. The histopathological

Table 1. Clinical features and middle ear lesions of nine "endemic deaf-mutes"[1]

Name Sex	Age Yrs.	Fam.[2]	Ht. cm[3]	"Cretin. features" Body[4]	Intellect[5]	Goiter[6]	Autopsy hr. postm.[7]	Audiol. exam[8]	Hypertr. bone changes[9]	Distort. windows[10]	Ossicle deform.[11]	Thick connect. tissue[12]
1.R.E. f	69	-	?	?	weak	++	24	A_1-e^6(r) A_1-f^6(l)	++	+	+	+
2.N.J. m	29	+dm	?	?	idiot	+	11	$e-h^5$(r) a^1-a^5(l)	+	+	+	+
3.K.M. f	52	+dm cr	118	typical	weak	+	26	e^1-c^5(r) c^1-e^5(l)	+	+	+	+
4.N.M. f	74	?	?	?	idiot	+	?	impossible	+	+	+	+
5.T.A. f	18	?	?	(-?)	(-?)	+	24	not done	++	+	+	
6.D.A. f	69	?(+) deb.	?	(-?)	weak	+	?	not done	+++	+	+	+
7.W.E. f	70	++dm/ deb.	?	?	weak	?	?	not done	+++	+	+	+
8.T.K. f	53	?	170	-	weak	+	8	convers. 100 cm	+++	+	+	+
9.K.F. m	38	+dm	"no."	-	intelligent	+	24	not done ("deaf")	+		+	+

1. Case evaluation by F. R. Nager:
   Typical endemic cretin (dwarfism, oligophrenia, deaf-mutism, goiter, motor abnormalities)-Case 3 (K.M.)
   "Endemic idiot" with congen.deaf-mutism, and goiter-Cases 2 (N.J.), 4 (N.M.), 6 (D.A.), 7 (W.E.), 8 (T.K.)
   Simple congen.deaf-mutism with goiter, normal intelligence and normal body build-Case 5 (T.A.), 9 (K.F.)

2. Family history: ? no clinical description in text
   - noncontributory
   +dm deaf-mutes or deaf in family
   cr cretin in family
   deb oligophrenia in family

3. Height in cm: ? no indication in text
   "no." in text no measure, but described as being of normal height

4. Description of the physical appearance in the text: ? no description
   - described as normal physically
   (-?) no clinical information about body build available to Nager - typical dwarfed, typical cretin

5. Description of the intellect in the text: **intelligent**, weak, idiot — mental status
   (-?) no information available to Nager

6. Presence and size of goiter

7. Time of autopsy in hours after death

8. Results obtained (or not) on audiologic examination:
   In case 1, 2, 3: range of hearing
   l = left ear
   r = right ear
   convers.100cm conversation understood at

9. Hypertrophic bone changes (hyperostosis) of promontorium

10. Distorted (eventually closed) round and oval windows

11. Deformation of the ossicles, particularly stapes

12. Thickened mucous membranes of the tympanic cavity

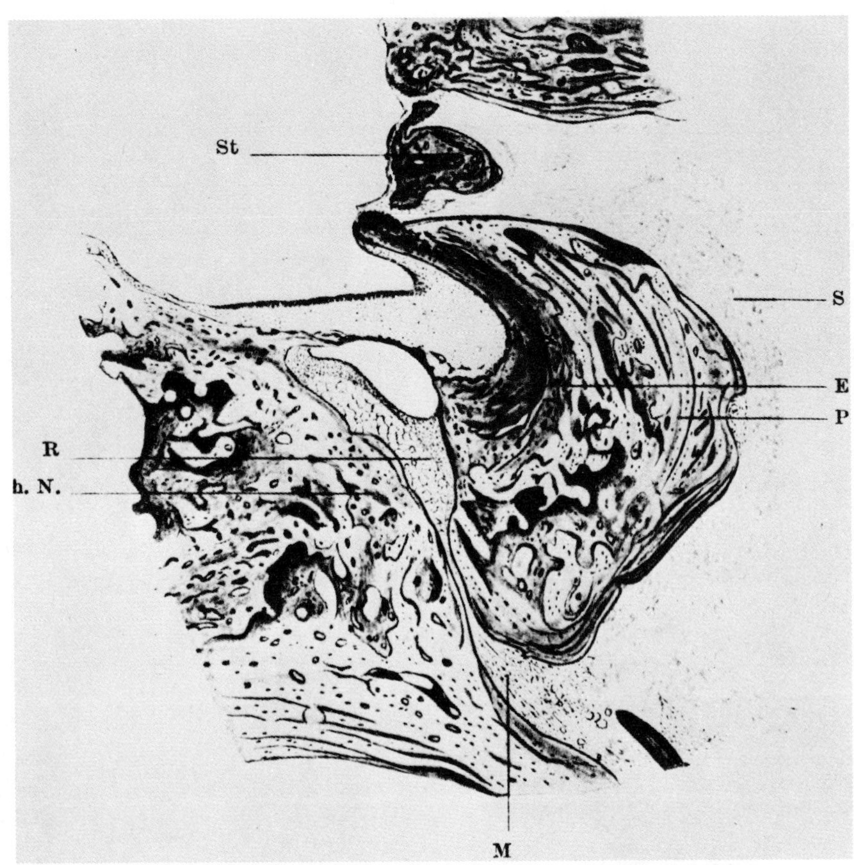

Fig. 1 Vertical section through window area of left petrous bone of a 69 yr old endemic deaf-mute (Case 1 in Table I and II). From Nager (5).

St distorted stapes
S acutely inflamed and thickened membrane of petrous bone
E enchondral labyrinthine capsule
P hyperostotic promontorium (thickened periostal labyr. capsule)
M tympanic mouth of the cochlear fossula
R cochlear fossula which is narrowed and filled with fat tissue
hN posterior wall of the cochlear fossula

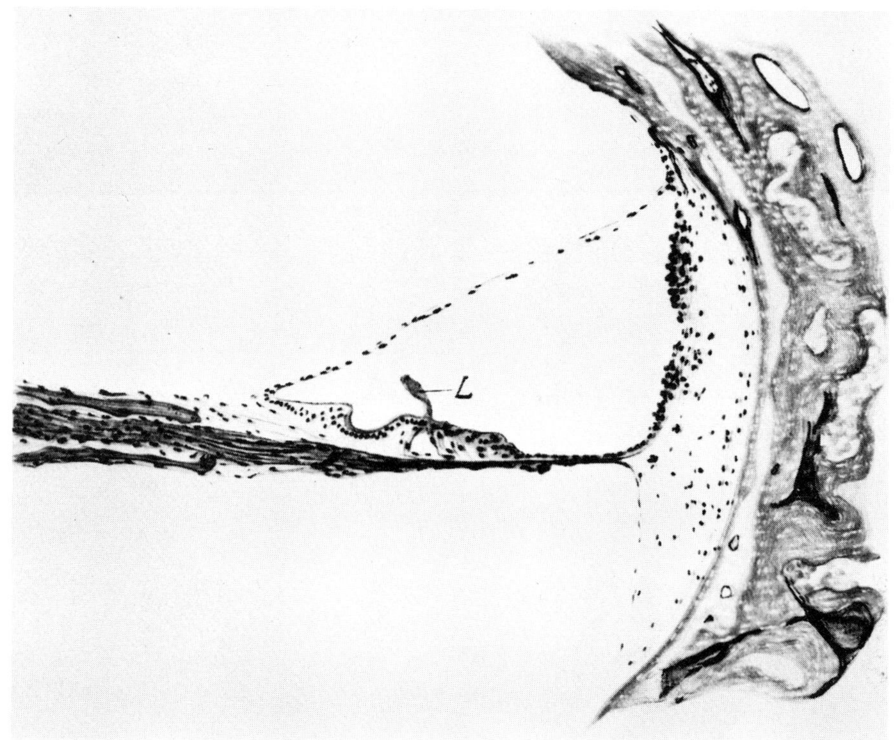

Fig. 2 Section through cochlea of endemic deaf-mute (70 yr old, same as Fig. 3). From Nager (5).

L hyaline streak between the tectorial membrane and the organ of Corti (tectorial membrane can scarcely be seen in the figure).

findings were discussed with great reservation by Nager (1), taking into account the importance of postmortem alterations and artifacts. The only specific derangement of endemic cretinism or deaf-mutism or both is, according to Nager (5), a hyaline streak between the tectorial membrane and the organ of Corti (Fig. 2).

Table 2. Histological findings in the inner ear of endemic deaf-mutes [F. R. Nager, 1921 (5)]

Case[1]	Hearing[2]	Histological fixatation[3]	Organ of Corti[4]	Spiral ganglion[5]	Vestib.[6]
1.R.E.	impaired	poor	flattened, irregular	atrophic	normal
2.N.J.	impaired	"fair"	partially absent or atrophic	reduced	normal
3.K.M.	impaired	unsatisfactory	flattened	much re-duced	normal
4.N.M.	?	unsatisfactory	normal	normal	normal
5.T.A.	?	"fair"	flattened	-	normal
6.D.A.	?	perfect	normal	reduced	normal
7.W.E.	?	unsatisfactory	cell masses hyaline streak	much re-duced	normal
8.T.K.	impaired	unsatisfactory	normal	normal	normal
9.K.F.	totally deaf	perfect	normal	normal	normal

1 Same cases as in Table I
2 Hearing evaluation according to the results summarized in Table I
3 Quality of histological fixation evaluated by Nager. In the original text there are no detailed descriptions of the different cell types
4 Evaluation of the organ of Corti
5 Evaluation of the spiral ganglia
6 Evaluation of the vestibular function by caloric testing

As may be seen in Table *2*, Nager also found some other alterations of the inner ear, such as flattened or atrophic organs of Corti and more or less pronounced atrophy or reduction of spiral ganglionic cells, but he was cautious in interpreting them. The morphologic changes described above have been reported by others, and all agree that changes vary considerably in severity, but that they are most specific for endemic cretinism with deafness.

DISCUSSION

One is surprised that the available information indicates that the principle lesions are uniformly located in the middle ear. Yet, with equal unanimity, the functional disturbance found by audiologic studies in endemic cretins, including our own (6), are described as receptive. The studies of Bargman and Gardner (7) and their chapter in this volume on otic lesions in congenitally hypothyroid chicks also show morphologic alterations in the inner ear (sensory hair cells of the accoustic papilla and cells of the spiral ganglion). One is tempted to the view that the basic defect of endemic deaf-mutism (in cretinous and non-cretinous individuals) is located in the inner ear, although there is no proof available. On the other hand, the changes in the middle ear, so typical for this condition,do not seem to be the main cause of this type of deafness, but rather are alterations mainly of the bone and are suggestive of a prenatal lesion. Finally, it may be mentioned that Siebenmann [quoted by Denker (3)] did not find any anomaly in the inner ear of a 13 yr old athyreotic ("sporadic") cretin.

SUMMARY

A review of the literature on the otic lesions in endemic cretinism and deaf-mutism is presented. The most typical and specific alterations described are in the middle ear and include a) hypertrophic bone changes of the promontorium, b) deformation of the ossicles with fixation of the stapes, c) distortions of the round and oval windows, and d) thickening of the mucous membrane of the tympanic cavity. The derangements of the inner ear are less specific and are not regularly found, in spite of the fact that endemic deafness has almost always been found to be perceptive. The definitive lesion of the inner ear may have been missed for technical reasons.

ACKNOWLEDGEMENTS

Figures 1 and 2 reprinted from Nager (5) by permission of the publishers, Springer-Verlag.

DISCUSSION BY PARTICIPANTS

ROSMAN: It is obvious that more detailed audiometric studies of cretins must be done. In addition, simple caloric tests of vestibular function could be done. Until this is done, it will be impossible to decide whether the damage is purely auditory or auditory and vestibular.

KOENIG: We examined about 12 of our cretins. Some of them were so frightened that we could get no data. In 10 we did audiometric tests. They had receptive-type hearing defects. Two of them had a middle-ear component. Nager in his review article (5) claims that he tested several endemic cretins with caloric tests and found normal vestibular function in all [Cf. also Table II, this chapter].

STANBURY: There is no central lesion that would cause such changes as are described for the middle and inner ear, are there?

ROSMAN: The changes that Dr. Koenig has described, predominantly bony changes, could be part of the general dysmorphic state of the cretin. Those changes may be unrelated to the pathogenesis of the deaf-mutism.

KOENIG: That is my impression. Throughout the literature they insist on how dramatic the bony changes were, and yet they insist that the otic lesion was receptive.

COSTA: Our otologists have found a high incidence of vestibular impairment in endemic cretins. Hearing loss and vestibular damage were not always commensurate; some patients with a "dead vestibule" possessed near normal hearing. The damage was generally bilateral; hearing loss was perceptive.

REFERENCES

1. Nager, F.R.: Weitere Beiträge zur Anatomie der endemischen Hörstörung. Z. Ohrenheilk. 80:107-174, 1921

2. Mayer, O.: quoted in Denker, A.: Die endemische Taubstumnheit. In: Hdb. Hals-Nasen-Ohrenheilkunde (A. Denker and A. Kahler, eds.). Vol. 8/III. Springer, Berlin, 1927. pp. 410-418.

3. Denker, A.: Die endemische Taubstummheit. In: Hdg. Hals-Nasen-Ohrenheilkunde (A. Denker and A. Kahler, eds.). Vol 8/III. Springer, Berlin, 1927. pp. 410-418.

4. Bircher, H.: *Der endemische Kropf und seine Beziehungen zur Taubstummheit und zum Cretinismus*. B. Schwabe, Basel, 1883.

5. Nager, F.R.: Die Beziehungen des endemischen Kretinismus zum Gehörorgan. In: *Hdb. Hals-Nasen-Ohrenheilkunde* (A. Denker and A. Kahler, eds.). Vol. 6/I. Springer, Berlin, 1926. pp. 617-635.

6. Koenig, M.P.: *Die kongenitale Hypothyreose und der endemische Kretinismus*. Springer, Berlin, 1968.

7. Bargman, G.J. and Gardner, L.I.: Otic lesions and congenital hypothyroidism in the developing chick. *J. Clin. Invest.* 46: 1828-1839, 1967.

SECTION 5
THE CENTRAL NERVOUS SYSTEM AND CRETINISM

THE NEUROPATHOLOGY OF CONGENITAL HYPOTHYROIDISM

N. Paul Rosman

Department of Pediatrics and Neurology, Boston University School of Medicine, Boston City Hospital, Boston, Massachusetts

INTRODUCTION AND REVIEW OF EARLIER STUDIES

While the association of congenital hypothyroidism with mental retardation has been recognized for many years (1), the pathophysiological mechanisms by which thyroid deficiency alters brain function are incompletely understood. The association is an important one, for the fundamental abnormality is biochemical and potentially reversible.

The anatomical basis for the mental subnormality that commonly accompanies congenital hypothyroidism is uncertain. Although the literature on the subject dates back to the 16th century, detailed pathological studies of the brains of patients have been surprisingly few and inconsistent with each other. The abnormalities recorded have included "vascular distention" (2), "reduction in brain weight" (3), "reduction in the cells of cerebral cortex" (4), "nerve cell loss and delayed myelinization" (5), "lack of development of cortical areas" (1), and "malformed convolutions with poor differentiation of the cortical layers" (6).

In one 18 month old cretin we found the brain to be well formed but very small, weighing only 570 gm (normal: 1,040 gm). The gyri were reduced in size, with a thin cortical ribbon and sparse underlying white matter. Microscopically, the neuronal population was decreased in all cortical layers. Similar changes were found in the cerebellum.

The variability of our observations and those of others emphasizes that no consistent pattern of brain lesions have been demonstrated. Clarification of this problem has been sought in the laboratory. Experimental animals have been made "hypothyroid" by a number of investigators and changes in the brains have been described. Morphological observations have included: a domed or disproportionately wide appearance to the brain, reduced brain weight, reduced numbers and dilatation of capillaries in the cerebral cortex, decreased size and increased density of cortical neurons, shorter and less frequently branched neuronal dendrites, decreased numbers of cortical axons (7,8,9,10,11), delayed disappearance of the cerebellar external granular layer (12), and retarded myelination of brain (13). Biochemical studies have been consistent with decreased numbers and reduced size of neurons in the rat cerebral cortex [as determined by increased DNA concentration with lowered RNA concentration per unit DNA (14)]. Quantitative histological determinations of nerve cell density have been confined almost exclusively to observations on the sensorimotor cortex (15). In the human cretin, one would anticipate no major difficulties in visual cortex (he is not blind), in auditory cortex (he very likely is not cortically deaf), in parietal cortex (he does not show other cortical sensory deficits) or in motor cortex (he does not invariably show pyramidal tract signs). Thus, the association cortex becomes highly suspect, but to date these areas have not been specifically studied. Biochemical studies have also shown reduced myelin content in brains of hypothyroid animals (16,17). Abnormal membranous bodies similar to those seen in Tay-Sachs disease in man have been found in electron micrographs of the visual cortex of hypothyroid rats (18).

All of these studies must be viewed with circumspection. The assumption has usually been made that the animal was hypothyroid at the time of study; in no instance have appropriate biochemical determinations, such as serum protein bound iodine, thyroxin or thyroid-stimulating hormone, been carried out. Thus there has been no confirmation or quantitation of the degree of the supposed hypothyroidism. Further, in virtually all of these studies there have been no adequate controls for poor nutritional intake. This is a serious deficiency, for Eayrs and Horn (19) and Horn (20) found a reduction in brain weight and axon density and an increased density of nerve cell bodies in malnourished animals. Benton _et al._ (21) have found impaired myelination in animals rendered nutritionally deficient in early life.

MATERIALS AND METHODS

NEURONAL CHANGES IN HYPOTHYROIDISM

The production of hypothyroidism was initially attempted by five separate methods using Sprague-Dawley rats: 1) Surgical thyroidectomy of newborn rats under anesthesia with cold (the mortality was prohibitively high, probably because of simultaneous removal of the parathyroid glands); 2) Administration of ^{131}I (200 microcuries) to pregnant female rats during the first half of pregnancy (this was abandoned because changes in the offspring could not be attributed solely to hypothyroidism. The lowered metabolic rate of the mother might have been deleterious to the fetuses. 3) In an attempt to induce hypothyroidism in the fetus without producing hypothyroidism in the mother, gravid rats were operated on under light ether anesthesia during the third week of pregnancy. The uterus was delivered through an abdominal incision and individual fetuses were injected intraperitoneally with 75 microcuries of ^{131}I through the uterine wall. The uterus was then replaced into the abdominal cavity, the incision closed and the mother allowed to deliver at term. The fetal loss with this method was about 30 percent of the injected fetuses. Since the fetal rat thyroid does not take up iodine until the 16th-17th day of a 21-day gestation (22), this method provided no significant advantage. 4) Administration of parenteral methimazole to pregnant female rats during gestation. (This method was effective, but the same objections as when pregnant mothers were given ^{131}I might be raised). 5) The intraperitoneal injection of ^{131}I (100 microcuries) to one-day old rats born to mothers maintained on an iodine-deficient diet (Nutritional Biochemicals Corp.) throughout the latter half of pregnancy [method of Goldberg and Chaikoff (23)]. This last method proved best for the studies reported here.

Accordingly, female rats at mid-term or near term of pregnancy were placed on an iodine-deficient diet and distilled water. Within 24 hours after birth, half of the pups of each litter were radiothyroidectomized by intraperitoneal injection of 100 microcuries of ^{131}I. The remaining pups each were injected intraperitoneally with 0.05 ml normal saline. All pups remained with their mothers until sacrificed.

The animals were weighed every other day. Two experimental animals and two control littermates were sacrificed by rapid exsanguination on each day. The thyroid gland was dissected from each animal and fixed in 10 percent formalin. Whole brains were removed and weighed. Each brain was cut sagitally; one half was fixed in formalin and the other was weighed and frozen for chemical analyses.

After fixation, the thyroid glands of rats from six to 31 days of age were embedded in paraffin. Eight-micra sections were cut and stained with hematoxylin-eosin.

The half-brains of animals sacrified on days 11, 14, 16, 19, 21, 22, 28 and 31 were embedded in paraffin, sectioned coronally at one mm intervals and stained with hematoxylin-eosin, cresyl violet, and by the Loyez method for myelin. Approximately 15 cross-sections of brain from each of eight pairs of animals were used for the study of myelination.

Biochemical studies were performed by Michael J. Malone, M.D. The frozen brain specimens were re-weighed on a Mettler balance and brought to room temperature in 19 volumes (ml per gm) of chloroform:methanol 2:1 (v/v). The specimens were homogenized in a ground glass homogenizer (Ten Broeck) and filtered. The filtrate was washed by addition of 0.2 volumes of 0.1 m KCl as described by Folch-Pi (24). The washed lower phase was separated and brought to a total volume of 10 ml by the addition of chloroform:methanol 2:1 (v/v).

Analyses were carried out on 1.0 to 0.5 ml aliquots of the washed total lipid extracts. Lipid hexose determinations were made by the anthrone method of Radin (25). Protein assays, an index of proteolipid content, were made by the method of Lowry (26). Lipid phosphorus determinations were carried out by the Bartlett modification of the Fiske-Subarow method (27). Measurements were expressed as mg per 100 gm of fresh weight.

NEURONAL CHANGES IN MALNUTRITION

Since it is well known that myelination is impaired in nutritionally deprived newborn rats (21,29,30) the question arose whether the changes in brains of hypothyroid animals might be specifically the result of thyroid hormone deficiency or might be secondary to malnutrition. Did hypothyroid animals, which weighed less than control littermates, compete less effectively for food and develop non-specific malnutritional changes in brain? In order to answer this question, malnourished rats were raised whose weights at all ages approximated those of the hypothyroid rats investigated during our earlier study.

Pregnant Sprague-Dawley white rats were fed an iodine-deficient diet (Nutritional Biochemicals Corp.) and distilled water beginning at midterm or near term of pregnancy. Within twenty-four hours after birth, the offspring from four to five litters were pooled. From this pool, groups of 20 newborns were placed with foster mothers. Since each foster mother had only a limited amount of milk for her large number of pups, the newborns became nutritionally deprived. A number of newborn rats were kept "in reserve" and used as necessary to supplement the malnourished groups. In this way, the mean body weights of these groups could be controlled; the more numerous the suckling rats, the lower their mean body weight.

The animals were weighed several times each week. Two malnourished animals were sacrified by rapid exsanguination every other day. Thyroid glands were removed, weighed on a Sartorius balance and fixed in formalin. Each brain was removed, weighed and cut sagitally; one half was fixed in formalin for histological study and one half was weighed and frozen for chemical analyses. Histological preparations of brains and thyroids and biochemical analyses of brains (proteolipid and lipid hexose determinations) were performed as reported elsewhere (31). Data obtained from these malnourished animals were compared with those from the investigations on neonatally thyroidectomized and control animals.

RESULTS

A. *HYPOTHYROID ANIMALS*

Body and Brain Growth. Total body weights of the hypothyroid rats were less than those of their control littermates, and this weight difference increased with age. The hypothyroid animals showed a cessation of body growth after 24 days. The brains of these animals were also smaller than those of their littermates, especially after 14 days. This difference increased with age, but at all ages the difference in brain weights was less marked than the disparity in body weights (Figs. 1, 2, 3).

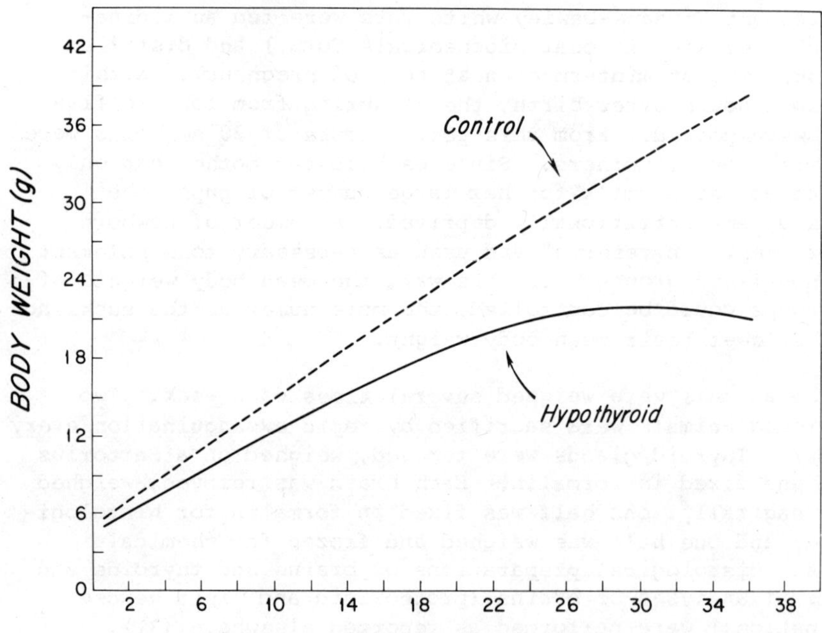

Fig. 1. Body growth in hypothyroid and control rats (31).

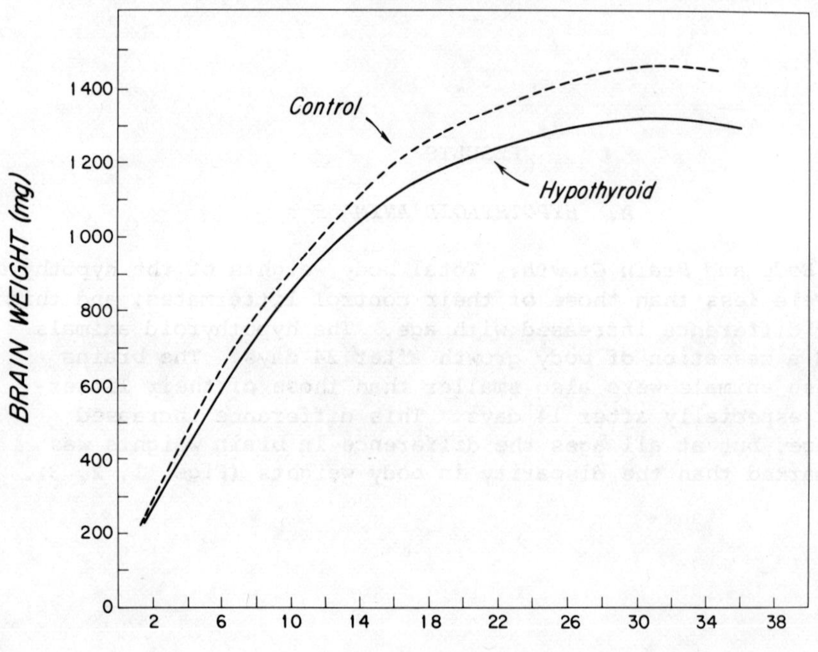

Fig. 2. Brain growth in hypothyroid and control rats (31)

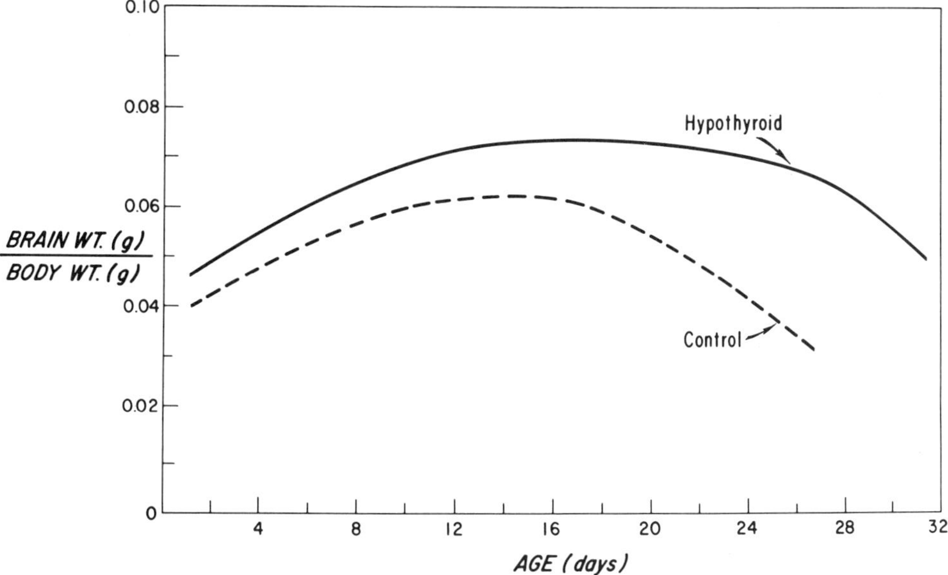

Fig. 3. Ratio of brain:body growth in hypothyroid and control rats (31).

Histological Studies of Thyroid Gland. The thyroid glands of all control animals were normal, with well-formed follicles. Colloid deposition was evident in specimens older than six days. Radiothyroidectomized rats from six days on showed total destruction of thyroid tissue with effacement of the normal follicular pattern and extensive cell loss. At eleven days most of the thyroid gland was replaced by connective tissue; at twenty-one days hyaline was present; at thirty-one days a foreign body giant cell reaction was noted. The parathyroid glands were histologically normal in both groups of animals.

Histological Studies of Brain. In sections stained for myelin by the Loyez method, a consistent distinction could be made after 14 days between hypothyroid and control specimens. The brains of hypothyroid animals showed less myelination when compared with those of their control littermates. Myelination of all tracts was approximately three to six days "delayed" in the hypothyroid animals. Myelination in the 19 day old hypothyroid animals resembled that in 16 day old controls; that in 28 day old hypothyroid animals was comparable to that in 22 day old controls. The sequence of myelination in different tracts was identical in both groups. The delay was present at each of the ages studied (14 days to 31 days). There was no histological evidence for active myelin breakdown (Figs. 4-7).

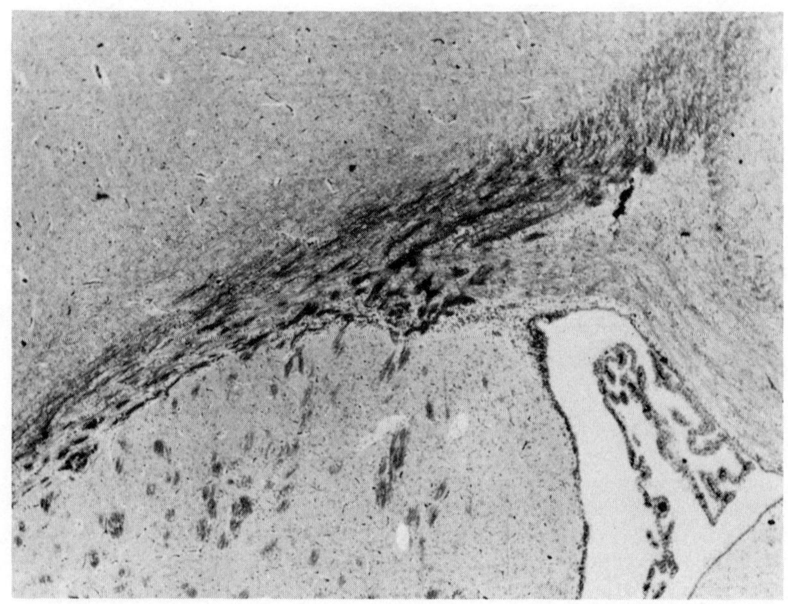

Fig. 4. 22 day old control rat. Coronal section of brain at level of corpus striatum. Normal myelination of radiation of corpus callosum. Loyez stain X40.

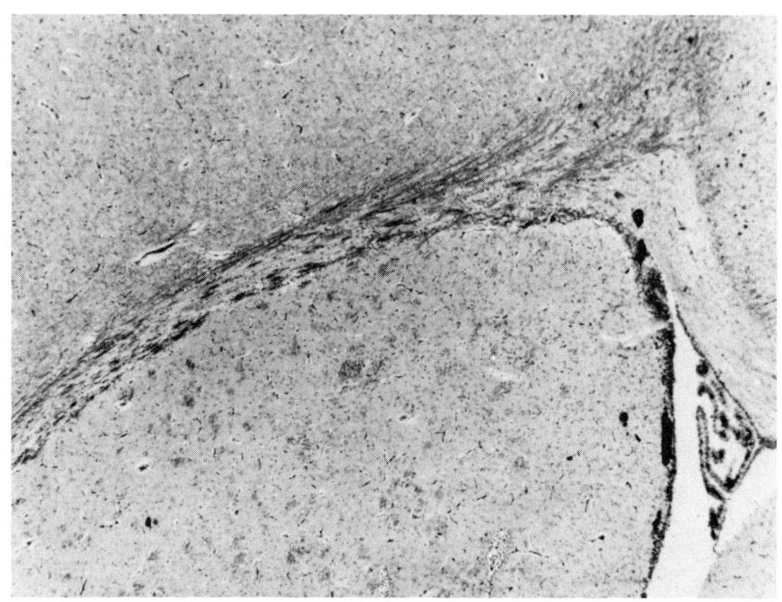

Fig. 5. 22 day old hypothyroid rat. Littermate of rat in Fig. 4. Coronal section of brain at level of corpus striatum. Considerably reduced myelination of radiation of corpus callosum. Loyez stain X40.

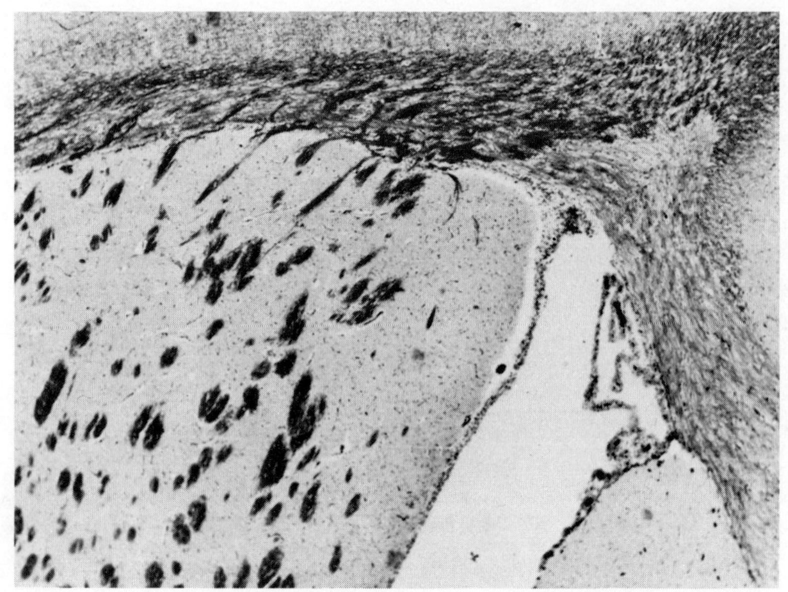

Fig. 6. 31 day old control rat. Coronal section of brain at level of corpus striatum. Normal myelination of corpus striatum and radiation of corpus callosum. Loyez stain X40.

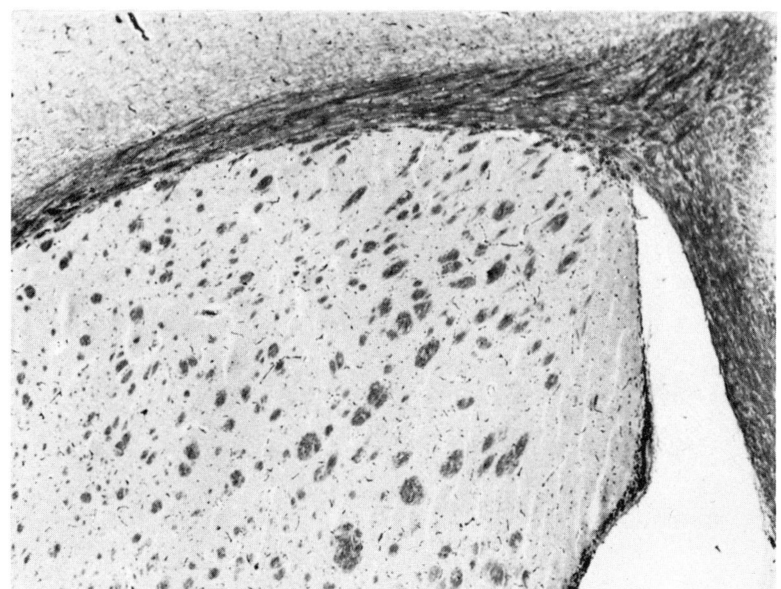

Fig. 7. 31 day old hypothyroid rat. Littermate of rat in Fig. 6. Coronal section of brain at level of corpus striatum. Considerably reduced myelination of corpus striatum and radiation of corpus callosum. Loyez stain X40.

A survey of brain sections stained with hematoxylin-eosin and cresyl violet disclosed a delay in the disappearance of the external granular layer of the cerebellar cortex in the hypothyroid animals. Otherwise, there was no apparent change in the number, appearance or arrangement of neurons in the hypothyroid animals at any age.

Biochemical Studies of Brain. Total lipid hexose (cerebroside and sulfatide) and proteolipid, which in the brain occur principally in myelin, differed significantly after 12 days between control and hypothyroid brains. In the latter, these biochemical indices of myelination were delayed in appearance and failed to reach the levels present in mature (31 day) control animals. The pattern of proteolipid increase followed a sigmoid curve of maturation between 12 and 24 days in the control animals. This critical period was delayed in the hypothyroid rats until

18-26 days, and total accumulation of the myelin lipids was decreased (Fig. 8).

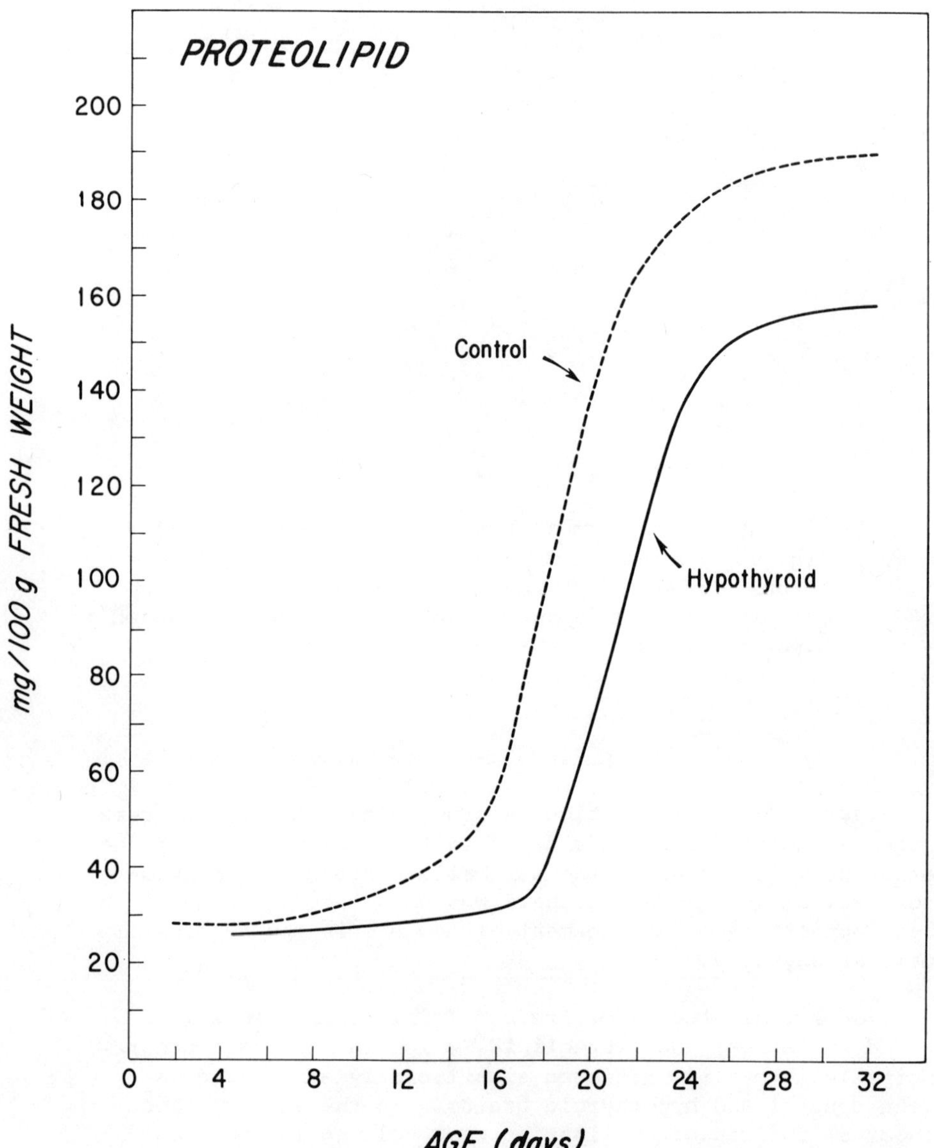

Fig. 8. Proteolipid content in brains of hypothyroid and control rats (31).

These differences were even more striking in the lipid hexose measurements, where the critical period in the hypothyroid rats was delayed until days 20 to 30 (Fig. 9.).

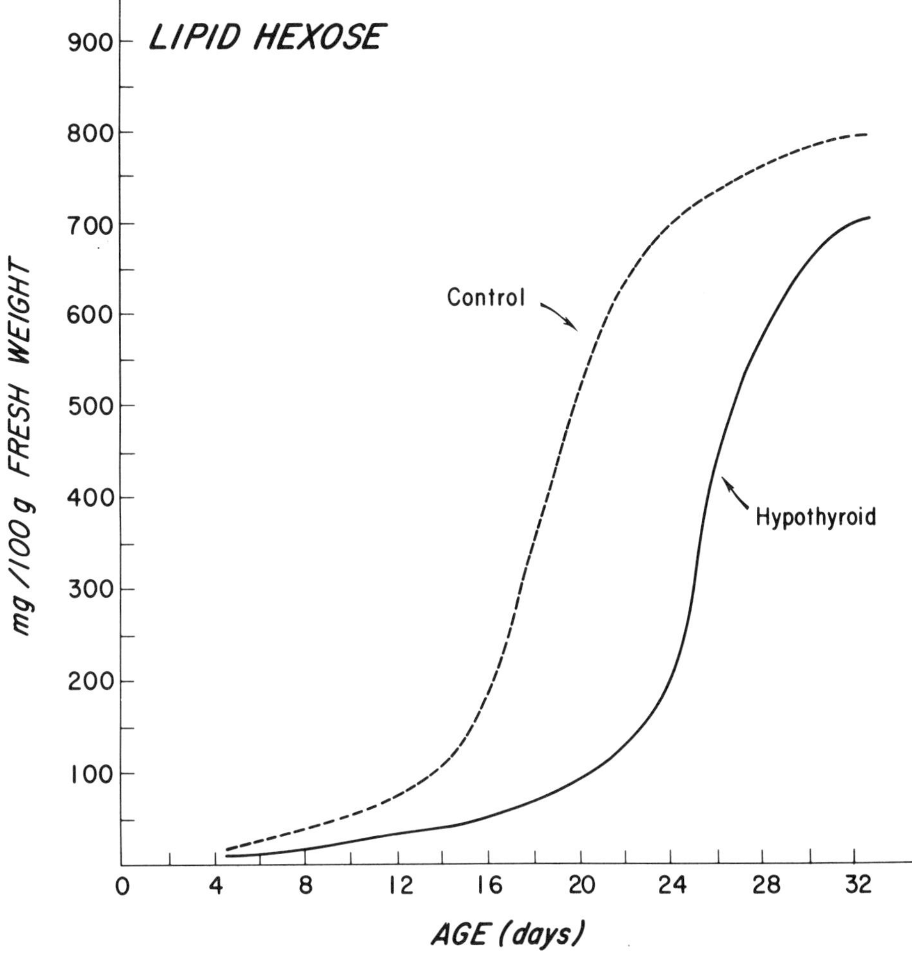

Fig. 9. Lipid hexose content in brains of hypothyroid and control rats (31).

B. *MALNOURISHED ANIMALS*

Body and Brain Growth. Mean total body weights of the malnourished animals were slightly lower than those of the hypothyroid rats of the same ages until the 28th day, after which they were slightly higher. There was no cessation of total body growth as in the hypothyroid animals after 24 days, and by the end of the experiment at 34 days, the malnourished curve had not leveled off. The wet weights of whole brains of the malnourished rats were approximately equal to those of the hypothyroid animals, slightly less until day 16, and then slightly greater. As in the hypothyroid animals, brain growth of the malnourished animals was not as severely retarded as was total body growth (Figs. 10,11).

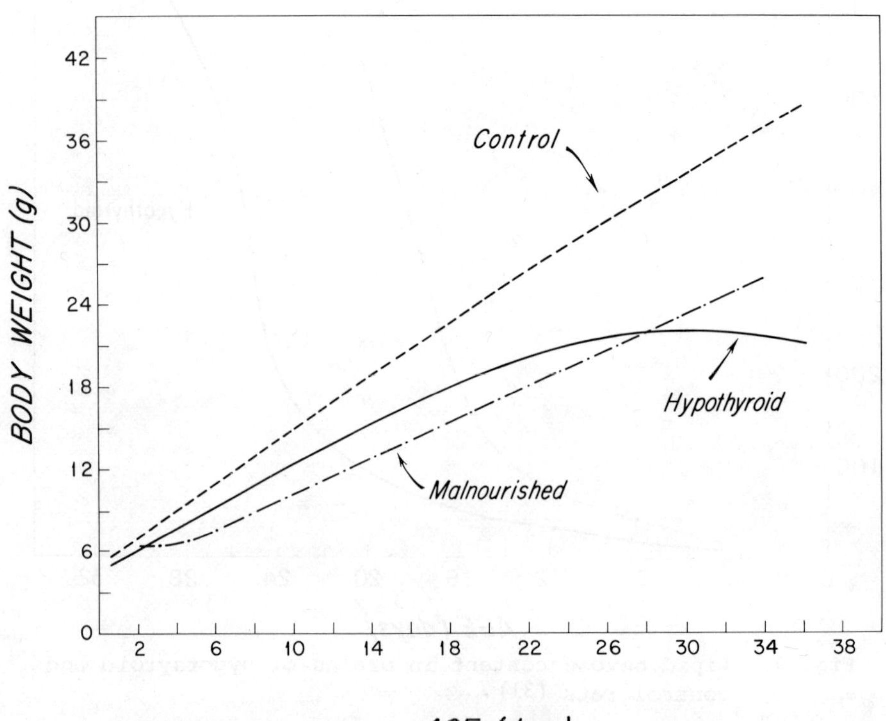

Fig. 10. Body growth in control, malnourished and hypothyroid rats.

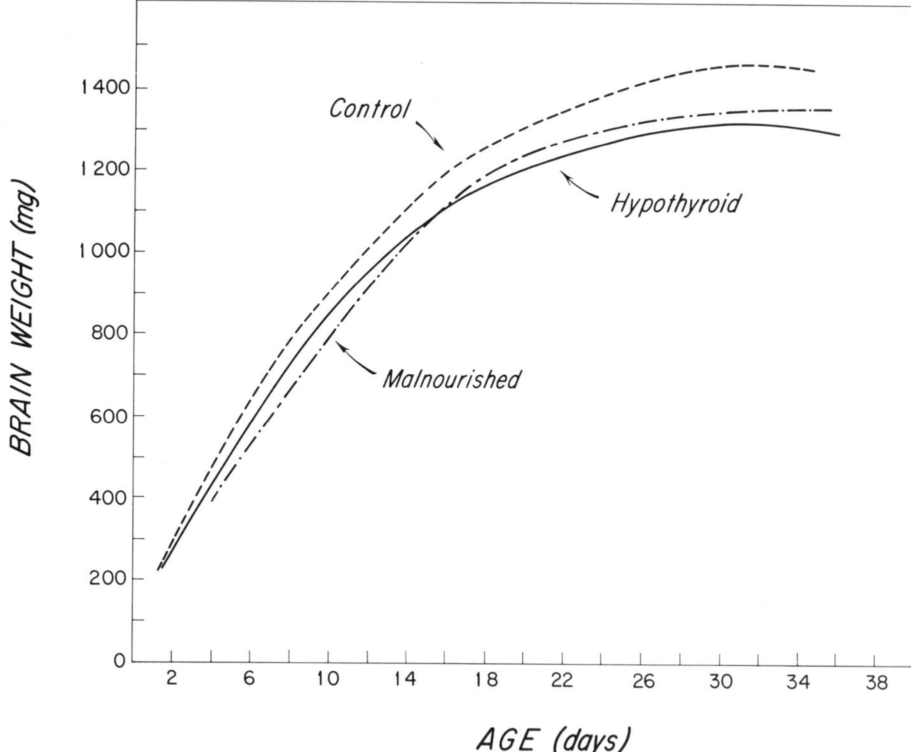

Fig. 11. Brain growth in control, malnourished and hypothyroid rats.

Histological Studies of Thyroid Gland. Thyroid glands from malnourished rats studied at 14 and 28 days were normal.

Histological Studies of Nervous System. Coronal sections of malnourished rat brains stained for myelin disclosed less myelin than did the control brains. These changes were obvious by 16 days of age and were present in all white matter tracts. At all ages, however, myelination in malnourished rat brains was greater than in the hypothyroid rat brains (Figs. 12,13).

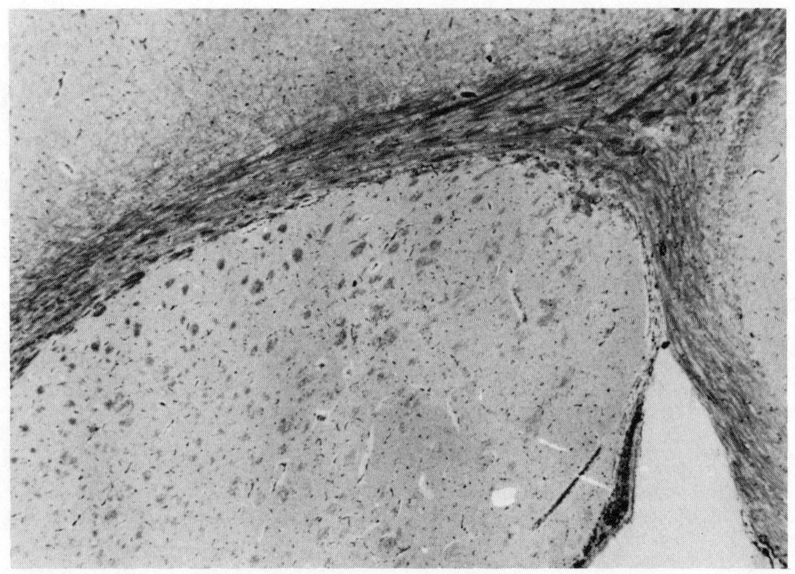

Fig. 12. 22 day old malnourished rat. Coronal section of brain at level of corpus striatum. Slightly reduced myelination of corpus striatum and radiation of corpus callosum. Loyez stain X40.

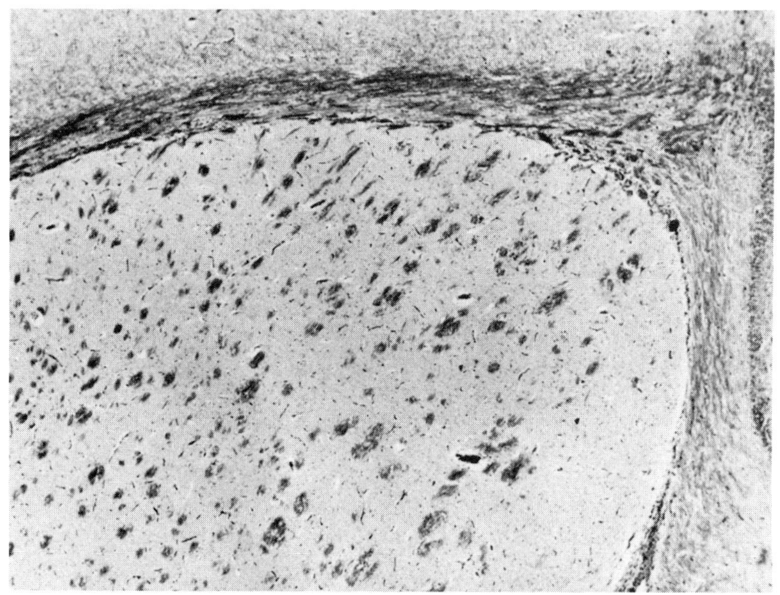

Fig. 13. 32 day old malnourished rat. Coronal section of brain at level of corpus striatum. Slightly reduced myelination of corpus striatum and radiation of corpus callosum. Loyez stain X40.

Biochemical Studies of Brain. Proteolipid was slightly greater in malnourished than in control brains until 15 days of age. From 16 to 28 days the appearance of proteolipid in malnourished brains followed a sigmoid curve, slightly below control values but well above the amounts present in hypothyroid brains. Thereafter, the proteolipid values in malnourished brains were somewhat higher than in the controls (Fig. 14).

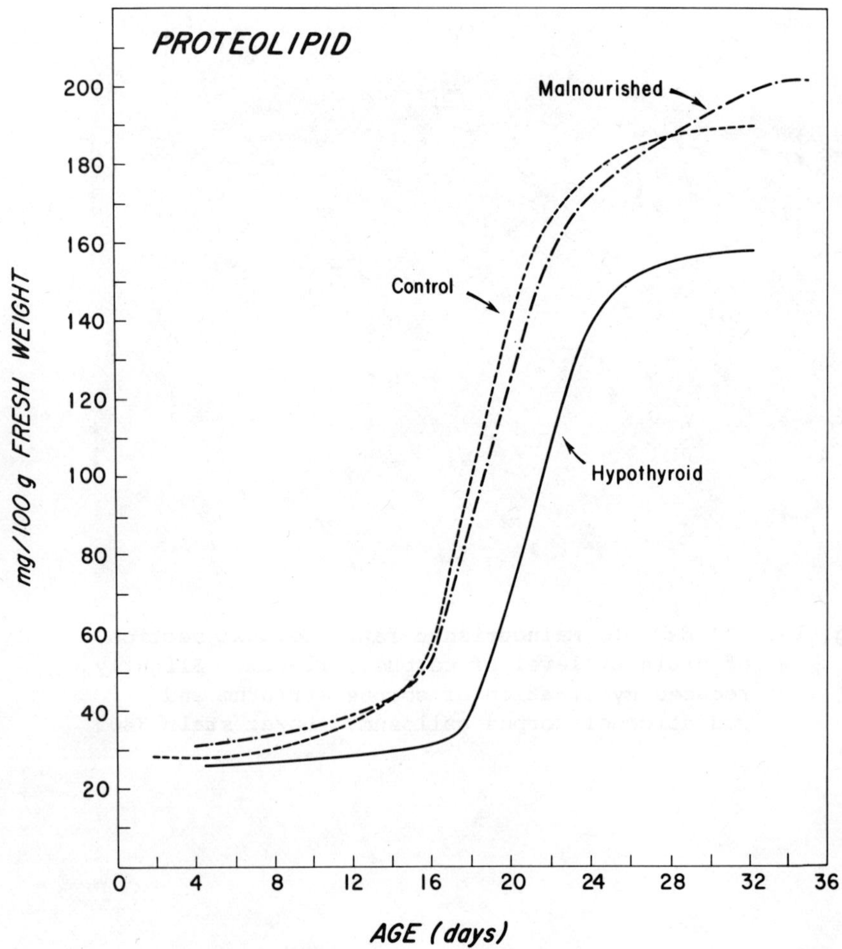

Fig. 14. Proteolipid content in brains of control, malnourished and hypothyroid rats.

Total lipid hexose (cerebroside and sulfatide) was slightly less in malnourished than in control brains until 19 days of age. Amounts of lipid hexose in malnourished brains then overlapped the control curve until 22 days, after which values from the malnourished brains were slightly elevated over control values. At all ages, lipid hexose content in the malnourished brains was considerably greater than in the hypothyroid brains (Fig. 15).

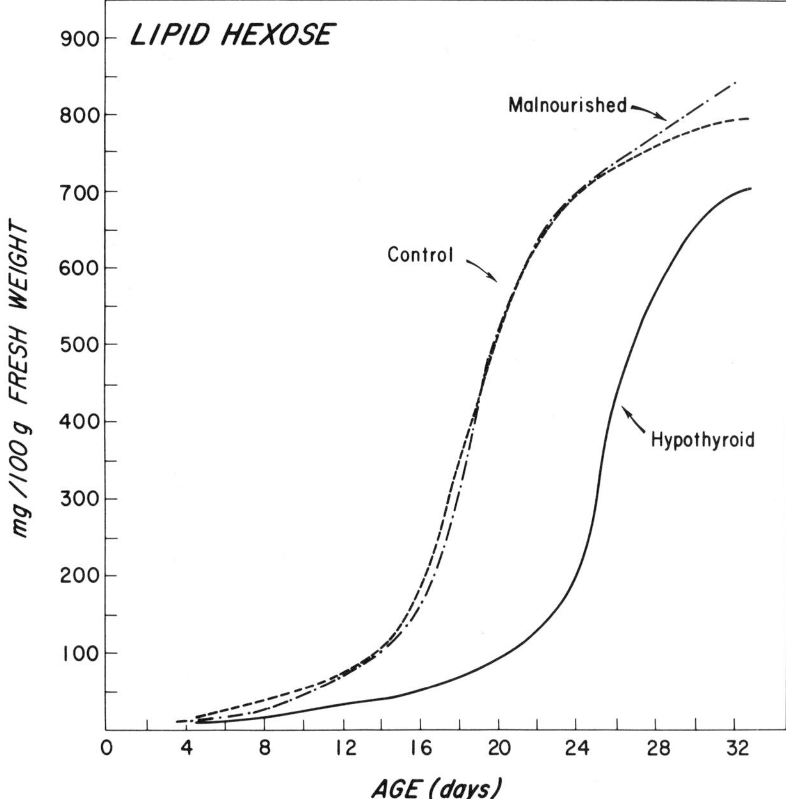

Fig. 15. Lipid hexose content in brains of control, malnourished and hypothyroid rats.

DISCUSSION

Maturation of the nervous system, in most mammal species, is incomplete at birth. A species-specific critical period in brain development marks the transition from immature to mature structure. This critical period is manifested morphologically by completion of most of the myelination of the brain (32). The transition is characterized biochemically by an increase in myelin lipids, such as cerebroside, sulfatide and proteolipid, which follow a sigmoid curve to mature brain levels (24).

Retardation of myelination can be effected by nutritional deprivation (33), by congenital or genetic disorders (34), and by metabolic deficiency states such as neonatal hypothyroidism (16,17). Accordingly we have studied the effect of hypothyroidism and of malnutrition in early life on myelination of brain, using a complementary morphological and biochemical approach.

Cerebral maturation in the hypothyroid animal has been assessed by a variety of methods. These include behavioral (35), neuropathological and biochemical studies (36). Much of the earlier work was of a cytohistological nature (11), and relatively little attention was given to myelinogenesis in spite of Barrnett's earlier observation of decreased myelin formation in the hypothyroid animal (13). Two recent studies of neonatal thyroid deficiency have shown that meylination, as judged by chemical parameters, is delayed (16,17). In neither investigation, however, was there an accompanying morphological study of brain.

The present investigation has shown that rats injected postnatally with radio-iodine were rendered hypothyroid, as evidenced by total destruction of thyroid tissue. These histopathological alterations were severe by the 11th day of age. Neonatal hypothyroidism retarded body growth more than brain growth, with cessation of overall weight gain after three to four weeks. These observations are in agreement with those of Rosenthal and Doljanski (37). Hypothyroidism also caused a delay in myelination of brain which was evident both by morphologic and biochemical criteria. The morphologic appearance of myelination correlated well with the companion biochemical criteria.

Myelin is a complex lipid and lipid-protein aggregate. It is formed by Schwann cells in the peripheral nervous system and by oligodendroglia in the central nervous system (38,39). Cerebroside, sulfatide and proteolipid have classically been regarded as myelin components. Cerebroside may be the most sensitive index of myelination (16). Recent investigations on "purified myelin" preparations have further established these complex lipid and lipid-protein aggregates as myelin sheath components (40). Proteolipid may represent the matrix material of the myelin lamellae.

Walravens and Chase (17) studied the effect of neonatal hypothyroidism on the accumulation of myelin sheath lipids in rat brain specimens at 18 days and found a reduction in cerebroside, sulfatide and cholesterol. Balázs et al. (16) found reduced cerebroside but normal cholesterol and phospholipid content in brain specimens from 35 day-old cretinous rats. Cuaron (41) also found no modification of lipid phosphorus accumulation in hyperthyroidism. Phospholipids, however, are relatively insensitive indices of myelination. Balazs et al. (16) suggest that the delayed myelination in hypothyroidism may be related either to altered metabolism of oligodendroglial cells or to decreased available axonal surface.

The deposition of myelin lipids defines the species-specific critical period in brain maturation, which, in the present study, occurred in control rats from 12 to 24 days. The accumulation of lipid hexose in developing brains of hypothyroid rats was more delayed than that of the proteolipid. The developmental sigmoid curve was shifted to the right and mature levels were never attained. In view of the postulated primary role of thyroxine in stimulating protein biosynthesis (42), our finding that neonatal ^{131}I-induced hypothyroidism had a greater effect on the accumulation of lipid hexose than on that of proteolipid was unexpected. An explanation may lie in the heterogeneity of the chloroform:methanol-soluble protein from whole brain. Gonzalez-Sastre (43) demonstrated that purified myelin protein consists of 26 percent basic protein, 63 percent proteolipid and 10 percent Wolfgram protein. The basic protein fraction may be the most sensitive index of myelination. Eng *et al.* (44) suggest that the myelin protein forms a template upon which myelin lipids are oriented. The basic protein fraction has been viewed as the structural feature of this template. Since the basic protein is present only in small amounts in the chloroform: methanol extract of whole brain, a selective effect on this fraction might not be detected by the present assay methods. If this is true, the influence of neonatal hypothyroidism might be seen to a greater extent in the lipid hexose determinations. A selective effect of neonatal hypothyroidism on the formation of basic protein is presently being investigated in purified myelin preparations.

Our earlier studies (31) and those reported here have shown that myelination in malnourished animals, as determined histologically, was intermediate between that in control animals and the more pronounced disturbance of myelinogenesis in the hypothyroid rats. This intermediate position was corroborated by the biochemical measurements of proteolipid and lipid hexose. These histological and biochemical differences between hypothyroid and malnourished brains indicate that the changes observed in hypothyroid animals could not be due solely to non-specific nutritional deprivation. The differences between hypothyroid and malnourished groups are further emphasized by the similar body weights of the two groups. In actuality, the mean body weights of the malnourished animals were less than those of the hypothyroid animals. In spite of this, myelination was greater in the former. Neonatal hypothyroidism thus exerts a specific effect, a delay in myelinogenesis which is distinct from that seen with non-specific nutritional deprivation.

Our data also show that brain growth is less affected by malnutrition than is general body growth. This relative priority enjoyed by brain over general somatic demands for available nutrients parallels the clinical observations of Stoch and Smythe (45,46).

Malnutrition, in contrast to thyroid deprivation, seemed to cause greater retardation of the accumulation of proteolipid than of lipid hexose in brain. The delay in synthesis of myelin constituents induced by neonatal hypothyroidism persisted throughout the period of study and may represent an irreversible effect. By contrast, in the later stages of development of malnourished animals, we found that the accumulation of myelin constituents increased abruptly and exceeded control values. This rise may reflect continued and even increased activity of myelin synthetic processes at that time. Malnutrition-induced delay in myelinogenesis seems to be a less severe insult than hypothyroidism and, in spite of the occurrence of malnutrition during a critical period of maturation, the pathological changes may not be irreversible.

These studies have been carried out on whole brain preparations. The measurements were complicated by the presence of major non-myelin constituents. This poses a particular problem in the case of very immature brains. In order to attempt more specific differentiation, complementary morphological and biochemical studies are presently being undertaken on purified myelin preparations from control, hypothyroid and malnourished animals.

SUMMARY

The effects of neonatal hypothyroidism on brain development have been studied by a combined morphological and biochemical approach. Hypothyroid rats showed a persistent histological retardation of myelination throughout the critical period of myelin formation. These morphological results correlated well with the chemical findings of reduced proteolipid and lipid hexose in brain.

In order to assess a possible role of malnutrition in the previously observed retardation of myelinogenesis caused by hypothyroidism, morphological and biochemical studies were also carried out on neonatally malnourished animals. The effects of neonatal hypothyroidism were shown to be significantly greater than the delayed myelinogenesis attributable to nutritional deprivation. Thus, the changes produced in maturing brains of neonatally thyroidectomized rats cannot be explained simply as non-specific nutritional deprivation.

ACKNOWLEDGEMENTS

This research was supported in part by a grant from the Charles H. Hood Dairy Foundation and Grant 5-RO1-NS-07751 from the U.S. Public Health Service, National Institute of Neurological Diseases and Stroke.

Figures 1-9 reprinted by permission from Neurology.

DISCUSSION BY PARTICIPANTS

HORNABROOK: I am inclined to believe that the neuropathology of the syndrome we are discussing arises far earlier in fetal life than that in most experiments that Dr. Rosman mentioned. The damage to the nervous system might occur during neuronal proliferation rather than during myelination. I know of no accurate histological descriptions of the brain in endemic cretinism.

PRETELL: I think Dr. Rosman's relating prematurity to spastic diplegia is interesting. I wonder how many of the newborns in the endemic area are premature. How often is spastic diplegia seen in prematures? Secondly, did you check thyroid function by any standard method in the experiment where only malnutrition was being investigated?

ROSMAN: Spastic diplegia is very frequent in prematurity. However, many prematures with or without spastic diplegia are intelligent. Famous examples include Churchill, Voltaire and Hugo. Nonetheless, the frequency of mental retardation is greater in premature infants than in those of normal birth weight. We did not do PBIs on our malnourished animals, but we have sera from them and these determinations could be done. The thyroid glands in those animals that we studied were histologically normal, and I would guess that the PBIs will also be normal. A problem in doing PBIs in rats is that they are normally low, so that one is working within a narrow range. Radioiodine uptake assay very likely will be a more sensitive test.

MOSIER: You were rather hard on the investigators who have not done PBIs. Do you have any reason to believe that if you give 100 microcuries of radioisotope that one is likely not to get hypothyroidism?

ROSMAN: Yes, on two bases. First, we studied 134 animals and it is apparent that the degree of thyroid destruction with a given dose of ^{131}I is variable. It is also apparent that the degree of myelinization of brain, determined histologically and biochemically, is variable in two littermates of the same body weight. I do not think you can equate the giving of radioactive iodine with clinical hypothyroidism. Probably most of the animals given this dose are hypothyroid, but it behooves the investigator to prove it.

HERSHMAN: There is both histochemical and hormone assay data showing that hypothyroid rats have decreased growth hormone in the pituitary and decreased secretion of growth hormone. Could your findings be explained by a lack of growth hormone?

ROSMAN: Your comment on growth hormone opens a whole range of possibilities. We simply have not done assays.

BALÁZS: There are a few reports on the effect of administration of growth hormone on the symptomatology of thyroid deficiency. As far as I know, there is only one paper (47) in which the claim is made that the success of the treatment with growth hormone in reversing the consequences of thyroid deficiency is similar in many respects to that of thyroid hormone therapy; other investigators have reported that growth hormone resulted in no or only slight improvement in the various parameters studied (48-50)

DELANGE: Are there critical periods for the effects you have found?

ROSMAN: Yes. If animals given radioactive iodine on day one are given replacement hormone within the first two weeks of postnatal life, these changes will be prevented. Such studies have been done by Eayrs (11) on neuronal populations. A disappointing aspect of many of Eayrs' anatomical studies has been the lack of accompanying photographs. Most of the neural development in the rat has occurred by three and one-half weeks of postnatal life, so that if, for example, the animals were made hypothyroid at six weeks, very little alteration would be produced.

MOSIER: With the large dose of radioactive iodine that you gave, would there be any effect on other tissue, such as the anterior pituitary?

DEGROOT: They probably get about 70 rads whole-body radiation.

PITTMAN: Iodine is concentrated in the choroid plexus, which might affect the brain.

KOENIG: Did you choose myelination because you thought it was the most important factor? I ask this question because Lotmar in 1929 and 1931 (51,52) did postmortem studies on the brains of endemic cretins and one athyreotic cretin. He concluded that the destruction or distortion he found occurred in the fifth or sixth fetal month. What you described would occur much later.

ROSMAN: I concentrated on myelination for several reasons: first, the motor defect. A spastic diplegia resulting from cerebral cortical lesions would involve a major portion of both cerebral cortices. Less extensive white matter involvement could produce the same deficit. Second, if one wants to study the cerebral cortex in this situation, one has two choices - to do cerebral cell counts (which can be a lifetime work) or to do biochemical assays. Third, Barrnett's studies dating back to 1948 (13) showed myelination to be impaired in hypothyroidism. Fourth, myelination is a very good marker of neural development. I am not suggesting that the primary brain lesion in hypothyroidism is necessarily an affection of myelin. If there is an abnormality in the cerebral cortex, and nerve cells die or fail to develop, myelin becomes secondarily affected. There was no evidence for active myelin breakdown in any of our animals, however. In summary, in hypothyroidism, myelinization is clearly delayed, but this could be secondary to impaired development of the cerebral cortex.

MOSIER: There has been work on the ratio of palmitic and oleic acids in brain lipids in the head-irradiated rat. After x-irradiation of the head at two days of age there is a delay in the maturation of the ratio (53).

ERMANS: Are these lesions reversible?

ROSMAN: Our studies suggest that in hypothyroidism the lesion may not be reversible, whereas in malnutrition the potential for reversibility is greater. To extrapolate to the clinical situation, it may be that malnutrition, if treated early, has a greater chance of being reversed than hypothyroidism. It is apparent clinically that cretins treated with appropriate therapy at an early age often do well, but sometimes do not. One wonders if there is a stage at which lesions occur and cannot be altered, despite replacement therapy.

I mentioned that we primed the mothers for the administration of radioactive iodine to the offspring by giving them an iodine-deficient diet provided by Nutritional Biochemicals Corporation. This is unfortified diet, and these animals don't grow well when compared with rats maintained on standard rat chow. We kept some animals on this iodine-deficient diet, noted the growth retardation, and at about four months of age noticed that they developed a profound paralysis of the hindlimbs. We obtained single-cell electrophysiological recordings from the hindlimb muscles of such animals at 35 days of age. The responses showed a lower amplitude and longer duration than those from control animals. These changes suggest an abnormality of muscle, and in particular, of muscle membrane. Pathologically one can see classical myopathic changes, with variability in muscle fiber shape and size, many small muscle fibers and muscle fiber necrosis. We are now studying seven different groups of animals on different diets:

1. Iodine-deficient diet.
2. Iodine-deficient diet supplemented with sodium iodide.
3. Iodine-deficient diet with supplemental vitamins.
4. Iodine-deficient diet with supplemental minerals.
5. Iodine-deficient diet with supplemental casein.
6. Iodine-deficient diet with all supplements but iodide.
7. Standard rat chow.

If iodide supplementation alone (group 2) prevents the development of the muscle changes, we will have shown something potentially important. Animals on an iodine-deficient diet (and by extension cretins on a low-iodine diet) may exhibit weakness in the lower limbs not only from central nervous system abnormalities, but also from muscle abnormalities.

REFERENCES

1. Smith, D.W., Blizzard, R.W. and Wilkins, L.: The mental prognosis in hypothyroidism of infancy and childhood. J. Pediatr. 19:1011, 1957.

2. Whipham, T.: Myxedema. Cerebral vascular change noted at autopsy. Lancet, I:709, 1885.

3. Mott, F.W.: The changes in the central nervous system in hypothyroidism. Proc. R. Soc. Med. 10:51, 1917.

4. Marinesco, M.G.: Contribution a l'étude des lesions du myxedeme congenital. (Idiotic myxodemateuse du Bourneville). Encephale, 19:265, 1924.

5. Benda, C.E.: Mongolism and Cretinism. Grune and Stratton, New York, 1946.

6. Beierwaltes, W.W., Carr, E.A., Raman, G., Spafford, N.R., Aster, R.A. and Lowrey, G.E.: Institutionalized cretins in the state of Michigan. J. Mich. State Med. Soc., 58:1077, 1959.

7. Eayrs, J.T. and Taylor, S.H.: The effect of thyroid deficiency induced by methyl thiouracil on the maturation of the central nervous system. J. Anat. 85:350, 1951.

8. Eayrs, J.T.: The vascularity of the cerebral cortex in normal and cretinous rats. J. Anat., 88:164, 1954.

9. Eayrs, J.T.: The cerebral cortex of normal and hypothyroid rats. Acta. Anat., 25:160-183, 1955.

10. Eayrs, J.T.: Effects of thyroid hormones on brain differentiation. Ciba Foundation Study Group #18, Little Brown and Co., Boston, 1964. pp. 60-74.

11. Eayrs, J.T.: Thyroid and central nervous development. In: The Scientific Basis of Medicine Annual Reviews, 1966. pp. 317-339.

12. Hamburgh, M., Lynn, E., and Weiss, E.P.: Analysis of the influence of thyroid hormone on prenatal and postnatal maturation of the rat. Anat. Rec. 150:147, 1964.

13. Barrnett, R.J.: Quoted in Pincus, C., Thimann, K.V., The Hormones. New York Acad. Press, 1948.

14. Geel, S.E. and Timiras, P.S.: The influence of neonatal hypothyroidism and of thyroxine on the ribonucleic acid and deoxyribonucleic acid concentrations of rat cerebral cortex. Brain Res. 4:135, 1967.

15. Eayrs, J.T. and Goodhead, B.: Postnatal development of the cerebral cortex in the rat. J. Anat., 93:385, 1959.

16. Balázs, R., Brooksbank, B.W., Davison, A.N., Eayrs, J.T. and Wilson, D.A.: The effect of neonatal thyroidectomy on myelination in the rat brain. Brain Res. 15:219-232 1969.

17. Walravens, P. and Chase, H.P.: Influence of thyroid on formation of myelin lipids. J. Neurochem. 16:1477-1484, 1969.

18. Cragg, B.G.: Synapses and membranous bodies in experimental hypothyroidism. Brain Res. 18:297-307, 1970.

19. Eayrs, J.T. and Horn, C.: The development of cerebral cortex in hypothyroid and starved rats. Anat. Rec. 121:53, 1955.

20. Horn, G.: Thyroid deficiency and inanition. Anat. Rec. 121:63, 1955.

21. Benton, J.W., Moser, W.W., Dodge, P.R. *et al*: Modification of the schedule of myelination in the rat by early nutritional deprivation. *Pediatr.* 38:801, 1966.

22. Speert, H., Quimby and Warner, S.C.: Radioiodine uptake by the fetal mouse thyroid and resultant effects in later life. *Surg. Gynocol. Obstet.* 93:230-242, 1951.

23. Goldberg, R.C. and Chaikoff, I.L.: A simplified procedure for thyroidectomy of the newborn rat without concomitant parathyroidectomy. *Endocrinology*, 45:64-70, 1949.

24. Folch-Pi, J.: Composition of the brain in relation to maturation In: *Biochemistry of the Developing Nervous System* (H. Waelsch, ed.). Academic Press, New York, 1955. pp. 121-136.

25. Radin, N.S.: Glycolipide determination. In: *Methods of Biochemical Analysis*. Vol. 6. Interscience, New York, 1958. pp. 163-189.

26. Lowry, O.H., Roseburg, N.J., Farr, A.L. and Randall, R.J.: Protein measurement with the Folin Phenol reagent. *J. Biol. Chem.* 193:265-275, 1951.

27. Bartlett, G.R.: Phosphorus assay in column chromatograph. *J. Biol. Chem.* 234:466-568, 1959.

28. Mordynsky, W.E.; King, G.A.; McDonald, T.A. and Murphy, W.M.: An ultramicro-method for PBI. *Clin. Chem.* 15:224, 1969.

29. Chase, H.P., Darsey, J. and McKhann, G.M.: The effect of malnutrition on the synthesis of a myelin lipid. *Pediatrics* 40:551, 1967.

30. Bass, N.H., Netsky, M.G. and Young, E.: II. Microchemical and histological study of myelin formation in the rat. *Arch. Neurol.* 23:303, 1970.

31. Rosman, N.P., Malone, M.J., Helfenstein, M. and Kraft, E.: The effect of thyroid deficiency on myelination of brain. *Neurology* 22:99-106, 1972.

32. Jacobson, S.: Sequence of myelinization in the brain of the albino rat. A. Cerebral cortex, thalamus, and related structures. *J. Comp. Neurol.*,121:5-29, 1963.

33. Winick, M.: Malnutrition and brain development. *J. Pediatr.* 74:667-679, 1969.

34. Prensky, A.L., Carr, S. and Moser, H.W.: Development of myelin in inherited disorders of amino acid metabolism. Arch. Neurol. 19:552-558, 1968.

35. Eayrs, J.T. and Lishman, W.A.: The maturation of behavior in hypothyroidism and starvation. Br. J. Anim. Behav. 3:17-24, 1955.

36. Cocks, J.A., Balázs, R., Johnson, A.L. and Eayrs, J.T.: Effect of thyroid hormone on the biochemical maturation of rat brain: Conversion of glucose-carbon into amino acids. J. Neurochem. 17:1275-1285, 1970.

37. Rosenthal, J. and Doljanski, F.: Biochemical growth patterns of normal and radiothyroidectomized rats. Growth 25:365, 1961.

38. Peters, A.: The structure of myelin sheaths in the central nervous system of Xenopus Laevis (Daudin). J. Biophys. Biochem. Cytol. 7:121-126, 1960.

39. Peters, A.: The formation and structure of myelin sheaths in the central nervous system. J. Biophys. Biochem. Cytol. 8:431-446, 1960.

40. O'Brien, J.S., Sampson, E.L., and Stern, B.: Lipid composition of myelin from the peripheral nervous system. J. Neurochem. 14:357-365, 1967.

41. Cuaron, A., Gamble, J., Myant, N.B. and Osorio, C.: The effect of thyroid deficiency on the growth of the brain and on the deposition of brain phospholipids in fetal and newborn rabbits. J. Physiol.(London) 168:613-630, 1963.

42. Sokoloff, L., Kaufman, S. and Gelboin, H.V.: Thyroxine stimulation of soluble ribonucleic acid bound amino acid transfer to microsomal protein. Biochem. Biophys. Acta 52: 410-412, 1961.

43. Gonzalez-Sastre, F.: The protein composition of isolated myelin. J. Neurochem. 17:1049-10-56, 1970.

44. Eng, L.F., Chao, F.C., Gerstl, B., Pratt, D., and Tavastjerna, M.G.: The maturation of human white matter myelin. Fractionation of the myelin membrane proteins. Biochemistry 7: 4455-4465, 1968.

45. Stoch, M.B., and Symthe, P.M.: Does undernutrition during infancy inhibit brain growth and subsequent intellectual development? Arch. Dis. Child. 38:546, 1963.

46. Stoch, M.B. and Symthe, P.M.: The effect of undernutrition during infancy on subsequent brain growth and intellectual development. S. Afr. Med. J. 41:1027, 1967.

47. Kraviec, L.; Garcia Argiz, C.A.; Gomez, C.J. and Rosman, J.H.: Hormonal regulation of brain development. III. Effects of triiodothyronine and growth hormone on the biochemical changes in the rat cerebral cortex and cerebellum of neonatally thyroidectimized rats. Brain Res. 15: 209-218, 1969.

48. Eayrs, J.T.: Protein annabolism as a factor ameliorating the effects of early thyroid deficiency. Growth 25: 175-189, 1961.

49. Hamburgh, M.: An analysis of the action of thyroid hormone on development based on in vivo and in vitro studies. Gen. Comp. Endocrinol. 10: 198-213, 1968.

50. Geel, S.E. and Timiras, P.S.: Influence of growth hormone on cerebral cortical RNA metabolism in immature hypothyroid rats. Brain Res. 22: 63-72, 1970.

51. Lotmar, F.: Entwicklungsstorungen in der Kleinhirnrinde beim endemische Kretinismus. Z. Neurol. 136: 412-435, 1931.

52. Lotmar, F.: Histopathologische Befunde in Gehirnen von endemische Kretinismus. Z. Ges. Neurol. Psychiatr. 146:1-53, 1933.

53. Schjeide, O.A.; Yamazaki, V.; Haack, K.; Ciminelli, E. and Clemente, C.: Biochemical and morphological aspects of radiation inhibition of myelin formation. Acta. Radiol. Ther. Phys. Biol. 5:185-203, 1966.

THE EFFECTS OF THYROID HORMONE ON PROTEIN SYNTHESIS IN THE CENTRAL NERVOUS SYSTEM OF DEVELOPING MAMMALS

John T. Dunn

University of Virginia School of Medicine

Charlottesville, Virginia

Protein synthesis has been one of the most active areas of biochemical research during the past decade. Its relation to the genetic code and the mechanisms by which this is translated were first worked out in bacteria, and quickly extended to the cells of higher organisms including mammals. It was recognized early that vertebrate hormones might exert their effects by alterations in the protein synthetic scheme, and a massive literature has sprung up concerning this topic. A number of hormones including insulin, growth hormone, TSH, estrogens, testosterone and thyroxine have been shown to have profound effects at this level [Reviewed in (1)].

The present chapter will consider some of the major effects of thyroid hormone and its deprivation on protein synthesis in the mammalian CNS. In the human brain, protein synthesis is at its most active around the time of birth and the months thereafter. This is also the period during which features of cretinism first appear. It is widely assumed, although not established, that endemic cretinism is the product of fetal or postnatal hypothyroidism. A central question here will be whether defective protein synthesis in neonatal hypothyroidism offers a reasonable explanation for some of the clinical features of endemic cretinism.

PROTEIN SYNTHESIS BY CYTOPLASMIC RIBOSOMES

GENERAL FEATURES

The major features of protein synthesis are well known and need not be described here in any detail [see (2) for review].

The components relevant to the subsequent discussion of the effects of thyroid hormones include:

1. DNA - This polynucleotide of large molecular weight is situated in the nucleus and bears the genetic code. Information contained in DNA controls the formation and structure of all three types of RNA.

2. mRNA (messenger RNA) - This polynucleotide (MW 200,000 or higher) carries directions on amino acid sequence from DNA to the ribosomes where peptides are formed. It is a small, but very important fraction of cellular RNA.

3. rRNA (ribosomal RNA) - This is a structural form of RNA. It is strongly associated with protein, has a high molecular weight, and represents about two-thirds of the RNA of the cell. Polyribosomes are aggregates of three to 10 or more ribosomes held together by a thread of mRNA, and are the units on which protein is synthesized.

4. tRNA (transfer RNA) - This represents about 10-20 percent of cellular RNA, is of small molecular weight (about 30,000), and transfers individual amino acids to ribosomes for incorporation into proteins, placing each amino acid correctly in the sequence as determined by mRNA. There is at least one tRNA and a specific amino acyl synthetase for each amino acid. The process of transfer requires GTP and Mg^{++}.

5. Amino acids - These are, of course, precursors of proteins. Their availability to protein synthesis in the cell may be affected by extracellular transport and supply, and this is particularly important when evaluating in vivo experiments on amino acid incorporation into proteins. Once in the cell, amino acids are transported to the site of protein synthesis by tRNA, a reaction requiring energy and specific amino acyl transferases.

EFFECTS OF THYROID HORMONE

Amino Acid Incorporation. This is the most common means of measuring protein synthesis. It obviously depends on the integrity of a number of components of the synthetic scheme.

In 1961 Sokoloff and Kaufman (3) studied the effects of thyroid hormone on amino acid incorporation by the rat liver. The administration in vivo of thyroxine (100 μg per day for 10 days) increased the incorporation of amino acids into protein by 42 percent, relative to controls, and hypothyroidism decreased incorporation by 28 percent. The assay involved a cell-free system to which mitochondria and microsomal suspensions were added. Similar experiments were done in vitro, using graded doses of L-thyroxine (3). While an effect was reported with concentrations as low as 10^{-7} M thyroxine, it was not until 10^{-5} M that an effect greater than 10 percent was obtained. The maximum effect of 77 percent was not obtained until $4X10^{-4}$ M. The increased incorporation was not dependent on RNA synthesis. From a number of experiments using different combinations of cell sap, microsomes, and mitochrondria from thyroxine-treated and control animals, the effect of thyroxine was localized to the mitochondrial fraction, and, more specifically, to a component which was acid-labile, heat-stable, and dialysable. On preliminary analysis this component was not GTP, ATP, glutathione, Mg, or K (4).

The experiments just cited were challenged by Tata (5), chiefly on the basis that the dose of L-thyroxine was too high. To rebut this criticism, Sokoloff (6) gave a single dose of triidothyronine (60 µg per 100 gm body weight) to euthyroid rats and, at varying times after injection, measured the incorporation in vitro of labelled amino acids into protein, both in the presence and absence of mitochondrial suspensions. Without mitochondria, incorporation was increased by about 23 percent over controls at 24 hr and was preceeded by increases in RNA content. When the same experiment was repeated in the presence of mitochondria, there was a prompt increase of about 20 percent in protein synthesis two hours after injection, and this rose steadily to about 40 percent by 27 hours. From these data, it was concluded that thyroid hormone in vivo affects protein synthesis in two ways. One involves an increase in cytoplasmic RNA, while the other, more rapid and about twice as great in effect, is dependent on a mitochondrial factor.

Protein synthesis in the brain was studied in a similar manner (7). Thyroxine, at a concentration of $6.5X10^{-5}$ M, increased the incorporation of amino acids into brain homogenates of 15 day old rats by 14 percent. In contrast, the brains of adult rats showed a decrease in synthesis of 21 percent. This latter result was not regarded as physiologically significant by these authors (4), and was not found in vivo. As was the case for liver, addition of the mitochondrial fraction was necessary for significant stimulation.

Others have examined the effects of hypothyroidism on amino acid incorporation into brain proteins. Balázs <u>et al</u>. (8), studying neonatally thyroidectomized rats at both 14 and 35 days of age, found a reduced incorporation of ^{14}C-leucine into all protein fractions of cerebral cortex homogenates (synaptosomal, mitochondrial, microsomal, nuclear, and supernatant) when the results were expressed as relative specific activity. Similar findings were reported with ^{3}H-phenylalanine at 15 and 30 days of age (9). In contrast, Andrews and Tata (10) found no effect of neonatal thyroidectomy on the incorporation in vitro of ^{14}C-leucine into protein by cerebral cortex slices of rats at two and 21 days after birth. No clear explanation for this discrepancy has emerged. It was suggested that the in vivo effect might reflect in part a decreased transport of amino acids from blood to the CNS, which would not affect the in vitro system.

DNA. The DNA content of the cerebral cortex of hypothyroid rats at 25-35 days of age is increased when related to wet tissue weight (11, 12, 13). This has been attributed to an increased packing density of cells in the hypothyroid animal. Balázs found no change in the overall cerebral content of DNA, but a decrease of 15 percent in the RNA:DNA ratio and of 20 percent in protein: DNA ratio at 35 days of age. Thyroxine was found to decrease the content of DNA (8). Andrews and Tata (10) reported no difference between hypothyroids and controls in either the DNA or RNA contents of cerebral cortex at 21 days of age.

Pyrimidine Incorporation into RNA. Balázs found no change in the relative specific activity of RNA after subarachnoid administration of ^{14}C orotic acid to thyroidectomized rats, and no change in the distribution of the label among the nuclear, supernatant, and microsomal fractions (13). Andrews and Tata (10) found no increase in similar experiments conducted in vitro on cortical slices. Thus, there is general agreement that the rate of incorporation of pyrimidines into RNA is not affected by hypothyroidism.

Total RNA Content. Several studies (11, 12, 13) have shown decreases in the total RNA content of cerebral cortex from hypothyroid rats. The magnitude of change, when related to DNA content, has ranged from about 17 percent (11) to 30 percent (12) at 25 days of age. The decrease was similar in both nuclear and cytoplasmic RNA (11). Andrews and Tata (10) found no change in RNA:DNA ratio in neonatally thyroidectomized rats when studied at four days, and an insignificant decrease (6 percent) when studied at 21 days. The experimental conditions were not strictly comparable, since the latter investigators used cortical slices rather than whole brains. More important, the age of the animals when assayed is critical: Balázs found no differences at 14 days but a significant decrease (14 percent) by 35 days (13).

The effects of thyroid hormones on the individual types of RNA have been more thoroughly studied in the liver than in the brain. Tata and Widnell (14) showed that a single injection of triiodothyronine (20 μg per 100 gm body weight) to thyroidectomized rats produced an increase in rapidly labelled nuclear RNA of 30-40 percent above control values within 3-4 hours, which reached 300 percent by 16 hours. The content of rRNA was increased by about 50 percent between 35-45 hours. Indirect evidence, based on enhanced polyU-directed incorporation of labelled amino acids by ribonucleoproteins, led to the suggestion that mRNA was decreased in thyroidectomized animals. The difficulty was emphasized of recognizing small increments in mRNA in the presence of large increases in rRNA.

Recent work involving a somewhat different system, that of amphibian metamorphosis, has indicated an effect of thyroxine on tRNA as well. Administration of the hormone decreased tRNA methylase activity, when assayed for ability to methylate a heterologous substrate (15). The consequent changes in the methylated bases of tRNA might be expected to affect protein synthesis by altering reactions involving tRNA. In addition, a novel tRNA for leucine was reported following hormone-induced metamorphosis in tadpoles (16). Thus, thyroxine may affect all three types of RNA.

Membranes. In secretory cells, ribosomes are attached to the membranes of the endoplasmic reticulum, apparently to expedite the packaging of proteins for export. This pattern is not limited to secretory cells and may be striking in the CNS during its period of rapid growth and development. Andrews and Tata (10) found that membrane-bound ribosomes from the brains of two-day old rats were six to seven times more active than free ribosomes in their ability to incorporate amino acids into protein in vitro. The rapid decrease seen in protein synthesis in the ensuing two weeks of life was more marked in the membrane-bound ribosomes than in the free. From information in adult rats that about 20 percent of the RNA in the cytoplasm is membrane-bound, it was suggested that over half of the protein synthesis in the cerebral cortex of the newborn rat takes place on membrane-bound ribosomes. In the same paper, it was noted that thyroidectomy had no effect on the rate of protein synthesis occurring on membranes. This would appear to be a different effect from that seen in the liver of hypophysectomized rats, where both triiodothyronine and growth hormone increased protein synthesis on the rough endoplasmic reticulum (17).

PROTEIN SYNTHESIS BY MITOCHONDRIA

GENERAL FEATURES

These have been recently reviewed by Ashwell and Work (18), and their paper should be consulted for details and references. Mitochondria appear capable of protein synthesis which is largely independent of that occurring on cytoplasmic ribosomes. This process follows in broad terms the universal mechanisms of protein synthesis already described, but there are unique features. DNA occurs principally in circular form and is synthesized by the mitochondria themselves, presumably under nuclear influence. Ribosomes are present within mitochondria and have proteins distinct from those of the cytoplasm. rRNA, tRNA, and mRNA have all been found in mitochondria and attributed to mitochondrial DNA. The DNA of the mitochondrion is insufficient to code for more than a limited number of proteins, and Ashwell and Work (18) have estimated that perhaps 5 percent of mitochondrial protein is synthesized by the mitochondrion itself. Mitochondria in higher organisms resemble bacteria in a number of ways, including details of protein synthesis, and it has been suggested that they are, in fact, degenerate bacteria adapted to intracellular life in the host (18).

EFFECTS OF THYROID HORMONE

There is an immense body of literature dealing with the effects of thyroid hormone on mitochondrial metabolism. Extensive review of this topic is outside the scope of the present discussion. Several reports deserve mention here, however, since they deal with the action of thyroxine at specific sites in mitochondrial protein synthesis.

Buchanan et al.(19) studied the incorporation of labelled leucine and isoleucine into protein by isolated mitochondria of rat liver in the presence of thyroxine added in vitro. Incorporation was increased by 10-15 percent at a thyroxine concentration of 2.5-5 μM, and by 84 percent at 50 μM. There was a parallel increase in water uptake by mitochondria up to 50 μM thyroxine, after which protein synthesis decreased despite further mitochondrial swelling. The use of various inhibitors and enzymes indicated peptide bond formation and absence of significant contamination with ribosomes or bacteria. The effects of thyroxine occurred within several minutes. Similar potency was observed with a number of related compounds, including D-thyroxine, L-triiodothyronine, 3,5-diiodo-3'isopropyl-L-thyronine, tetraiodothyroacetic acid, and tetraiodothyropropionic acid. Buchanan et al. (19) concluded that thyroid hormone increased protein synthesis by producing structural alterations in mitochondria. These results conflict with those of Roodyn et al. (20), who found no increase in the incorporation of valine by rat liver mitochondria with the addition of 10μM triiodothyronine in vitro. This discrepancy has been attributed to differences in methods of mitochondrial isolation (19). The administration of triiodothyronine in vivo increased the amino acid incorporation and RNA content of isolated mitochondria, while thyroidectomy depressed these values (20).

In a different study, the turnover rates of protein and of DNA from isolated mitochondria of heart and liver were found slower in hypothyroid rats than in normals (21). In the heart, thyroxine given to normal rats in vivo produced a decreased rate of degradation of mitochondrial protein. In the liver, the turnover of newly synthesized DNA in mitochondria was increased after thyroxine administration when compared with the DNA synthesized prior to thyroxine. In another report (22) the administration of triiodothyronine in vivo appeared to double the ratios of both DNA and RNA to protein in mitochondria isolated from rat liver. Thus the effect on mitochondrial DNA differed from that on nuclear DNA, while the changes in RNA levels were similar for both cytoplasm and mitochondria.

Work on the effects of thyroid hormones on mitochondrial protein synthesis is limited, and attended by a host of experimental problems. The amounts of thyroxine used in studies in vitro are large relative to its concentration in serum under euthyroid conditions. Also, it is difficult to interpret the equal potency in vitro of thyroxine analogs which are ineffective in vivo. Nevertheless, the few reports at hand do suggest that thyroxine and its deprivation affect protein synthesis in mitochondria as well as in cytoplasmic ribosomes. Further work is urgently needed in this area.

TYPES OF PROTEINS SYNTHESIZED

There are hundreds of proteins in the brain, only a handful of which are well-characterized. The focus in this section will be on two groups - enzymes and myelin proteins - in which an effect of thyroid hormone has been implicated.

ENZYMES

Levels of a number of enzymes have been studied in normal and hypothyroid animals. We shall consider here only several which may have particular relevance to abnormal development in hypothyroidism.

Cholinesterase and acetyl cholinesterase are associated with neurotransmission, and have been found to increase in parallel with the development of the young brain. They were found decreased by about a third in rats hypothyroid from birth when studied at 22 days of age in comparison with normal (23).

Succinate dehydrogenase, an enzyme of the Krebs cycle, is associated with mitochondria, and Balázs (8) has offered evidence that it is associated with synaptosomal mitochondria in the CNS. Neonatal thyroidectomy in rats resulted in depressed enzyme levels as early as 10 days of age and persisted into adulthood. At 20 days of age, levels were less than half those of euthyroid rats. By contrast, the activity of glutamate dehydrogenase, which is largely associated with non-synaptosomal mitochondria, was not reduced (8).

Glutamate decarboxylase is concentrated in the synaptosomal fraction. It was decreased by about 16 percent in neonatally thyroidectomized rats when compared with controls at 24 days of age (8).

GABA transaminase is located principally in mitochondria, and promotes the production of glutamate. Neonatal thyroidectomy produced a marked depression by 10 days of age, and this persisted into adulthood (12).

Na^+-K^+- activated ATPase is highly localized to synaptosomes. Its activity is decreased in the cerebral cortex by neonatal thyroidectomy while the Mg^{++}-activated ATPase is not. Changes in the former enzyme are accompanied by an increase in cerebral Na^+ and a decrease in K^+, and have been attributed to a depressed Na^+-K^+ pump. Geel and Timiras (23) have suggested that changes in ions may represent a major effect of thyroid hormone on protein synthesis in the brain, since this process is quite sensitive to ionic levels.

Aspartyl amino transferase promotes the synthesis of glutamate and is associated with mitochondria (18). Its activity is decreased to about half that of control levels by 20 days of age in neonatally thyroidectomized rats (12).

Alpha-glycerophosphate dehydrogenase is thought important to the synthesis of central myelin, by providing glycerol phosphate for myelin lipids. Thyroidectomy of one-day old rats lowered enzyme activity by 60 percent (24).

A number of other enzymes have been studied and found unchanged as a result of neonatal thyroidectomy (8). A common feature of the enzymes which are depressed by hypothyroidism is their association with synaptosomes and with mitochondria.

PROTEINS OF CENTRAL MYELIN

Shooter and Einstein (25) have recently reviewed this subject.

The three major proteins are a proteolipid protein, a basic protein (also called encephalitogenic protein), and an acidic proteolipid protein. Their relative proportions in the brain are 5:3:2. About a third of the proteolipid protein is lipid. The remainder is protein which is high in neutral and aromatic residues, low in charged residues, and has a molecular weight of about 12,500. The basic protein has a molecular weight of about 17,000 and a high content of basic amino acids. It has been the focus of considerable research because its administration produces an experimental allergic encephalomyelitis. Its amino acid sequence has been reported and the encephalitogenic fragment isolated. Little is known about the third protein, the acidic proteolipid protein.

The functions of these proteins are poorly understood. The basic protein is absent during the first few months after birth in humans. Its appearance corresponds to the synthesis of cholesterol and cerebrosides, which are the two major lipid components of myelin (26). Levels of the basic protein are highest during active myelination.

Mitochondria appear to play a major role in the synthesis of proteolipids of myelin. Klee and Sokoloff (27) studied the incorporation of ^{14}C-leucine into proteins of adult and immature rat brains, using a crude mitochondrial fraction which also contained myelin fragments and nerve endings, but was largely free of microsomal contamination. Incorporation of isotope into proteolipid protein was about 8 times greater than that of total protein when studied at 10 days of age. By 25 days of age the specific activity of proteolipid was the same as that of total protein. The 'proteolipid protein' in this study represented a neutral chloroform-methanol extract and probably included at least some of the basic protein as well.

A similar study by Tolani and Mokrasch (28) showed that a crude mitochondrial fraction from rat brain was twice as active as the nuclear fraction, and seven times as active as the microsomal one, when measured by incorporation of ^{14}C-amino acids into proteolipid protein. On subfractionation of this mitochondrial preparation the activity of the mitochondrial fraction was equal to that of nerve endings, and both were much more active than vesicles or myelin. Ribonuclease did not affect incorporating ability.

The importance of thyroid hormone to normal myelin formation has been emphasized by Balázs (8). Neonatal thyroidectomy results in a decreased concentration of myelin and a disproportionate decrease in the lipids associated with myelination, chiefly cerebrosides. One can conjecture that neonatal hypothyroidism might result in a decreased synthesis of myelin proteins, chiefly proteolipid, by the mitochondria of developing brain cells. To our knowledge, there has not been direct experimental examination of this possibility. It would also be important to see whether hypothyroidism affects each of the myelin proteins to the same degree and in the same manner.

DISCUSSION

Table I summarizes some of the experimental data on the effects of thyroid hormone and its deprivation on protein synthesis in the developing CNS. This type of compilation is risky, since an arrow in the table may appear much more clear-cut than the experimental data it tries to represent. It is immediately apparent that there are large gaps in knowledge both of protein synthesis in the CNS and of its alteration by thyroid hormones. As already pointed out, there are several instances in which definite conflicts emerge from comparisons of different reports. Perhaps this is to be expected in view of the complexity of the processes being studied and the indirect techniques available for their examination.

With these limitations in mind, we can still make some tentative conclusions about thyroid hormones and the developing CNS:

1. Thyroid hormone appears to stimulate amino acid incorporation into proteins by cytoplasmic ribosomes in vivo and by mitochondria both in vivo and in vitro.

2. Neonatal hypothyroidism decreases protein synthesis in vivo, but perhaps not in vitro.

3. Myelin proteins are probably synthesized by mitochondria and are among the major proteins affected by thyroid hormones.

4. In the developing CNS, thyroid hormones may have their major impact at the level of mitochondrial protein synthesis.

5. Defective protein synthesis is a reasonable mechanism for at least some of the effects of hypothyroidism on CNS development.

Table 1. Some effects of thyroid hormone on protein synthesis (entries refer to mammalian brain unless otherwise specified).

	Hormone Added	Hypo-thyroid
1. Amino acid incorporation		
a. by cytoplasmic ribosomes		
(1) in vivo	↑[liver (5)]	↓(8,9)
(2) in vitro	-	O (10)
b. by ribosomes plus mitochondria		
(1) in vivo	↑ (7)	↓(7)
(2) in vitro	↑ (7)	-
c. by isolated mitochondria		
(1) in vivo	↑ (20)	↓(20)
(2) in vitro	↑ (19)	-
2. DNA content		
a. nuclear	↓ (8)	↑(11, 12, 13)
b. mitochondrial	↑ [liver (22)]	-
3. Pyrimidine incorporation into RNA	O (10)	O (13)
4. RNA		
a. cytoplasmic		
(1) total content	-	↓(11, 12, 13)
(2) mRNA content	↑ [liver (14)]	?↓ [liver (14)]
(3) rRNA content	↑ [liver (14)]	-
(4) tRNA	Δ [amphibia (15, 16)]	-
b. mitochondrial	↑ [liver (20)]	↓ [liver (20)]
5. Membrane-bound ribosomes	↑ [liver (17)]	O[brain (10)]
6. Enzymes		
a. cholinesterase	-	↓(23)
b. succinate dehydrogenase	-	↓(8)
c. glutamate decarboxylase	-	↓(8)
d. GABA transaminase	-	↓(12)
e Na+-K+activated ATPase	-	↓(23)
f. aspartyl amino transferase	-	↓(12)
g. α-glycerophosphate dehydrogenase	-	↓(24)
7. Myelin proteins	↑ (27)	-

Symbols: ↑, increased; ↓, decreased; O, no change; Δ, qualitative change; -, data not available.

It remains to relate these conclusions to endemic cretinism in humans. There are, of course, severe ethical and logistical limitations to the study of protein synthesis in the CNS of human infants, and it is not surprising that we depend on experimental animals for a picture of this process. There is every reason to believe that the general features of protein synthesis in the developing CNS are comparable between humans and other mammals. There are, however, significant differences from one species to another in the chronological relationships among the various anatomic, biochemical, and neurophysiological components of development (29).

Most of the work already described has been done in the rat. This species has the major spurt of brain growth occurring well after birth, with a maximum at about 10-15 days of age. This period is preceded by one of neuronal growth and increase in glial cells. Myelination in the rat begins at about 10 days of age. Protein synthesis is most active near the time of birth and declines rapidly, reaching adult levels by about 21 days. The incorporation of labelled amino acid into protein in two-day old rats was at least 10 times greater than at three weeks (10).

In humans the peak period of brain growth and development begins during the last several months of gestation and reaches a peak shortly before birth (30). Significant myelination does not begin until the first few weeks after birth. Dobbing (31) has suggested that in man any adverse influences on development (including hypothyroidism) will be most effective shortly before birth and during the several months thereafter. As already mentioned, this is also the time during which features of endemic cretinism may first be apparent.

From these considerations, it seems possible that the clinical syndrome of endemic cretinism could result, at least in part, from the effects of thyroid deficiency on protein synthesis in the developing CNS. To establish this, however, will require proof of hypothyroidism during the critical period of brain growth and some direct quantitation of protein synthesis in the CNS. Since we are dealing with humans rather than experimental animals, neither of these conditions is likely to be satisfied except by chance observation. For the present, efforts in this area should be towards more detailed animal research. Particular emphasis should be given to the precise effects of thyroxine on protein synthesis and to an evaluation of other factors which may affect this process, especially iodine deficiency, malnutrition, and genetic disposition.

SUMMARY

From this review, thyroxine appears to stimulate protein synthesis in cytoplasmic ribosomes in vivo and in mitochondria both in vivo and in vitro. Neonatal thyroidectomy reduces protein synthesis in vivo but perhaps not in vitro. Proteins associated with mitochondria, especially enzymes and myelin proteins, appear particularly susceptible to the effects of thyroidectomy. Defects in protein synthesis may explain at least some of the consequences of neonatal hypothyroidism. Extension of the findings in experimental hypothyroidism to endemic cretinism in humans is tempting but not yet supported by direct evidence.

ACKNOWLEDGEMENTS

The author is the recipient of a Research Career Development Award from the National Institutes of Health.

DISCUSSION BY PARTICIPANTS

BALÁZS: The effect of thyroid deficiency in infancy on the incorporation rate of labelled amino acids into cerebral proteins has been studied in different laboratories and the results are controversial. Andrews and Tata found that the rate, determined in vitro, was normal in brain slices of thyroid deficient rats. On the other hand, it has been observed by Geel _et al_. (32) and confirmed by us (8) and by others (33) that the incorporation rate rate was reduced when determined in vivo. Thus there is an impor-that difference in techniques used in the experiments of Andrews and Tata (10) in comparison with the other groups (8,32,33), which raises the question whether or not, in this particular case, the in vitro studies reflect the in vivo situation. When the rate of amino acid incorporation into protein is studied during development in the brain of _normal_ animals a remarkable difference is observed depending on whether the rate is determined in vitro or in vivo. In vivo, the rate, which is relatively constant from birth till nine days, increases significantly between nine and 12 days and it starts to decrease only after the age of 21 days (34,35). On the other hand, the in vitro incorporation rate into protein decreases dramatically during the first 21 days after birth: For example, when the rates are calculated from Fig. 1 of Andrews and Tata (1) as a percentage of the value at 2 days of age, they are about 26 percent at 10 days and 10 percent at 21 days. Thus the drastic reduction in the rate of amino acid incorporation into brain proteins in vitro is in contrast to the findings in vivo and it may result from factors other than the rate of protein synthesis proper. The operation of such factors was indicated by the observations of Guroff *et al*. (36): these authors observed in vitro an apparent decrease with age in the rate of cerebral RNA synthesis which correlated with an increase in the activity of an enzyme concerned in the hydrolysis of the labelled precursor used. It appears that with our present methods the rate-limiting reactions in the processes of protein or RNA synthesis are not the same in vitro and in vivo, and thyroid hormones may have influenced in vivo a rate-limiting reaction which is not any longer the rate-determining step in vitro. It is evident that in vitro investigations are vital in elucidating the basic mechanisms involved in protein synthesis. However, when the results obtained in vitro are used to draw conclusions with respect to in vivo situations, such as the effects of hormones, it must be ascertained that possible artifacts due to the in vitro conditions do not mask the real effects.

DUNN: What do you think the effect on the circulation is? Is that an important effect?

BALÁZS: I do not think so. The entry of leucine into brain tissue is apparently unimpeded, and leucine was the precursor in the studies of both Andrews and Tata (10) and ourselves (8). When the labelling of cerebral protein is corrected on the basis of the specific radioactivity of free leucine either in the blood or in the tissue, the results show a reduction in the rate of incorporation in the hypothyroid animals compared with controls.

REFERENCES

1. Manchester, K.L.: Sites of hormonal regulation of protein metabolism. In: *Mammalian Protein Metabolism*, Vol. IV (H.N. Munro, ed.). Academic Press, New York, 1970. pp. 229-298.

2. Baglioni, C. and Colombo, B.: Protein synthesis. In: *Metabolic Pathways*, Vol. IV (D.M. Greenberg, ed.). Academic Press, New York, 1970. pp. 277-351.

3. Sokoloff, L. and Kaufman, S.: Thyroxine stimulation of amino acid incorporation into protein. *J. Biol. Chem.* 236:795-803, 1961.

4. Sokoloff, L: The mechanism of action of thyroid hormones on protein synthesis and its relationship to the differences in sensitivities of mature and immature brain. In: *Protein Metabolism of the Nervous System* (A. Lajtha, ed.). Plenum Press, New York, 1970. pp. 367-382.

5. Tata, J.R., Ernster, L., Lindberg, O., Arrhenius, E., Pedersen, S. and Hedman, R.: The action of thyroid hormones at the cell level. Biochem. J. 86:480 -428, 1963.

6. Sokoloff, L., Roberts, P.A., Januska, M.M. and Kline, J.E.: Mechanisms of stimulation of protein synthesis by thyroid hormones in vivo. Proc. Natl. Acad. Sci. 60:652-659, 1968

7. Gelber, S., Campbell, P.L., Deibler, G.E. and Sokoloff, L.: Effects of L-thyroxine on amino acid incorporation into protein in mature and immature rat brain. J. Neurochem. 11: 221-229, 1964.

8. Balázs, R., Cocks, W.A., Eayrs, J.T. and Kovács, S.: Biochemical effects of thyroid hormones on the developing brain. In: Homones in Development (M. Hamburgh and E.J.W. Barrington, eds.). Appleton-Century-Crofts, New York, 1971. pp. 357-379.

9. Szijan, I., Kalbermann, L.E. and Gomez, C.J.: Hormonal regulation of brain development. IV. Effect of neonatal thyroidectomy upon incorporation in vivo of L-[^{3}H]phenylalanine into proteins of developing rat cerebral tissues and pituitary gland. Brain Res. 27:309-318, 1971

10. Andrews, T.M. and Tata, J. R.: Protein synthesis by membrane-bound and free ribosomes of the developing rat cerebral cortex. Biochem. J. 124:883-889, 1971.

11. Geel, S.E. and Timiras, P.S.: The role of thyroid and growth hormones on RNA metabolism in the immature brain. In: Hormones in Development (M. Hamburgh and E.J.W. Barrington, eds.). Appleton-Century-Crofts, New York, 1971. pp. 391-401.

12. Gomez, C.J.: Hormonal influences of the biochemical differentiation of the rat cerebral cortex. In: Hormones in Development (M. Hamburgh and E.J.W. Barrington, eds.). Appleton-Century-Crofts, New York, 1971. pp. 417-435.

13. Balázs, R., Kovács, S., Teichgräber, P., Cooks, W.A. and Eayrs, J.T.: Biochemical effects of thyroid deficiency on the developing brain. J. Neurochem. 15:1335-1349, 1968.

14. Tata, J.R. and Widnell, C.C.: Ribonucleic acid synthesis during the early action of thyroid hormones. Biochem. J. 98:604-620, 1966.

15. Sharma, O.K., Kerr, S.J., Lipshitz-Wiesner, R. and Borek, E.: Regulation of the tRNA methylases. Fed. Proc. 30:167-176, 1971.

16. Tonoue, T., Eaton, J. and Frieden, E.: Changes in leucyl-tRNA during spontaneous and induced metamorphosis of bullfrog tadpoles. Biochem. Biophys. Res. Commun. 37:81-88, 1969.

17. Tata, J.R. and Williams-Ashman, H.G.: Effects of growth hormone and tri-iodothyronine on amino acid incorporation by microsomal subfractions from rat liver. Eur. J. Biochem. 2:366-374, 1967.

18. Ashwell, M. and Work, T.S.: The biogenesis of mitochondria. Ann. Rev. Biochem. 39:251-290, 1970.

19. Buchanan, J., Primack, M.P. and Tapley, D.F.: Relationship of mitochondrial swelling to thyroxine-stimulated mitochondrial protein synthesis. Endocrinology. 87:993-999, 1970.

20. Roodyn, D.B., Freeman, K.B. and Tata, J.R.: The stimulation by treatment in vivo with tri-iodothyronine of amino acid incorporation into protein by isolated rat-liver mitochondria. Biochem. J. 94:628-641, 1965.

21. Gross, N.J.: Control of mitochondrial turnover under the influence of thyroid hormone. J. Cell Biol. 48:29-40, 1971.

22. De Leo, T., Barletta, A. and Di Meo, S.: Effects of testosterone and of tri-iodothyronine on the levels of mitochondrial DNA and RNA from rat liver. Life Sci. [II] 8:747-755, 1969.

23. Geel, S.E. and Timiras, P.S.: The role of hormones in cerebral protein metabolism. In: Protein Metabolism of the Nervous System (A. Lajtha, ed.). Plenum Press, New York, 1970. pp. 335-353.

24. Schwark, W.S., Singhal, R.L. and Ling, G.M.: Metabolic control mechanisms in mammalian systems. XIII. Thyroid hormone control of glycerophosophate dehydrogenase activity in rat cerebral cortex and cerebellum. Can. J. Physiol. Pharmacol: 49:598-607, 1971.

25. Shooter, E.M. and Einstein, E.R.: Proteins of the nervous system. Ann. Rev. Biochem. 40:635-652, 1971.

26. Einstein, E.R., Dalal, K.B. and Csejtey, J.: Biochemical maturation of the central nervous system. II. Protein and proteolytic enzyme changes. Brain Res. 18:35-49, 1970.

27. Klee, C.B. and Sokoloff, L: Amino acid incorporation into proteolipid of myelin *in vitro*. *Proc. Natl. Acad. Sci.* 53: 1014-1021, 1965.

28. Tolani, A.J. and Mokrasch, L.C.: Incorporation of ^{14}C-amino acids into proteolipid protein of subcellular fractions from rat brain, heart and liver. *Life Sci.* 6:1771-1774, 1967.

29. Himwich, W.A.: Biochemical and neurophysiological development of the brain in the neonatal period. *Int. Rev. Neurobiol.* 4: 117-159, 1962.

30. Davison, A.N. and Dobbing, J.: The developing brain. In: *Applied Neurochemistry* (A.N. Davison and J. Dobbing, eds.). Blackwell, Oxford, 1968. pp. 253-286.

31. Dobbing, J.: Vulnerable periods in developing brain. In: *Applied Neurochemistry* (A.N. Davison and J. Dobbing, eds.). Blackwell, Oxford, 1968. pp. 287-316.

32. Geel, S.E., Valcana, T. and Timaras, P.S.: Effect of neonatal hypothyroidism and of thyroxine on L-[^{14}C]leucine incorporation in protein *in vivo* and the relationship to ionic levels in the developing brain. *Brain Res.* 4: 143-150, 1967.

33. Dainat, J., Rebière, A. and Legrand, J. Influence de la deficience thyroïdienne sur l'incorporation in vivo de la L-[^{3}H]leucine dans les proteines du cervelet chez le jeune rat. *J. Neurochem.* 17:581-586, 1970.

34. Patel, A.J. and Balázs, R.: Manifestation of metabolic compartmentation during the maturation of the rat brain. *J. Neurochem.* 17:955-971. 1970.

35. Balázs, R. and Richter, D.: Effects of hormones on the biochemical maturation of the brain. In: *Biochemistry of the Developing Brain* (W.A. Himwich, ed.). Dekker, New York, in press.

36. Guroff, G.; Hogans, A.F. and Udenfriend, S.: Biosynthesis of ribonucleic acid in rat brain slices. *J. Neurochem.* 15: 489-497, 1968.

EFFECTS OF HORMONES AND NUTRITION ON BRAIN DEVELOPMENT

R. Balázs

Medical Research Council Neuropsychiatry Unit

Carshalton, Surrey, England

In contrast to the reversible mental changes sometimes associated with dysfunction of endocrine glands in the adult, permanent changes seem to result from hormonal imbalance during certain periods of the development of the central nervous system (CNS). Cretinism is by far the best documented illness in this class, and it is associated with severe mental retardation. Model experiments with laboratory animals are valuable for investigating the neurological mechanisms underlying these pathological conditions.

Attempts to relate these observations to the processes of human development and pathology must allow for species differences, in both the complexity of the nervous system and the development of the CNS. In most of the studies reviewed here, the animals were exposed to adverse influences soon after birth; they were usually rats and mice, which are immature at birth compared with man. Thus the effects of various postnatal treatments on the development of the CNS of experimental animals and man cannot be strictly compared. Furthermore, there are marked species differences in the development of the neuroendocrine system; for example, the thyroid gland starts to function in man at the end of the first trimester of pregnancy (1), while in the rat this occurs when about 80 percent of gestation is over (2). There are, however, important similarities in the postnatal development of the CNS of experimental animals and man.

The postnatal development of the CNS in the rat is characterized by the extensive differentiation of the nerve cells, expanding the neuronal processes, and thus laying the foundation of the intricate interneuronal connections (3,4); by the formation and migration of "microneurons" which complete the cellular complement of the neuronal networks in many regions (5), and by the massive myelination of central tracts (6). There is evidence that even in man these processes, as well as the functional development of the CNS, continue well into the postnatal period. In some parts of the brain, including the cerebral cortex, extensive dendritic arborization occurs during the first 1 1/2-2 yr after birth (Fig. 1).

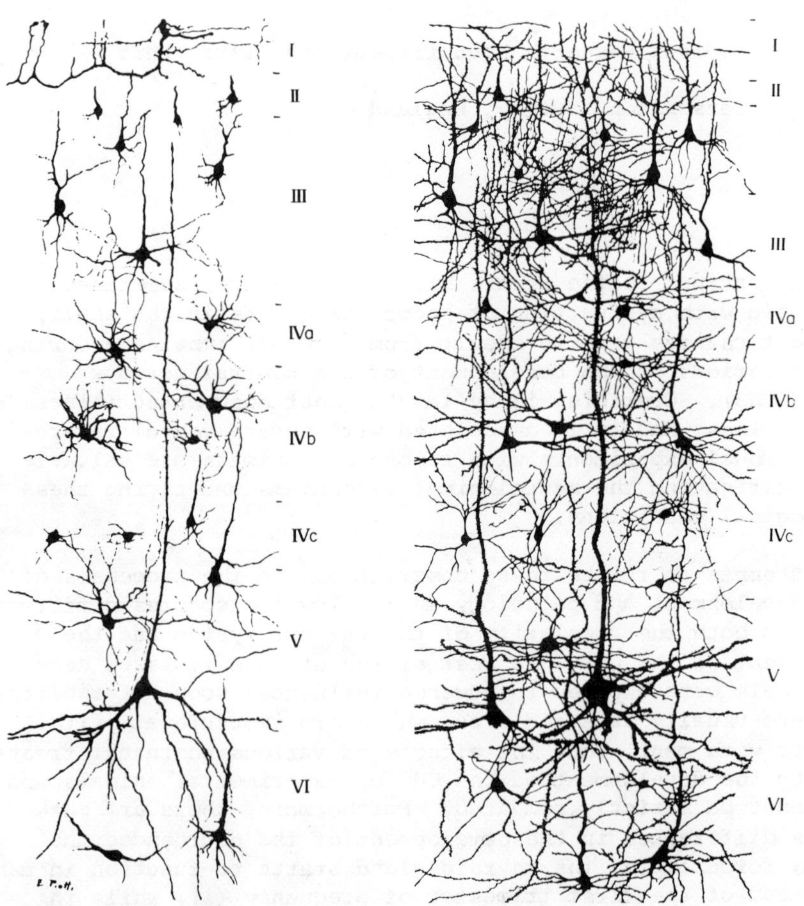

Fig. 1. Dendritic arborization in the visual cortex in man at birth (left) and two years after birth (right). [From Conel (7)].

Because there must be a relationship between synapse formation and available neuronal receptor surface, the timing of the formation of nerve terminals, and thus of interneuronal connections, must be similar. It is known that in man also myelination in the brain continues after birth (8). Furthermore, recent observations suggest the need to reconsider the belief that neurogenesis is completed in man before birth. There is appreciable postnatal cell formation in the human brain (9,10); in the first 1 1/2 years after birth the cells increase in number about three-fold in the cerebrum and six-fold in the cerebellum. In the cerebellum the most abundant cell types are microneurons (5), and so the great increase in number indicates that in this part of the human CNS postnatal cell formation must involve nerve cells as well as glial cells. In the rat and other species studied, postnatal neurogenesis in the cerebellum takes place in a germinal zone (the external granular layer), the width of which is related partly to the number of dividing cells and partly to the rate of emigration of newly formed cells to their final location in the deeper parts of the cerebellar cortex. In man, the external granular layer is relatively wide at birth and then persists for several months: migrating cells disappear from the deeper zones of the cerebellum only about 1 1/2 years after birth (8). In the forebrain the germinal matrix is the subependymal layer in the lateral ventricles, and there is evidence that remnants of this layer are found in man throughout infancy (11). In experimental animals the origin of microneurons, which are ultimately localized in the hippocampus or olfactory lobes, has been traced to the subependymal layer (5). These nerve cells are formed at about the same time as the microneurons in the cerebellum. Thus, in view of the evidence from other species, it is expected that in man also microneurons are formed in different parts of the brain, as well as in the cerebellum after birth.

I shall now describe evidence indicating that in experimental animals permanent impairment of brain function can result from adverse influences, such as hormonal imbalance or nutritional deprivation, operating during certain periods of the postnatal development of the CNS. The conclusions drawn also seem to be applicable to man, with certain limitations. Whereas the regulatory mechanisms of the mother provide protection for the fetus, they are not yet fully developed in the infant and this may lead to the special vulnerability of brain, both in experimental animals and in man, during the postnatal period of brain development.

POSTNATAL CELL FORMATION

The rapid growth of brain in the rat during the first three weeks after birth is due partly to an appreciable formation of new cells (Fig. 2). With certain limitations a good approximation to cell number is given by DNA estimations: there are tetraploid cells in the CNS (12) but their number is relatively small.

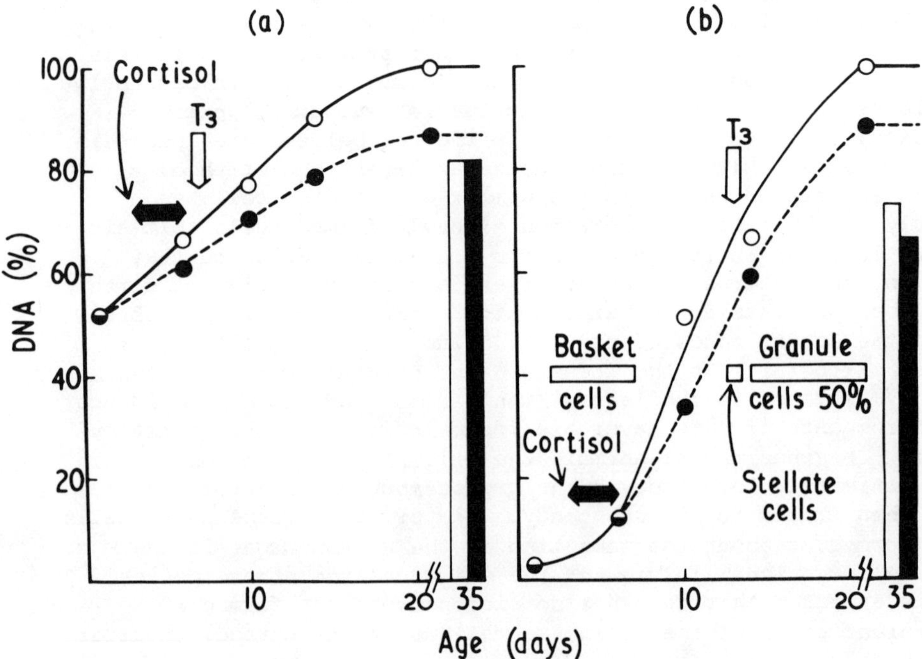

Fig. 2. Effects of adverse conditions on the postnatal increase in cell number in the cerebrum (a) and cerebellum (b) in the rat. The ordinates represent the total amount of DNA per brain region expressed as a percentage of the values at the age of 21 days (which is similar to the adult values) in the cerebrum and the cerebellum respectively. The experimental conditions were as follows: <u>nutritional deprivation</u> - the mothers received about 50 percent of the normal food from the 6th day of gestation until the 21st day of parturition. o - Control, and • - the young of undernourished mothers. The results are taken from Patel and Balázs (38). <u>Treatment with thyroid hormone</u> (T_3) - 25 μg. T_3 was given at the day of birth followed by 0.5-1.5 μg every

(Fig. 2 Continued)

second day. The vertical arrows indicate the time when the effect of T_3 on cell number become significant, and the reduction in final cell number is shown by the open columns which give the amount of DNA at 35 days of age. [From Balázs et al. (18)]. Treatment with cortisol - 0.2 mg was given daily during the period indicated by the horizontal arrow. The DNA content was significantly reduced during the time of the treatment. The closed columns represent the values of DNA in the brain of 35 day-old cortisol-treated rats [from Balázs (27); Cotterrell et al. (30)]. The blocks in (b) indicate the time of the differentiation peak of the postnatally formed neurons in the cerebellar cortex; the period is also shown when approx. 50 percent of the granule cells are formed. These results are taken from Altman (5).

For example there are about 300 diploid granule cells per tetraploid Purkinje cell in the rat cerebellum (5). Another source of error is the presence of extranuclear DNA in the cells, but the amounts of both mitochondrial DNA (13) and the "membrane-bound" DNA are very small in comparison with the nuclear DNA (14). Finally, the amount of DNA gives an estimate of cell number, but further histological information is needed to identify the types of cells which are formed.

The results showed that with respect to the final assembly of the total cell population, the development of the cerebellum is delayed compared with the cerebrum (Fig. 2). At birth, cell number is about 50 percent of the adult value in the cerebrum, whereas it is only 3 percent in the cerebellum, and the period of relatively rapid increase in cell number lasts about a week longer in the cerebellum. There are also qualitative differences: in the cerebrum, with the exception of microneurons in certain regions, most nerve cells are formed prenatally, but in the cerebellum they are mostly formed postnatally [exceptions are the Purkinje cells and the large neurons in the deep cerebellar nuclei, as well as the Golgi cells which are formed around the time of birth (5)].

It is characteristic of the CNS that cell proliferation takes place predominantly at certain germinal sites, such as the subependymal layer of the forebrain ventricles and the external granular layer of the cerebellum (5). The cerebellum, because of its late development and layered structure, offers special

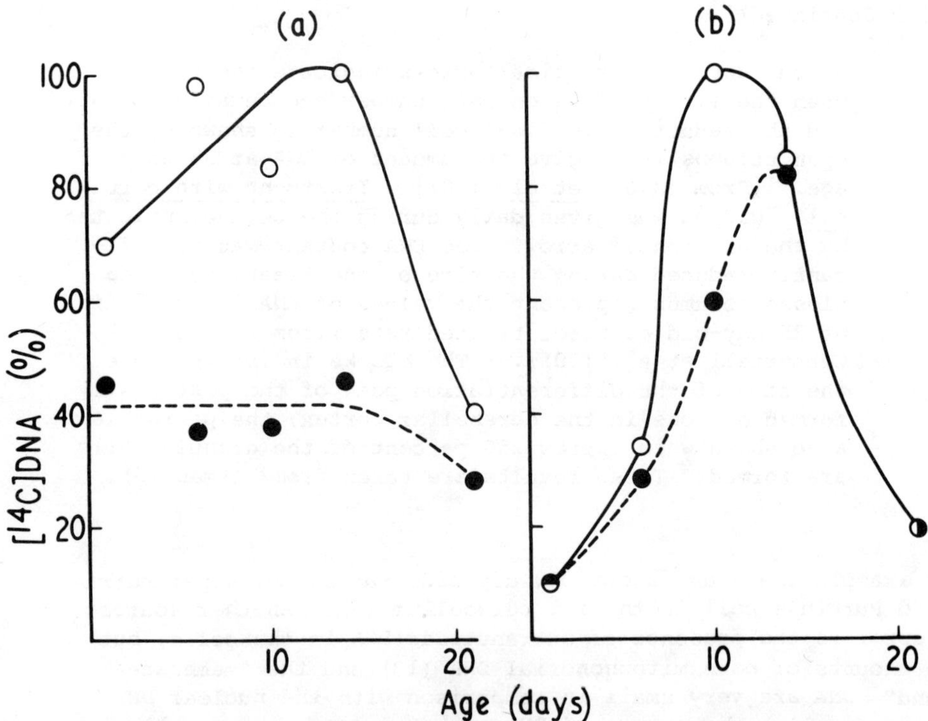

Fig. 3. Effect of undernutrition on the synthesis of [^{14}C]-DNA in (a) the cerebrum and (b) cerebellum at 30 min. after a subcutaneous injection of [2-^{14}C] thymidine (59 mCi/mmole; dose 20 μCi/100 g body wt.) The results are expressed as a percentage of the maximal labelling of DNA in the cerebrum and cerebellum respectively. o - Control, and ● - the young of undernourished mothers. [From Patel and Baláz̓s (38)].

advantages for the study of cell proliferation in the CNS. During the first few days after birth, the number of stem cells increases; this is reflected morphologically in the enlargement of the external granular layer and biochemically in the 'lag' period preceding rapid cell formation (Fig. 2). In the rat the germinal layer disappears, after progressive reduction in size, by about 21 days after birth; this is the time when the adult level of DNA is reached in the brain.

EFFECTS OF THYROID HORMONES AND CORTICOSTEROIDS

Investigations in our laboratory showed that thyroid hormones affect cell proliferation in the brain. After neonatal radiothyroidectomy the increase in cell number was retarded in the cerebellum (15). At the age of 14 days there was a 25 percent reduction in cell number compared with the normal situation, which, however, was reached at 35 days. Morphological observations are consistent with these results: the involution of the external granular layer is delayed in the cerebellum of thyroid deficient rats (16, 17).

We found that treatment with thyroid hormone (tri-iodothyronine, T_3) in early life resulted in a permanent deficit in cell number in the brain (18). T_3 affected cell formation rather than cell destruction: less [^{14}C]thymidine was incorporated into DNA than in controls (19). The results indicated that treatment with T_3 led to a premature termination of postnatal cell formation: in comparison with controls, the reduction in the labelling of DNA was more marked towards the end of the period of massive cell formation (50 percent) than at the peak of cell multiplication [10-20 percent (19)],and the dissolution of the external granular layer of the cerebellum was advanced (20).

It seems that the earlier cessation of extensive cell proliferation in the brain of rats treated with T_3 is related to the advancement of the biochemical differentiation of the cells (Fig. 4). The functional development of the CNS was also accelerated, as indicated by the time of appearance of innately organized behavior (21). However, when the T_3 treated rats mature their performance in tests of adaptive behavior seems to be impaired in comparison with controls (21). In the rat postnatal cell formation also involves microneurons, not only in the cerebellum but in other parts of the brain, such as the hippocampus and olfactory lobe. Altman (5) has suggested that microneurons formed after birth modify the structural and functional organization of the developing nervous system to an extent which depends on environmental influences. Balázs et al. (18) have proposed that the impairment of adaptive behavior caused by neonatal treatment with thyroid hormone is related to the resulting deficit of microneurons in certain regions of the brain. Other factors may also be involved: permanent changes in the neuroendocrine system were observed (22-24). It must also be considered that, if the accelerated maturation triggered by thyroid treatment is not completely synchronized throughout the CNS, dysfunction may follow.

Postnatal cell formation in the brain is also influenced by corticosteroids (25,26). Both the deposition of cells and the incorporation of [^{14}C]thymidine into DNA were severely inhibited in the rat brain during the period of treatment with cortisol in the first few days of life, showing that cortisol interferes with cell formation (27-29). Mitotic activity, however, is restored soon after the cessation of treatment with cortisol and there was a tendency to compensate the initial cell deficit by an increase in mitotic activity towards the end of the period of postnatal cell proliferation (30). Nevertheless, the results showed that massive cell formation ceased at more or less the same age as in normal rats.

The results showed that the reduction in final cell number was similar after treatment with cortisol or with thyroid hormone (Fig. 2). On the other hand, the behavioral consequences of the two treatments seem to differ (Table 1). The appearance of certain features of innately organized behavior is retarded by cortisol but accelerated by T_3 (31). Furthermore, in contrast to T_3-treated rats, the performance of animals treated with corticosteroids is normal in tests of adaptive behavior, although an impairment in motor coordination and emotional control has been observed (32). Thus an explanation based simply on a reduction in the number of microneurons cannot account for the observed effects of hormonal imbalance in early life. However, corticosteroids and thyroid hormone, in the conditions of treatment used, affected cell formation at different times after birth. Cell multiplication was inhibited throughout the brain by corticosteroids, chiefly during the time of treatment, that is the first five days of life, whereas it was affected by thyroid hormone only after a delay of about a week in the cerebrum or two weeks in the cerebellum.

There is a chronological order in the formation of the different types of nerve cells in the CNS (33). Postnatal neurogenesis was studied in detail recently in the rat cerebellum and it was found that the 'birthday' of the basket cells is at two to six days and that of the stellate cells at 13 days, whereas about half of the granule cells develop during the third week after birth (Fig. 2). There is also evidence with respect to the sites of the synaptic contacts and the functions of the various microneurons in the cerebellum (34). Thus the stellate cells make synaptic contacts on the terminal branches of the Purkinje cells, whereas the terminals of the basket cell, which is the other inhibitory cell formed after birth, are strategically localized on the Purkinje cell bodies near the axon hillock. It is evident that the functional consequences of the deletion of a basket cell are more drastic than those of the loss of a stellate cell.

Table 1. Effects of thyroid hormone or corticosteroids on brain development

	Treatment: Thryoid hormone	Treatment: Corticosteroids
Postnatal cell formation	Reduced (18)* (premature termination)	Reduced (25-27,30) (Inhibition during the period of treatment, 1-5 days after birth)
Biochemical differentiation (conversion of glucose carbon into amino acids)	Advanced (41)	Normal (27,28) **(In comparison with controls, the age curve did not differ significantly, but a slight retardation was noted in the period 10-14 days after birth).**
Appearance of innately organized behavior	Advanced (21,31)	Retarded (31)
Performance in tests of adaptive behavior	Impaired (21)	Normal (32)

* Numbers in parentheses are reference numbers

The cerebellum has been considered in more detail because, although it is not the critical part of the CNS with respect to adaptive behavior, knowledge of neurogenesis and the functional role of the different type of nerve cells in the cerebellum is relatively advanced. However, the implications are probably valid for other parts of the CNS in which microneurons are formed after birth. It has therefore been proposed that the different behavioral effects of corticosteroids or thyroid hormones depend on the time when treatment interferes with cell formation, which determines the cell types affected in different parts of the brain (27,29). This hypothesis may be applicable to other conditions, such as the effects of undernutrition (35,36) and amino acid imbalance (37) which also interfere with cell formation in the brain in rat and other species, including man (9).

EFFECT OF UNDERNUTRITION

Undernutrition deserves special attention: it may be a complicating factor not only in the model experiments described above, but also in human pathology. For example, it has been documented in the present volume that undernutrition is a serious problem in parts of the world where cretinism is endemic.

In a recent investigation rats received approximately 50 percent of their usual food intake from the sixth day of pregnancy throughout lactation, and the young were studied during the suckling period (38). This food restriction during pregnancy had only small overall effects; compared with controls the number of animals per litter was similar, and body and brain weights of newborn rats were only reduced by about 10 percent and four percent respectively. However, growth was seriously retarded after birth; at 21 days of age the weights of the body, cerebrum and cerebellum were respectively 65 percent, 15 percent, and 25 percent less than in the controls. Cell number in terms of DNA estimation was reduced only after birth, and although the age curves in both the cerebrum and the cerebellum were significantly different from controls, the differences were relatively little (Fig. 2).

In contrast to the relatively small effect of undernutrition on the postnatal increase in cell number, mitotic activity, measured by estimating the incorporation of [^{14}C]thymidine DNA, was markedly affected. The reduction in the labelling of DNA was even more severe than indicated by Fig. 3. In comparison with controls cell multiplication was reduced throughout the body, and [^{14}C]thymidine was removed from the blood more slowly. Thus, more

^{14}C was left in the precursor pool of the brain of experimental animals 1/2 hour after the injection of [^{14}C]thymidine, although the dose given per unit body weight was the same as in controls. When the labelling of DNA was corrected on the basis of the concentration of acid-soluble ^{14}C, the values were (as a percentage of control), at six days when inhibition was most severe, 17 percent in the cerebrum and 30 percent in the cerebellum. At 21 days they were 54 percent in the cerebrum and 73 percent in the cerebellum.

These results therefore showed that the reduction in the formation of DNA was not accompanied by a similar decrease in the extent of deposition of DNA in the brain of undernourished animals. One explanation for this is that in normal development cells are destroyed and formed at the same time, and that in the undernourished animal the massive retardation in mitotic activity is compensated by a reduction of cell loss. Other observations supported the view that cell destruction occurs in the brain during normal development: when the rate of deposition of DNA (cells) was expressed relative to the rate of labelling of DNA (mitotic activity) the values of the cerebrum were, depending on age, 30-80 percent less than in the cerebellum (38), although the lengths of the cell cycle and of DNA synthesis seem to be similar in the germinal sites of these two brain parts (80, 81). It is also known that during certain periods in embryogenesis cell loss accompanies new cell formation in the nervous system (39).

To summarize this section, it seems that mitotic activity in the CNS is sensitive to the maintenance of the metabolic balance, and that various unrelated influences result in a decrease in postnatal cell formation. The functional consequences of the interference with cell formation, that is the type of cell which is affected, depend on time. It seems that the final assembly of cells is affected not only by a reduction in the number of certain types of cells, but also by interference with the processes underlying cell destruction in the developing brain. The plasticity of the developing CNS is demonstrated by the different mechanisms which can counteract the ill-effects of an insult. For example, the retardation in cell formation may be compensated by a prolongation of the period of massive cell proliferation, as in thyroid deficiency, or by a reduction in the number of cells lost after birth, as in undernutrition. Nevertheless, the plasticity of the developing CNS has limitations, and cell number is not always restored to normal.

"BIOCHEMICAL DIFFERENTIATION" OF THE BRAIN

Adverse influences during the early postnatal period may affect not only the formation of new cells but also differentiation within the CNS. As a consequence of differentiation, the cells of a given organ attain a unique biochemical constitution. The coordination of the different metabolic pathways associated with glucose metabolism in the brain is well reflected in the fate of labelled glucose, which is a function of the age of the animal (40,41). Gaitonde and Richter (42) found that glucose carbon was converted rapidly into amino acids in the brain of adult animals. At 10 days of age, however, only 10-20 percent of the ^{14}C in the tissue was incorporated into amino acids and the values characteristic of the adult (60-70 percent) were reached during the following one to two weeks (Fig. 4 upper). Analysis of the results indicated that the developmental changes in the conversion of glucose carbon into amino acids result from quantitative and qualitative changes in the energy-yielding metabolism of the brain (41) - the glucose flux is about twice as high in the adult as in the immature brain. The pool size of glutamate, which is the most important single "trap" for the metabolized glucose carbon in the brain, is doubled, and the capacity for oxidizing a wide range of substrates is replaced by a predominant utilization of glucose. These biochemical changes occur during the period of rapid growth of neuronal processes (3,4), and there is independent evidence for an inter-relationship (for references, see ref. 41). As a result of the development of the metabolic compartment associated with neuronal processes the apparently homogeneous metabolic pattern is replaced by the heterogeneous pattern characteristic of the adult brain (Fig. 4 lower).

The metabolic heterogeneity of the brain was first observed by Waelsch's group (reviews 43-45). Briefly, it has been found that at short times after the administration of labelled amino acids or fatty acids to an animal the specific radioactivity of glutamine in the brain was higher than that of glutamate. Since glutamine is formed from glutamate the results indicate that a small and highly active pool of glutamate is the precursor of a major part of glutamine, i.e. glutamate and the associated tricarboxylic acid cycles are compartmented in brain tissue. Fig. 4 shows that metabolic compartmentation of glutamate develops during the same period as the maturation of glucose metabolism in terms of the rapid conversion of glucose carbon into amino acids, and the evidence has recently been summarized indicating that both phenomena are related to the metabolic properties of the expanding neuronal processes (46,47).

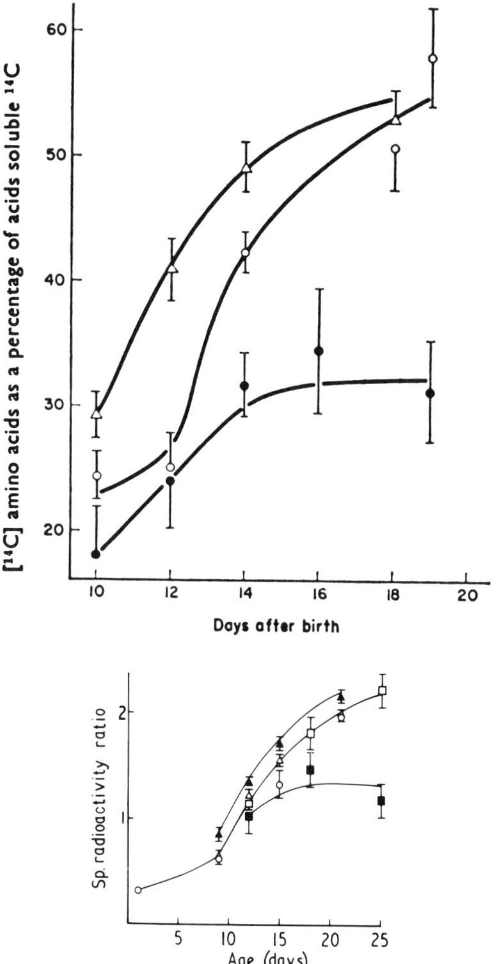

Fig. 4. Effect of thyroid hormone on the biochemical differentiation of the forebrain. (Upper) Conversion of glucose carbon into amino acids at 20 min after the intraperitoneal injection of 10-20 μCi [U-^{14}C]glucose per 100 g body wt.: o - Control, Δ- T_3-treated rats (cf. Fig.2), and ● - rats radiothyroidectomized at birth. The results are taken from Cocks et al. (41). (Lower) Metabolic compartmentation of glutamate. The ordinate represents the glutamine/glutamate specific radioactivity ratio at 10 min after subcutaneous injection of 10 μCi of [U-^{14}C]leucine per 100 g body wt. Open symbols - control: ▲ - T_3-treated rats, and ■ - rats radiothyroidectomized at birth. The data are taken from Patel and Balázs (47).

Studying the effects of thyroid hormone on brain development, we have used the conversion of glucose carbon into amino acids and the metabolic compartmentation of glutamate as markers for the "biochemical differentiation" of the brain (41,46,47). Our results showed that the biochemical maturation of the brain was advanced by treatment with thyroid hormone and retarded by neonatal thyroid deficiency. Since both biochemical markers studied are related to the development of the neuronal processes it seems that thyroid hormone is involved in the regulation of neuronal differentiation.

This conclusion is supported by morphological observations: the formation of dendritic spines on nerve cells is advanced by treatment with thyroid hormone in infancy (48,49). In contrast the dendritic arborization of the nerve cells is severely retarded in the thyroid deficient rat (16,50,51; Fig. 5). Eayrs (50) has postulated that as a result the probability of interneuronal connections is reduced, and recent developments in technology have facilitated the demonstration of the retardation in nerve termination formation in the brain of thyroid-deficient animals. The first indications of this effect were provided by biochemical studies. Hamburgh and Flexner (52) showed that the activity of succinate dehydrogenase, a mitochondrial enzyme which seems to be relatively concentrated in mitochondria derived from nerve terminals, is permanently reduced in the brain by neonatal thyroidectomy. On the other hand, the activity of glutamate dehydrogenase, a mitochrondrial enzyme which is not concentrated in synaptosomal mitochondria, was unaffected by thyroid deficiency (15). There is further evidence of a selective reduction in synaptosomal enzymes. Glutamate decarboxylase is enriched in the synaptoplasm whereas lactate dehydrogenase is uniformly distributed in the cytoplasm, and the activity of the former enzyme, but not the latter, was found to be significantly reduced in the brain of thyroid-deficient rats (15,53). Balázs *et al.* (15) proposed that the selective reduction in the activity of enzymes such as glutamate decarboxylase and succinate dehydrogenase, which are relatively concentrated in synaptosomes, is related to a decrease in the number of nerve terminals in the brain of thyroid-deficient rats. Ultrastructural studies have shown that the number of terminals per nerve cell is indeed reduced in the visual cortex of thyroid-deficient rats (54).

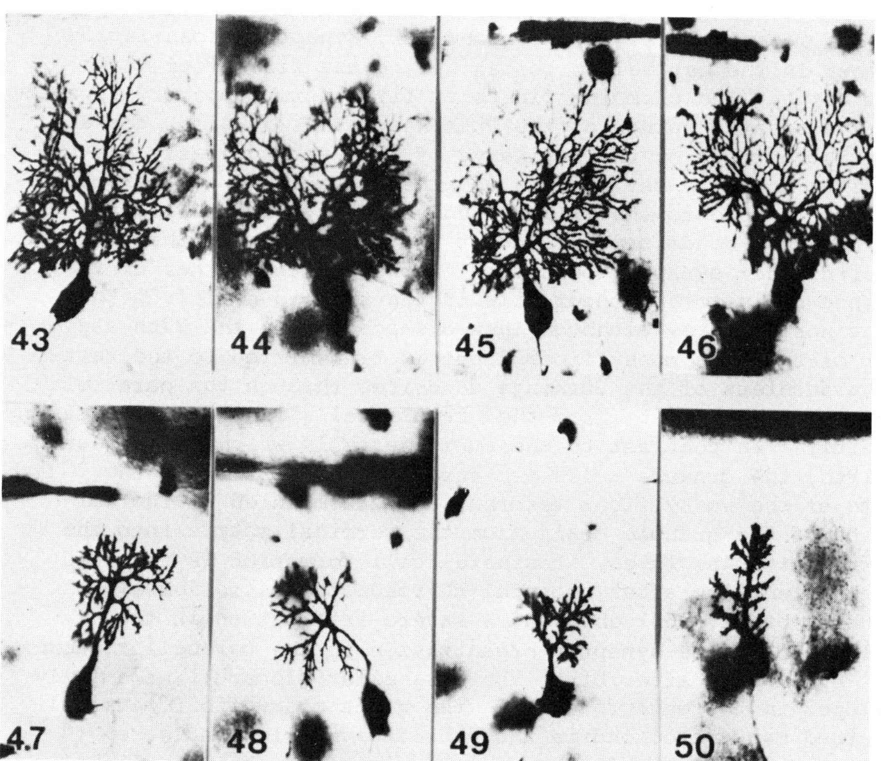

Fig. 5. Dendritic arborization of the Purkinje cells in the cerebellum of 14-day-old normal (upper row) and thyroid deficient rats (lower row) Golgi-Cox preparations. The results are taken from Legrand (16).

The development of synaptic organization in the cerebellar cortex has been studied recently by Hajos *et al.* (55). The axons of the Purkinje cells are the only fibers which leave the cerebellar cortex, and the Purkinje cells receive inputs directly from the climbing fibers and indirectly through the granule cells from the mossy fibers (34). In the rat, synaptic organization develops in the cerebellar cortex during the first four weeks after birth. The climbing fibers at first form temporary synapses with the somatic spines of the Purkinje cells (56,57). These synaptic contacts on the perikarya of the Purkinje cells disappear by the 16th day of life and the contacts of the climbing fibers move up onto the primary and secondary branches of the Purkinje cell dendrites. Hajos *et al.* (55) observed that the climbing fiber synapses persisted on the somatic spines of the Purkinje cells for a longer time in the thyroid-deficient than in the normal rats, although they disappeared by the 27th day after birth. The mossy fiber input is transmitted to the tertiary branchlets of the Purkinje dendrites through the parallel fibers which originate from the granule cells in the cerebellar glomeruli. In contrast to the Purkinje cells which are present at birth, the granule cells are formed after birth, and the growth of the mossy fiber terminals is accompanied by the emigration of the granule cells from the germinal matrix into the internal granular layer. Postnatal cell formation is retarded in the cerebellum after neonatal thyroidectomy (cf. above), and Hajós *et al.* (55) observed a severe retardation in the development of the synaptic organization in the cerebellar glomeruli. By 27 days after birth the cerebellar glomeruli were fully developed in the euthyroid rat: the giant mossy fiber terminals contained many mitochondria and synaptic vesicles and were surrounded by the terminal dendritic digits of the granule cells, each digit forming a synapse with the mossy terminal "rosette". In the thyroid-deficient rat at the same age, the mossy terminal rosettes were much smaller, the dendrites of the granule cells were often not split into terminal digits, and each dendritic trunk formed multiple synapses with the mossy terminal. In comparison with controls, glial processes occupied a larger area of the cerebellar glomeruli. It seems that thyroid deficiency in infancy results in the longer persistence of an immature "wiring" pattern in the cerebellum, in which the anatomical situation favors the dominance of the climbing fiber-Purkinje cell circuit over the mossy fiber-granule cell-Purkinje cell circuit.

PERIOD OF THYROID SENSITIVITY: COMPARISON OF EFFECTS OF THYROID DEFICIENCY AND UNDERNUTRITION

There seems to be a limited period when brain development is sensitive to thyroid hormones (for reviews see 58, 59). This is reflected in the age-dependence of the reversal of the biochemical and functional manifestations of thyroid deficiency by replacement therapy - in the rat, treatment is only successful when started before the age of 10-14 days (17,21,60). These results indicate that thyroid hormone is involved in the regulation of brain development during the period which precedes the extensive differentiation of nerve cells.

It is difficult to pinpoint the corresponding thyroid-sensitive period in the development of the human brain. Relative to either birth or life-span the thyroid gland starts to function earlier in man than in the rat. However, in both species extensive differentiation of nerve cells occurs during the early postnatal period (3,4,7,8). The possibility of the success of early remedial treatment in man is further increased by the observations indicating that the 'ontogenetic clock' is slower than normal in the brain of thyroid-deficient animals - both the period of cell proliferation and that of synaptic organization are prolonged (15,17,51,55). Thus, in terms of the developmental stage of the CNS, the hypothyroid subjects are "younger" than their chronological age would indicate.

Thyroid hormones may act directly on the cells in the CNS since they are taken up by brain tissue and by nerve cells in particular (61). Although the symptoms observed in experimental thyroid deficiency are reversed by remedial treatment when it is started at the right time, it is difficult to exclude the involvement of other factors, such as undernutrition or hypothermia, which are associated with the hypothyroid state (17,48). However, it seems that there are differences in the effects of undernutrition or thyroid deprivation on brain development (Table 2). The final cell number is less than normal after nutritional deprivation but it is normal in thyroid deficiency. The reduction in the rate of cell deposition is compensated by a prolongation of the period of massive cell proliferation in the brain of thyroid-deficient rats. In contrast, cell proliferation seems to stop at about the normal time in the undernourished animals, and the severe reduction in mitotic activity is counteracted by a decrease in cell loss. Average cell size is less than normal in the brain after neonatal thyroidectomy and this is related chiefly to a decreased expansion of the neuronal processes. Cell size is little affected by food deprivation, suggesting that dendritic arborization and nerve terminal formation are similar to normal.

In agreement with this view, it was observed that, in contrast to thyroid deficiency, undernutrition did not cause a delay either in the differentiation of Purkinje cells or in the appearance of cerebellar glomeruli (60). This conclusion is further supported by observations of certain enzymatic activities. There

Table 2. Effects of thyroid deficiency and undernutrition on brain development

	THYROID DEFICIENCY	UNDERNUTRITION
Brain weight	Reduced (15)*	Reduced (35,38,72)
Final cell number	Unaffected (15)	Reduced (35,38)
Period of postnatal cell formation	Prolonged -Cerebellum (15,16,17)	Unaffected - This is deduced from the observations that the deficit in cell number observed after post-weaning rehabilitation (36,64) is similar to that found at the end of the period of food restriction (38).
Mitotic activity		Reduced (38)
Cell loss		Reduced (38) - However, a selective loss of nerve cells which are formed before birth has been reported (65).
Cell size	Reduced (15)	Unaffected (38). A slight increase in cell size in the cerebellum of rehabilitated mice was noted (66).
Neurons:		
formation of dendrites	Reduced (50,51)	Normal - The Purkinje cells in cerebellum were studied (60).
formation of nerve terminals	Reduced (15,54)	
synaptic organization	Retarded - The development of the synaptic contacts of the climbing fibers and mossy fibers was studied in the cerebellum (55)	Normal - The development of the cerebellar glomeruli (mossy fiber input) was studied only with light microscopy (60).
Glia (myelination):		
amount of myelin	Reduced (62,67)	Reduced (36)
age when peak of [^{35}S] sulfatide synthesis is reached	Delayed (67)	Unaffected (68)
myelin structure	Unaffected	Impaired
	The thickness of myelin sheath per unit axonal diameter was determined in fibers of sciatic nerve and cervical spinal cord (60).	
Enzymes:		
glutamate decarboxylase	Reduced (15,53)	Unaffected - Determined only after rehabilitation; the activity per unit weight was increased, but it was normal when expressed per brain (69).
acetylcholine esterase	Reduced (52,70)	Transient reduction (71-73)
succinate dehydrogenase	Reduced (53,52)	Unaffected (71). Transient reduction (72,73).
Rate of protein synthesis	Reduced (74,75)	Unaffected - Determined only 24 hr after injection of [^{14}C]amino acids in mice (76).
Rate of RNA synthesis	Unaffected (15,75,77)	Transient reduction - Determined only 24 hr after injection of [^{3}H]orotic acid in mice (76).
Biochemical differentiation:		
maturation of glucose metabolism	Retarded (41)	Retarded (80)
Behavior:		
innately organized behavior	Retarded (21)	Retarded (78).
adaptive behavior	Impaired (21)	Impaired - Some investigators did not find a significant impairment (66,79).

*Numbers in parentheses are reference numbers

**In (84) the enzyme activity was determined at the end of the suckling period and in (69) only after rehabilitation. In contrast, when animals received protein-deficient diet after weaning, the enzyme activity was decreased and this was restored to normal on rehabilitation (85). [Added in proof] is evidence for relative enrichment of glutamate decaroylase in the cytoplasm of synaptosomes, and of succinate dehydrogenase in the synaptosomal mitochondria. These enzymic activities were less than normal in the brain of thyroid-deficient animals, but were either unaffected or only transiently influenced by nutritional deprivation. Acetylcholinesterase, which is probably relatively concentrated in post-synaptosomal membranes, behaved similarly.

Information about the effects of these treatments on the development of glial cells is more or less restricted to myelination, which can be taken, with certain limitations, as a marker of oligodendroglial function. Although in both conditions the amount of myelin deposited is less than normal, it seems that in the CNS the effects of thyroid deficiency are more severe than those of undernutrition. When the incorporation of ^{35}S into brain sulphatides was followed as an index of myelination, labelling reached a peak later in thyroid-deficient rats than in underfed or control rats. However, the retardation of myelination is not necessarily caused by altered oligodendroglial metabolism, but may result from a decrease in axonal density (62). This view is supported by the observation that the growth of fibers in the sciatic nerve and in cervical spinal cord was delayed in thyroid deficiency while, in terms of fiber diameter, myelination was normal. On the other hand, undernutrition affected the growth of myelinated fibers less than did hypothyroidism, but the myelination of the fibers was retarded.

The rate of protein synthesis is reduced in the brain of thyroid deficient rats _in vivo_ and the defect seems to involve the translation of the genetic message, since the rate of RNA synthesis is not correspondingly affected. Although a more detailed analysis would be needed, the effects of undernutrition are apparently different: the labelling of proteins was not affected at 24 hr after the injection of a mixture of [^{14}C]amino acids in the brain of 21-day-old mice, but the rate of incorporation of [^{3}H]orotic acid into RNA was significantly reduced.

The biochemical differentiation of the brain, assessed by the development of glucose metabolism and metabolic compartmentation, is severely retarded after neonatal thyroidectomy. A significant retardation of the maturation of glucose metabolism has also been observed recently in our laboratory with brain of undernourished animals (82). In thyroid deficiency the retarded development of the CNS is associated with a delay in the appearance of innately organized behavior. The functional consequences of abnormal brain development seem to be permanent, since when the animals grow up their performance in tests of adaptive behavior is impaired. Undernutrition also results in a retardation in the appearance of innately organized behavior. Observations concerning adaptive behavior are still controversial: some investigators reported that the performance of animals undernourished in infancy was normal whereas others claimed an impairment.

The results therefore indicate that the effects of thyroid deprivation on brain development are not mediated through undernutrition. Conversely, although undernutrition may lead to a decrease in thyroid function (63), it is unlikely that the observed effects are due to hypothyroidism. Nevertheless, it must be considered that in parts of the world where endemic cretinism is common, undernutrition is also a serious problem, and thus thyroid and nutritional deprivations may occur together. This may seriously impair the compensating faculties of the developing nervous system, leading to an aggravation of the functional consequences of the deficiencies.

SUMMARY

Transient changes in hormonal balance or temporal nutritional deprivation can influence the organization of the central nervous system leading to permanent changes in brain function. In animals such as the rat, which are relatively immature at birth, brain development is especially vulnerable during the early postnatal period, when the regulatory mechanisms of the infant are not yet fully developed. This applies also to man: neuronal differentiation extends well into the postnatal period, and there is reason to believe that microneuron formation also occurs, as in the rat, after birth.

Insults may affect the development of the brain by interfering with postnatal cell formation (e.g. treatment with thyroid hormone or corticosteroids and undernutrition). Behavioral consequences seem to depend on the timing of the event, which determines the type of nerve cells affected in different parts of the brain. Insults may also influence the differentiation of nerve cells in the central nervous system. The results indicate that thyroid hormones are involved in the regulation of processes associated with the growth of dendrites and axons: neuronal maturation is accelerated after treatment with thyroid hormones and is retarded in thyroid deficiency.

To correct the symptoms observed in neonatal thyroid deprivation replacement treatment must be started in the rat before the 14th day of age, which in the normal animal is near the end of the period of postnatal cell formation in the forebrain and is less than midway in the age course of the biochemical and morphological manifestations in neuronal maturation. The corresponding developmental stage in man would include the early postnatal period. Thus the implications from animal experiments are that the chances of therapeutic success are good if the treatment of the thyroid-deficient infant is started soon after birth.

The comparison of the results of undernutrition and thyroid deficiency on brain development indicated that the effects of thyroid deprivation are not mediated through undernutrition and vice versa. The sites of action of either condition on the developmental processes seem to be different. Thus when nutritional and thyroid deprivation occur together, brain function must be severely impaired by the reduction of the compensating faculties of the developing nervous system.

DISCUSSION BY PARTICIPANTS

HETZEL: Shall we return to the question of the lesion in hearing loss in cretinism?

BALÁZS: I think the sorts of changes in synaptic organization we have found in the cerebellum of thyroid deficient animals also occur in other parts of the central nervous system. The cerebellum is simply the easiest structure in which to study the effect. On the basis of the clinical observations I have heard in this symposium, it may be of interest to investigate the effects of thyroid deficiency on the development of synaptic organization in the central structures associated with hearing.

STANBURY: You can't discard the bony and hair cell changes that Gardner studied. Certainly something is happening locally in the middle ear.

QUERIDO: The lesions, if they arise during fetal life, probably have to occur midway in the first trimester. We are looking for something that could happen to the auditory system in the first trimester.

HORNABROOK: I fit Dr. Balázs's report with clinical observations this way: Perhaps damage may occur in the same way to other areas than the cerebellum at other stages of uterine life. Certainly there does not seem to be any doubt clinically that there must be eighth nerve damage as well as more extensive damage. There is no evidence of cerebellar damage, but I do not think that is important because we may be dealing with a different phase of development.

KOENIG: Does not the perceptive type of deafness in rubella, which according to the otolaryngologists is similar to deaf-mutism seen in endemic cretinism, occur in the first trimester of pregnancy? What Dr. Balázs described occurs later.

BALÁZS: In the experiments I have described the anomalous conditions, such as abnormal thyroid state, were initiated at a relatively late stage of development, and this was one of the reasons why we studied in more detail the cerebellum, which is a late-developing part of the CNS. However, I would suggest that when the abnormal conditions arise at an earlier stage, the effects on the maturation of parts of the CNS whose development is relatively advanced will be similar to those observed in the present studies in the cerebellum. I think that the nerve cells respond to these conditions in a more or less general fashion. It would appear that thyroid hormones are not necessary for the expression of the genetic potential of the nerve cells, but they are needed for the proper timing of the differentiation of the nerve cells, and they are somehow involved in the quantitative aspects of formation of neuronal processes.

STANBURY: The damage must be primarily after the third month, because all the evidence has it that the human fetus is athyreotic until about the twelfth week.

QUERIDO: We don't have any information on the first weeks of pregnancy. The placenta to fetus ratio is so excessive that the fetus is really bathing in blood, and under those conditions transfer of T_3 could occur, which could be very effective.

HERSHMAN: It is possible that unmeasurable amounts of T_3 of maternal origin are influencing development.

PHAROAH: That would mean the fetus is dependent on maternal hormone in the first three months, but the myxedematous mother does not produce a neurologically damaged child.

STANBURY: There is only one such case that is really well documented.

PHAROAH: Why isn't there a lower birth rate in iodine-deficient areas, if there is such a degree of hypothyroidism there?

IBBERTSON: There is little evidence that real hypothyroidism interferes with fertility. I have personally managed three hypothyroid women through pregnancy and each has produced a normal infant.

DELANGE: In Idjwi the hypothyroid women did not get pregnant because sexual development was retarded. There was no menarche.

BECKERS: In the Uele, where women had low PBIs, normal children were born.

FIERRO: In Ecuador a woman with a PBI of 0.8, a typical cretin, had a cretin infant.

PHAROAH: I had a patient with a PBI of 0.8 during pregnancy who had normal twins.

PRETELL: We had a case in which the mother had a T_4 of 1.8. She was a cretin, but clinically didn't look like a myxedematous cretin. Her baby had nine micrograms of T_4. He now looks normal.

PITTMAN: Price and Netsky reported what are called "cerebellar myxedema bodies" (83). They presumably occur in the adult myxedema. They were said to be specific for myxedema and presumably occurred after the brain was fully developed. The authors made a point of their being digested with diastase, indicating glycogen content.

ACKNOWLEDGEMENTS

The author gratefully acknowledges the collaboration of Mrs. M. Cotterrell, Drs. F. Hajós and A. J. Patel in the previously unpublished studies reported in the present paper. Gratitude is express to Dr. D. Richter for his advice and encouragement.

Figure 1 republished from (7) by permission of Harvard University Press; Figure 5 from Arch. Anat. Micr. Morph. Exp. by permission of Masson et cie; Figure 4 (upper) from J. Neuro-Chem, and Figure 4 (lower) from Biochem. J. by permission of the editor.

REFERENCES

1. Andersen, H.: The influence of hormones on human development. In: Human Development (F. Falkner, ed.). Saunders, Philadelphia, 1966. pp. 184-221.

2. Deanesly, R.: Foetal endocrinology. Br. Med. Bull. 17: 91-95, 1961.

3. Eayrs, J.T. and Goodhead, B.: Postnatal development of the cerebral cortex in the rat. J. Anat. 93:385-402, 1959.

4. Aghajanian, G.K. and Bloom, F.E.: The formation of synaptic junctions in developing rat brain: a quantitative electron microscopic study. Brain Res. 6:716-727, 1967.

5. Altman, J.: DNA metabolism and cell proliferation. In: Handbook of Neurochemistry, Vol. 2, Structural Neurochemistry (A. Lajtha, ed.) Plenum Press, New York, 1969, pp. 137-182.

6. Davison, A.N. and Dobbing, J.: The developing brain. In: Applied Neurochemistry (A.N. Davison and J. Dobbing, eds.). Blackwell, Oxford, 1968. pp. 253-286.

7. Conel, J.C.: The Postnatal Development of the Human Cerebral Cortex. Harvard Univ. Press, Cambridge, Mass., 1939-1967. 8 vols.

8. Larroche, J.-C.: The development of the central nervous system during intrauterine life. In: Human Development (F. Falkner, ed.). Saunders, Philadelphia, 1966. pp. 257-276.

9. Winick, M.: Malnutrition and brain development. J. Pediatr. 74:667-679, 1969.

10. Dobbing, J.: Undernutrition and the developing brain. The relevance of animal models to the human problem. Am. J. Dis. Child. 120:411-415, 1970.

11. Schwarz, H., Goolker, P. and Globus, J.H.: The normal histology of infants' brains with particular reference to anatomic changes in the brain in intestinal intoxication of infants. Am. J. Dis. Child. 43:889-913, 1932.

12. Lentz, R.D. and Lapham, L.W.: A quantitative cytochemical study of the DNA content of neurons of rat cerebellar cortex. J. Neurochem. 16:379-384, 1969.

13. Balázs, R. and Cocks, W.A.: RNA metabolism in subcellular fractions of brain tissue. J. Neurochem. 14:1035-1055, 1967.

14. Lerner, R.A., Meinke, W. and Goldstein, D.A.: Membrane-associated DNA in the cytoplasm of diploid human lymphocytes. Proc. Natl. Acad. Sci. USA 68:1212-1216, 1971.

15. Balázs, R., Kovács, S., Teichgräber, P., Cocks, W.A. and Eayrs, J.T.: Biochemical effects of thyroid deficiency on the developing brain. J. Neurochem. 15:1335-1349, 1968.

16. Legrand, J.: Analyse de l'action morphogénétique des hormones thyroïdiennes sur le cervelet du jeune rat. Arch. Anat. Microsc. Morphol. Exp. 56:205-244, 1967.

17. Hamburgh, M.: An analysis of the action of thyroid hormone on development based on in vivo and in vitro studies. Gen. Comp. Endocrinol. 10:198-213, 1968.

18. Balázs, R., Kovács, S., Cocks, W.A., Johnson, A.L. and Eayrs, J.T.: Effect of thyroid hormone on the biochemical maturation of rat brain: postnatal cell formation. Brain Res. 25:555-570, 1971.

19. Kovács, S., Cocks, W.A. and Balázs, R.: Incorporation of [2-^{14}C] thymidine into deoxyribonucleic acid of rat brain during postnatal development: effect of thyroid hormone. Biochem. J. 114:60P, 1969.

20. Tusques, J.: Recherches expérimentales sur le rôle de la thyroïde dans le développement du système nerveux. Biol. Med. (Paris) 45:395-413, 1956.

21. Eayrs, J.T.: Developmental Relationships between brain and thyroid. In: Endocrinology and Human Behaviour (R.P. Michael, ed.). Oxford Univ. Press, London, 1968. pp. 239-255.

22. Eayrs, J.T. and Holmes, R.L.: Effect of neonatal hyperthyroidism on pituitary structure and function in the rat. J. Endocrinol. 29:71-81, 1964.

23. Bakke, J.L. and Lawrence, N.: Persistent thyrotropin insufficiency following neonatal thyroxine administration. J. Lab. Clin. Med. 67:477-482, 1966.

24. Kovács, S., Cocks, W.A. and Balázs, R.: Effect of thyroid hormone administration on the incorporation of [1-^{14}C]-leucine into protein of rat pituitary and hypothalamus during development. J. Endocrinol. 45:IX-X, 1969.

25. Howard, E.: Effects of corticosterone and food restriction on growth and on DNA, RNA and cholesterol contents of the brain and liver in infant mice. J. Neurochem. 12:181-191, 1965.

26. Howard, E.: Reductions in size and total DNA of cerebrum and cerebellum in adult mice after corticosterone treatment in infancy. Exp. Neurol. 22:191-208, 1968.

27. Balázs, R.: Effects of hormones on the biochemical maturation of the brain. In: Influence of Hormones on the Nervous System (D.H. Ford, ed.). Karger, Basel, 1971. pp. 150-164.

28. Cotterrell, M.: The effect of growth hormone and corticosteroid treatment on the biochemical maturation of rat brain. M. Phil. Thesis: Council for National Academic Awards, London, 1971.

29. Balázs, R. and Cotterrell, M.: Effect of hormonal state on cell number and functional maturation of the brain. Nature (Lond.), 236:348-350, 1972.

30. Cotterrell, M., Balázs, R. and Johnson, A.L.: Effects of corticosteroids on the biochemical maturation of rat brain: postnatal cell formation. J. Neurochem., in press.

31. Schapiro, S., Salas, M. and Vukovich, K.: Hormonal effects on ontogeny of swimming ability in the rat: assessment of central nervous system development. Science 168:147-151, 1970.

32. Howard, E. and Granoff, D.M.: Increased voluntary running and decreased motor coordination in mice after neonatal corticosterone implantation. Exp. Neurol. 22:661-673, 1968.

33. Prestige, M.: On numbers and neurones. In: The Brain in Unclassified Mental Retardation, Ciba Foundation Study Group No. 3 (J.B. Cavanagh, ed.). Churchill, London, in press.

34. Eccles, J.C., Ito, M. and Szentágothai, J., The Cerebellum as a Neuronal Machine, Springer, Berlin, 1967.

35. Winick, M. and Noble, A.: Cellular response in rats during malnutrition at various ages. J. Nutr. 89:300-306, 1966.

36. Dobbing, J.: Effects of experimental undernutrition on development of the nervous system. In: Malnutrition, Learning and Behaviour (N.S. Scrimshaw and J.E. Gordon, eds.). M.I.T. Press, Cambridge, Mass., 1968. pp. 181-202.

37. Chase, H.P. and O'Brien, D.: Effect of excess phenylalanine and of other amino acids on brain development in the infant rat. Pediatr. Res. 4:96-102, 1970.

38. Patel, A.J. and Balázs, R.: Effect of undernutrition on postnatal cell formation in the rat brain. (in preparation)

39. Hamburger, V. and Levi-Montalcini, R.: Proliferation, differentiation and degeneration in the spinal ganglia of the chick embryo under normal and experimental conditions. J. Exp. Zool. 111:457-501, 1949.

40. Balázs, R.: Carbohydrate metabolism. In: Handbook of Neurochemistry, Vol. 3, Metabolic Reactions in the Nervous System (A. Lajtha, ed.). Plenum Press, New York, 1970. pp. 1-36.

41. Cocks, J.A., Balázs, R., Johnson, A.L. and Eayrs J.T.: Effect of thyroid hormone on the biochemical maturation of rat brain: conversion of glucose-carbon into amino acids. J. Neurochem. 17:1275-1285, 1970.

42. Gaitonde, M.K. and Richter, D.: Changes with age in the utilization of glucose carbon in liver and brain. J. Neurochem. 13:1309-1316, 1966.

43. Berl, S. and Clarke, D.D.: Compartmentation of amino acid metabolism. In: Handbook of Neurochemistry, Vol. 2, Structural Neurochemistry (A. Lajtha, ed.). Plenum Press, New York, 1969. pp. 447-471.

44. Van den Berg, C.J.: Glutamate and glutamine. In: Handbook of Neurochemistry, Vol. 3, Metabolic Reactions in the Nervous System (A. Lajtha, ed.). Plenum Press, New York, 1970. pp. 355-379.

45. Balázs, R. and Cremer, J.E., eds.: Metabolic Compartmentation in the Brain. Macmillan, London, in press.

46. Patel, A.J. and Balázs, R.: Manifestation of metabolic compartmentation during the maturation of the rat brain. J. Neurochem. 17:955-971, 1970.

47. Patel, A.J. and Balázs, R.: Effect of thyroid hormone on metabolic compartmentation in the developing rat brain. Biochem. J. 121:469-481, 1971.

48. Schapiro, S.: Some physiological, biochemical, and behavioral consequences of neonatal hormone administration: cortisol and thyroxine. Gen. Comp. Endocrinol. 10:214-228, 1968.

49. Legrand, J. and Bout, M.-C.: Influence de l'hypothyroïdisme et de la thyroxine sur le development des épines dendritiques des cellules de Purkinjé dans le cervelet du jeune rat. C. R. Acad. Sci. (Paris) 271:1199-1202, 1970.

50. Eayrs, J.T.: The cerebral cortex of normal and hypothyroid rats. Acta Anat. (Basel) 25:160-183, 1955.

51. Legrand, J.: Variations, en fonction de l'age, de la réponse du cervelet a l'action morphogénétique de la thyroïde chez le rat. Arch. Anat. Microsc. Morphol. Exp. 56:291-307, 1967.

52. Hamburgh, M. and Flexner, L.B.: Biochemical and physiological differentiation during morphogenesis. XXI. Effect of hypothyroidism and hormone therapy on enzyme activities of the developing cerebral cortex of the rat. J. Neurochem. 1:279-288, 1957.

53. García Argiz, C.A., Pasquini, J.M., Kaplún, B. and Gómez, C.J.: Hormonal regulation of brain development. II. Effect of neonatal thyroidectomy on succinate dehydrogenase and other enzymes in developing cerebral cortex and cerebellum of the rat. Brain Res. 6:635-646, 1967.

54. Cragg, B.G.: Synapses and membranous bodies in experimental hypothyroidism. Brain Res. 18:297-307, 1970.

55. Hajós, F., Patel, A.J. and Balázs, R.: Effect of thyroid deficiency on the synaptic organization of the rat cerebellar cortex. (in preparation)

56. Larramendi, L.M.H. and Victor, T.: Synapses on the Purkinje cell spines in the mouse. An electronmicroscopic study. Brain Res. 5:15-30, 1967.

57. O'Leary, J.L., Inukai, J. and Smith, J.M.: Histogenesis of the cerebellar climbing fiber in the rat. J. Comp. Neurol. 142:377-392, 1971.

58. Eayrs, J.T.: Age as a factor determining the severity and reversibility of the effects of thyroid deprivation in the rat. J. Endocrinol. 22:409-419, 1961.

59. Balázs, R.: Biochemical effects of thyroid hormones in the developing brain. In: Cellular Aspects of Neural Growth and Differentiation, UCLA Forum in Medical Science No. 14 (D.C. Pease, ed.). Univ. Calif. Press, Berkeley, 1971. pp. 273-311.

60. Legrand, J.: Comparative effects of thyroid deficiency and undernutrition on maturation of the nervous system and particularly on myelination in the young rat. In: Hormones in Development (M. Hamburgh and E.J.W. Barrington, eds.). Appleton-Century-Crofts, New York, 1971. pp. 381-390.

61. Ford, D.H.: Central nervous system-thyroid interrelationships. Brain Res. 7:329-349, 1968.

62. Balázs, R., Brooksbank, B.W.L., Davison, A.N., Eayrs, J.T. and Wilson, D.A.: The effect of neonatal thyroidectomy on myelination in the rat brain. Brain Res. 15:219-232, 1969.

63. Mulinos, M.G. and Pomerantz, L.: Psuedo-hypophysectomy. A condition resembling hypophysectomy produced by malnutrition. J. Nutr. 19:493-504, 1940.

64. Guthrie, H.A. and Brown, M.L.: Effect of severe undernutrition in early life on growth, brain size and composition in adult rats. J. Nutr. 94:419-426, 1968.

65. Dobbing, J., Hopewell, J.W. and Lynch, A.: Vulnerability of developing brain: VII. Permanent deficit of neurons in cerebral and cerebellar cortex following early mild undernutrition. Exp. Neurol. 32:439-447, 1971.

66. Howard, E. and Granoff, D.M.: Effect of neonatal food restriction in mice on brain growth, DNA and cholesterol, and on adult delayed response learning. J. Nutr. 95: 111-121, 1968.

67. Walravens, P. and Chase, H.P.: Influence of thyroid on formation of myelin lipids. J. Neurochem. 16:1477-1484, 1969.

68. Chase, H.P., Dorsey, J. and McKhann, G.M.: The effect of malnutrition on the synthesis of a myelin lipid. Pediatrics 40:551-559, 1967.

69. Adlard, B.P.F., Dobbing, S., Lynch, A., R. Balázs, and Reynolds, A.P.: Effect of undernutrition in early life on glutamate decarboxylase activity in the adult brain. Biochem. J., in press.

70. Geel, S.E. and Timiras, P.S.: Influence of neonatal hypothyroidism and of thyroxine on the acetylcholinesterase and cholinesterase activities in the developing central nervous system of the rat. Endocrinology 80:1069-1074, 1967.

71. Sereni, F., Principi, N., Perletti, L. and Sereni, L.P.: Undernutrition and the developing rat brain. I. Influence on acetylcholinesterase and succinic acid dehydrogenase activities and on norepinephrine and 5-OH-tryptamine tissue concentrations. Biol. Neonat. (Basel) 10:254-265, 1966.

72. Adlard, B.P.F. and Dobbing, J.: Vulnerability of developing brain. III. Development of four enzymes in the brains of normal and undernourished rats. Brain Res. 28:97-107, 1971.

73. Adlard, B.P.F. and Dobbing, J.: Elevated acetylcholinesterase activity in adult rat brain after undernutrition in early life. Brain Res. 30:198-199, 1971.

74. Geel, S.E., Valcana, T. and Timiras, P.S.: Effect of neonatal hypothyroidism and of thyroxine on L-[^{14}C]-leucine incorporation in protein in vivo and the relationship to ionic levels in the developing brain of the rat. Brain Res. 4:143-150, 1967.

75. Balázs, R., Cocks, W.A., Eayrs, J.T. and Kovács, S.: Biochemical effects of thyroid hormones on the developing brain. In: Hormones in Development, (M. Hamburgh and E.J.W. Barrington, eds.). Appleton-Century-Crofts, New York, 1971. pp. 357-379.

76. Lee, C-J.: Biosynthesis and characteristics of brain protein and ribonucleic acid in mice subjected to neonatal infection or undernutrition. J. Biol. Chem. 245:1998-2004, 1970.

77. Geel, S.E. and Timiras, P.S.: Influence of growth hormone on cerebral cortical RNA metabolism in immature hypothyroid rats. Brain Res. 22:63-72, 1970.

78. Smart, J.L. and Dobbing, J.: Vulnerability of developing brain. II. Effects of early nutritional deprivation on reflex ontogeny and development of behaviour in the rat. Brain Res. 28:85-95, 1971.

79. Baird, A., Widdowson, E.M. and Cowley, J.J.: Effects of calorie and protein deficiencies early in life on the subsequent learning ability of rats. Br. J. Nutr. 25: 391-403, 1971.

80. Fujita, S.: Quantitative analysis of cell proliferation and differentiation in the cortex of the postnatal mouse cerebellum. J. Cell. Biol. 32:277-287, 1967.

81. Lewis, P.D.: A quantitative study of cell proliferation in the subependymal layer of the adult rat brain. Exp. Neurol. 20:203-207, 1968.

82. Balázs, R. and Patel, A.J.: Factors affecting the biochemical maturation of the brain. In: Neurological Aspects of Maturation and Ageing (D.H.Ford, ed.) Progr. Brain Research Elsevier, Amsterdam (in press).

83. Price, T.R. and Netsky, M.G.: Myxedema and ataxia; cerebellar alterations and "neural myxedema bodies". Neurology (Minneap.) 16:957-962, 1966.

84. Rajalakshmi, R.; Ali, S.Z. and Ramakrishnan, C.V.: Effect of inanition during the neonatal period on discrimination, learning and brain biochemistry. J. Neurochem. 14:29-34, 1967.

85. Rajalakshmi, R., Govindarajan, K.R. and Ramakrishnan, C.V.: Effect of dietary protein content on visual discrimination learning and brain biochemistry in the albino rat. J. Neurochem. 12:261-271, 1965.

DEVELOPMENT OF THE THYROID CONTROL SYSTEM

Jerome M. Hershman and Fleurette Kram Hershman

Metabolic Research Laboratory, Birmingham Veterans Administration Hospital, and Division of Endocrinology and Metabolism, Department of Medicine, University of Alabama, Birmingham, Alabama

The role of thyroid hormone in the development of the human fetus has not been defined clearly. The neurologic abnormalities of the cretin suggest that thyroid hormone exerts a crucial role in the development of the central nervous system, but the stage of fetal development at which thyroid hormone affects the brain remains unknown. This review concerns the development of the hypothalamic-pituitary-thyroid control system primarily in the human fetus. In the developmental history of an endocrine gland, three different phases may be distinguished: (1) the first morphological differentiation of a recognizable gland from its embryological primordium; (2) the biochemical capacity for the production of a specific hormone; and (3) functionally significant synthesis and release of hormone into the blood stream (1).

THYROID GLAND

The human fetal thyroid gland has the capacity to make thyroglobulin at 4.2 weeks of gestation (2), at which time the thyroid is a bud-like mass of cells either still attached to the pharyngeal floor or just detached and not yet invaded by vascular mesenchyme. The synthesis of the protein thyroglobulin precedes the capacity for its iodination; iodination has been demonstrated at 11 weeks of gestation (2,3). The beginning of colloid formation occurs at 10 to 11.5 weeks of gestation in the human fetal thyroid (4,5). This is the stage when the ratio of thyroid weight to body weight attains the mature level and the time when the follicles begin to accumulate colloid in their central lumina (5).

The iodinated thyroglobulin of the 11 week fetus has the full spectrum of organically bound, iodinated products including significant amounts of T_4 and T_3 (4). Thyroxine has been found in serum at 11 weeks of gestation, indicating that it is secreted within a few days of the initiation of synthesis (6). Free thyroxine is low initially, increases progressively, and nearly reaches term serum levels at 18-20 weeks (6).

In a study of 13 fetuses obtained at therapeutic abortions (ages 12.6 to 19 weeks gestation), the mean thyroid uptake of the fetus 24 to 48 hours after the administration of ^{131}I to the mother was 2.1 percent per gm thyroid (range 0.2 to 4); the ^{131}I uptake per gm thyroid did not vary with age within this range of ages, as shown in Fig. 1. The total thyroid uptake

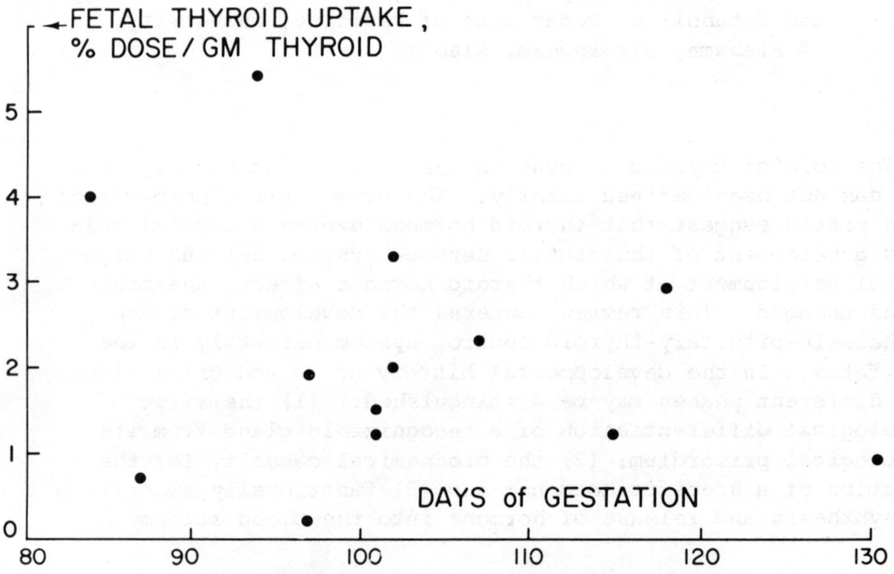

Fig. 1. Fetal thyroid uptake (% dose/gm thyroid) 24 to 48 hours after the administration of ^{131}I to the mother shown in relation to the gestational age of the fetus calculated from crown-rump length.

increased with the age and weight of the thyroid. These results are similar to those reported by Evans et al. (7). Comparison of the fetal thyroid uptake with that of the mother per unit weight of thyroid showed that the fetal thyroid had a higher uptake than the maternal thyroid in 12 of 13 pairs (Fig. 2). Although estimates of the maternal thyroid size by palpation for these calculations were not likely to be very accurate, none

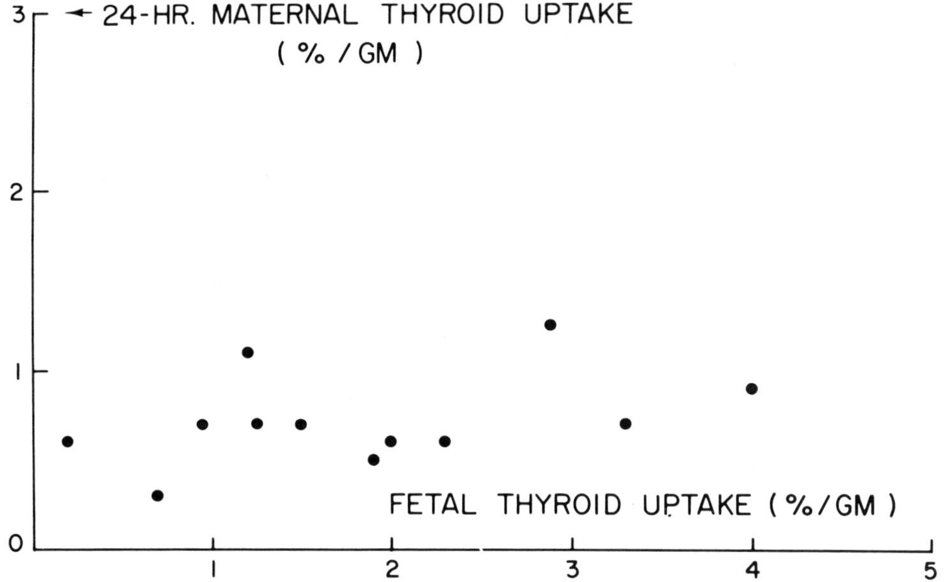

Fig. 2. Maternal thyroid uptake per gram thyroid (size estimated by palpation) plotted against the fetal thyroid uptake (% dose given to the mother/gm fetal thyroid).

of the maternal glands was enlarged beyond the size expected for a normal pregnancy. The high functional activity of the fetal thyroid per unit of mass suggests that the thyroid cells are both competent and efficient after 12 weeks of gestation.

PITUITARY THYROTROPIN

Although the cytologic differentiation of the pituitary begins at about eight weeks gestation, histochemical evidence of thyrotropin formation does not occur until 13 weeks (8). Gitlin and Biasuccio found immunochemical evidence of growth hormone in pituitaries of nine to 10.5 weeks; thyrotropin was not detectable in these glands, but was found in a 14 week pituitary (9). Fukuchi *et al.* recently showed that thyrotropin was detectable in the human pituitary at 12 weeks of gestation (10). The content increased progressively, reaching one-tenth of adult pituitary content at 32 weeks gestation. Recent studies of the pituitary content of TSH in 19 fetuses in our laboratory gave similar results; TSH was detectable by radioimmunoassay as early as 10.6 to 11 weeks of gestation (Fig. 3).

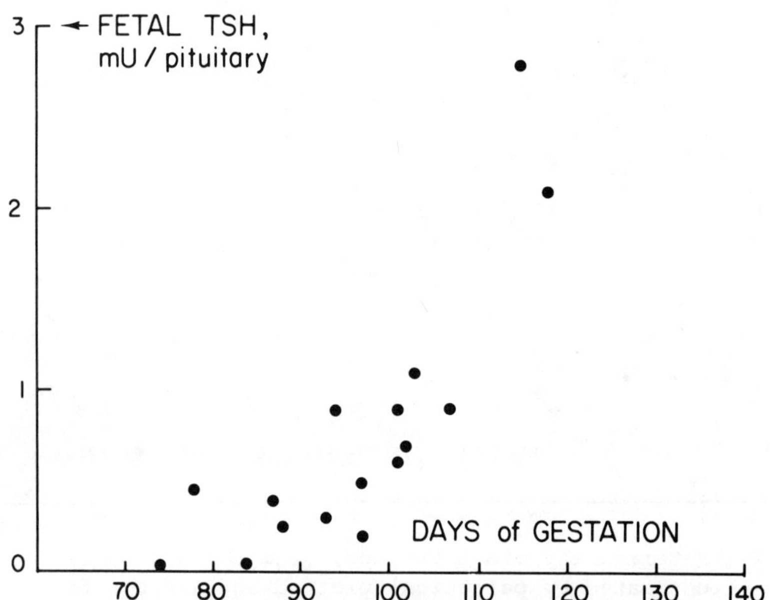

Fig. 3. Fetal pituitary TSH measured by radioimmunoassay at various gestational ages for 19 fetuses.

TSH has been detected in serum at 12 weeks gestation (6,11), and increases in an irregular manner therafter; fetal levels exceed maternal levels at 22 to 38 weeks. Serum TSH levels at birth exceed maternal levels (11-13), and rise abruptly within one hour after birth, preceding and probably initiating the neonatal increase in thyroid hormone seen at one to two days of life (12). The onset of synthesis and secretion of thyroid hormone and thyrotropin in the fetus are very closely associated. This suggests that secretion of a functionally significant amount of thyroid hormone is dependent on thyrotropin.

Jost showed that the thyroid of rats differentiates follicles and attains its typical histologic structure in the absence of the pituitary (1), but it remains smaller than controls, as in infants lacking a pituitary (14). The thyroids of decapitated rat and rabbit fetuses show reduction of radioiodine uptake and of thyroxine release and synthesis (1). Propylthiouracil given to the mother is transferred to the fetus and causes goiter unless the fetus is decapitated (1). Antithyroid treatment and fetal thyroidectomy both cause enlargement of the fetal pituitary which is prevented by administering thyroxine to the fetus. In summary these studies show that, in the absence of the pituitary gland, differentiation of the thyroid takes place but thyroid function is considerably reduced and that the response of the fetal thyroid to physiologic stimuli is dependent on thyrotropin. Further, the data suggest that in the absence of thryotropin, the fetal thyroid does not secrete enough hormone to influence other organs (1).

Thyroid-stimulating activity has been extracted from normal placentas (15,16). This thyrotropin, human chorionic thyrotropin, is similar to human pituitary thyrotropin in molecular size but differs from it immunologically. The content of chorionic thyrotropin in individual full-term human placentas varies markedly (17). Another thyrotropin of larger size and different immunologic activity has been found in urinary extracts of normal women and in the serum and tissue of women with hydatidiform mole (18). Recently we have isolated the larger placental thyrotropin from normal placentas (19). Hennen and his colleagues reported the detection of significant amounts of human chorionic thyrotropin in the serum of pregnant women with highest levels in the first trimester (16); but we have not been able to confirm this even with a sensitive immunoassay for chorionic thyrotropin (19). Whether placental thyrotropin enters the fetal circulation and influences the fetal thyroid has not been established. Another possible role for placental thyrotropin is stimulation of the maternal thyroid to increase secretion of maternal thyroid hormone and thereby increase transport of maternal thyroid hormone to the fetus, but this concept remains speculative.

HYPOTHALAMUS AND THYROTROPIN-RELEASING FACTOR (TRF)

Studies in encephalectomized rats with intact pituitaries show little reduction of thyroid function and indicate the capacity of the fetal pituitary to respond to alterations of thyroid feedback in the absence of the hypothalamus (1). However, the thyroid function of these animals is not completely normal. In human anencephalic monsters, the thyroid gland is normal in weight and in histologic structure in contrast with the atrophy seen in the infant without a pituitary (1,14). These data are compatible with Reichlin's concept that the hypothalamus, through its secretion of thyrotropin-releasing hormone, regulates the "set point" of the pituitary secretion of TSH but does not turn it off (20). In contrast with TSH, which does not cross the rat placenta in either direction, the synthetic tripeptide, TRF (L-pyroglutamyl-L-histidyl-L-proline amide) stimulates the maternal thyroid when injected into the fetus and the fetal thyroid when injected into the mother (21). This raises the possibility that maternal (or fetal) TRF may play a role in initiating the secretion of thyrotropin.

Fig. 4 summarizes the development of the hypothalamic-pituitary-thyroid system showing the initial time of hormonogenesis and secretion of thyroid hormone and pituitary TSH. Data on the role of the hypothalamus in this aspect of man's development are lacking. This should be a fruitful area for further research.

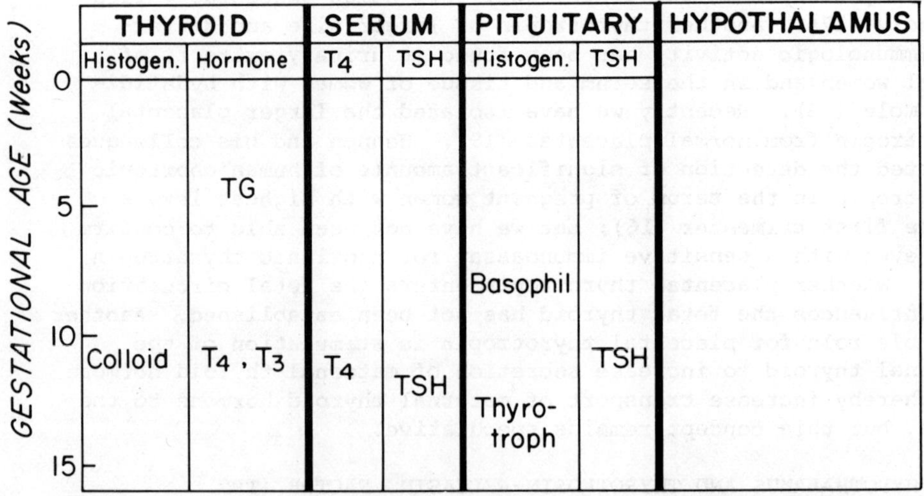

Fig. 4. Diagram of the histogenesis and hormogenesis of the hypothalamic-pituitary-thyroid control system. The possible role of the placenta is not shown.

SUMMARY

The parallel functional development of the human fetal pituitary and thyroid suggests that the onset of secretion of thyroid hormone is dependent on thyrotropin. The roles of the hypothalamic secretion of thyrotropin-releasing factor and of placental thyrotropin have not been adequately evaluated in the development of the thyroid control system of man.

ACKNOWLEDGEMENTS

The authors are grateful for the excellent technical assistance of Anne L. Bailey, Willard R. Starnes, and Pamela Switzer and the secretarial assistance of Mary K. Miles.

This work was supported by USPHS Research Grant HD05487 from the National Institute of Child Health and Human Development and VA Research Funds

DISCUSSION BY PARTICIPANTS

COSTA: We have found thyrotropic activity in the hypophyses of three-month human fetuses by biological methods. The excretion of thyroxine from the fetal thyroid and the TSH serum activity occurred nearly at the same point. We made these studies in Yugoslavia when legal abortion was done by "sectio parva"; the age of the fetus was deduced from the crown-rump length. We are now studying the problem of chorionic TSH. In the serum of both the mother and the fetus we have found a higher level of TSH when measured by biological methods than when measured by radioimmunoassay. If maternal sera and amniotic fluids are tested both in a human homologous and in a heterologous (bovine) radioimmunoassay, the maternal sera do also cross react in the heterologous radioimmunoassay while the amniotic fluids interfere in the bovine system only. These results suggest that the high TSH activity of the maternal sera is supported both by hypophyseal and by chorionic TSH, while the latter only is responsible for the TSH activity of the amniotic fluid.

HERSHMAN: That would fit with the data reported by Hennen (16) who found high levels of biologic activity that could also be detected in an immunoassay for chorionic thyrotropin, but not in the human TSH immunoassay. There is another problem. The bioassay for TSH, the mouse bioassay of McKenzie, gives a higher activity, when one uses the human standard, than does the immunoassay (13). This was also reported by Miyai, et al. (22) in their studies of pituitary content of TSH in human fetuses. They found five times as much activity by bioassay as by immunoassay, and we also found this discrepancy. That does muddy the issue of whether the differences would be due to another thyrotropin or whether there is a problem comparing bioassay with immunoassay data. I have been unable to confirm the data of Hennen. The amounts of biologic activity that I have been able to detect at various stages of pregnancy would just correspond roughly to the amounts we can find by immunoassay for human pituitary TSH. In other words, we do not find anything suggesting that there would be large quantities of thyrotropin in the serum. If anything, I think that the quantitites are relatively small and perhaps within the physiologic range of thyrotropic activity, rather than there being large amounts of TSH activity arising from the placenta. I think also that we are missing, with the chorionic TSH immunoassay, the large molecular weight stimulator. That does not cross-react at all in the immunoassay for TSH, and would not in the heterologous assay of Lemarchard-Beraud.

IBBERTSON: You mentioned the lack of evidence of chorionic thyrotrophin in the fetal circulation. Have you in fact tried your assay with fetal serum?

HERSHMAN: We have looked at a couple of them and have not found it, but have not made a good search.

PRETELL: Your data show that the fetal gland is more active than the maternal gland in taking up iodine. It has also been said that the thyroxine turnover rate in the fetal system is much more rapid than in the maternal. What would be the requirements of iodine in the fetal gland to synthesize thyroid hormones for its own use?

HERSHMAN: I could make no quantitative estimate. Fisher and Oddie (23) show an extremely high thyroxine turnover in newborns in relation to body size. Our data would show that the fetal thyroid is more avid for radioiodine, but ours are static measurements. We could not estimate thyroxine turnover. The comparison is fetus versus mother, and the fetus seems to have higher uptake.

IBBERTSON: Fisher (24) estimates 35 μg per day of T_4 turnover for the average 7.5 lb. infant.

HERSHMAN: That is just slightly under the adult rate.

STANBURY: You alluded to the set point of the pituitary-thyroid loop and its possible modulation by TRF. I think this is an important point conceptually. The control of the thyroid is more complex than a single loop system. If it were that simple, we would have no trouble determining the set point. There is evidence that the thyroid is not only controlled by TSH, but, to a limited degree, by the amount of iodine within the thyroid, and perhaps by the amount of T_4 directly within the thyroid. The secretion of TRF, unless it is different from other systems in the body, has its own feedback loop, perhaps with the pineal body and perhaps with higher centers involved. The whole is a complex system of feedback loops. The engineers will tell you that if you upset one loop in such systems the others will tend to compensate. Perhaps we should speak not of set point, but of equilibrium point.

COSTA: How was the blood of human fetuses obtained in the studies you reported?

HERSHMAN: In most of the studies, it was obtained from the cord. In some cases it was obtained by cardiac puncture.

COSTA: We have found transplacental passage of thyroxine already during the third month of fetal life. In these experiments radiothyroxine was administered intravenously to the mother, and two days later it was demonstrated chromatographically in the cord blood. The thyroids of the mother and of the fetus had been previously saturated with iodine. We do not know the amount of the hormone crossing the placenta, or whether it is biologically important.

DEGROOT: Do you think one can argue from the low levels of free thyroxine in three-month fetuses that thyroid hormone is not very important up to that point? Does the importance of the hormone in development parallel the level of the free T_4, or is that too simplistic?

HERSHMAN: Speculating teleologically, the system certainly gets turned on at that point and is presumably doing something. As to what is happening beforehand, we have not ruled out the possibility of maternal thyroid hormone getting across in small quantitites and affecting the embryo or fetus at very early stages.

DELANGE: Fisher showed me data from sheep just last week which indicated that there is negligible passage of T_4 from the mother to the fetus during pregnancy. Secondly, T_4 does not seem to be necessary to induce fetal growth in terms of weight. The mothers were normal, the fetuses thyroidectomized.

STANBURY: The thyroidectomy is probably done after the fetus has completed most of its differentiation. You could postulate active transport across the placenta. There is active iodine transport across the placenta, according to Logothetopoulos and Scott (25). This was in guinea pig, rabbit, and rat.

DEGROOT: There is active transport of gamma globulin across the placenta; other proteins are not concentrated.

REFERENCES

1. Jost, A., and Picon, L.: Hormonal control of fetal development and metabolism. Adv. Metab. Dis. 4:123-184, 1970.

2. Gitlin, D., and Biasucci, A.: Ontogenesis of immunoreactive thyroglobulin in the human conceptus. J. Clin. Endocrinol. Metab. 29:849-853, 1969.

3. Olin, P., Vecchio, G., Ekholm, R. and Almqvist, S.: Human fetal thyroglobulin: characterization and in vitro biosynthesis studies. Endocrinology 86:1041-1048, 1970.

4. Shepard, T.H.: Onset of function in the human fetal thyroid: biochemical and radioautographic studies from organ culture. J. Clin. Endocrinol. Metab. 27:945-958, 1967.

5. Shepard, T.H., Andersen, H. and Andersen, H.J.: Histochemical studies of the human fetal thyroid during the first half of fetal life. Anat. Rec. 149:363-380, 1964.

6. Greenberg, A.H., Czernichow, P., Reba, R.C., Tyson, J. and Blizzard, R.M.: Observations on the maturation of thyroid function in early fetal life. J. Clin. Invest. 49:1790-1803, 1970.

7. Evans, T.C., Kretzschmar, R.M., Hodges, R.E. and Song, C.W.: Radioiodine uptake studies of the human fetal thyroid. J. Nucl. Med. 8:157-165, 1967.

8. Rosen, F., and Ezrin, F.: Embryology of the thyrotroph. J. Clin. Endocrinol. Metab. 26:1343-1345, 1966.

9. Gitlin, D., and Biasucci, A.: Ontogenesis of immunoreactive growth hormone, follicle-stimulating hormone, thyroid-stimulating hormone, luteinizing hormone, chorionic prolactin and chorionic gonadotropin in the human conceptus. J. Clin. Endocrinol. Metab. 29:926-935, 1969.

10. Fukuchi, M., Ionue, T., Abe, H. and Kumahara, T.: Thyrotropin in human fetal pituitaries. J. Clin. Endocrinol. Metab. 31:565-569, 1970.

11. Fisher, D.A., Hobel, C.J., Garza, R. and Pierce, C.A.: Thyroid function in the preterm fetus. Pediatrics 46:208-216, 1970.

12. Fisher, D.A., and Odell, W.D.: Acute release of thyrotropin in the newborn. J. Clin. Invest. 48:1670-1677, 1969.

13. Hershman, J.M. and Pittman, J.A., Jr.: Utility of the radioimmunoassay of serum thyrotrophin in man. Ann. Intern. Med. 74:481-490, 1971.

14. Reid, J.O.: Congenital absence of the pituitary gland. J. Pediatr. 56:658-664, 1960.

15. Hershman, J.M., and Starnes, W.R.: Extraction and characterization of a thyrotropic material from the human placenta. J. Clin. Invest. 48:923-929, 1969.

16. Hennen, G., Pierce, J.G., and Freychet, P.: Human chorionic thyrotropin: further characterization and study of its secretion during pregnancy. J. Clin. Endocrinol. Metab. 29:581-594, 1969.

17. Hershman, J.M., and Starnes, W.R.: Placental content and characterization of human chorionic thyrotropin. J. Clin. Endocrinol. Metab. 32:52-58, 1971.

18. Hershman, J.M., Higgins, H.P., and Starnes, W.R.: Differences between thyroid stimulator in hydatidiform mole and human chorionic thyrotropin. Metabolism 19:735-744, 1970.

19. Hershman, J.M., and Starnes, W.R.: Big and little placental thyrotropins: interconversion and function. Program of the 53rd Meeting of The Endocrine Society, San Francisco, June 26, 1971, p. 131.

20. Reichlin, S.: Control of thyrotropic hormone secretion. In: Neuroendocrinology. Vol. I (L. Martini and W.R. Ganong, eds.). Academic Press, New York, 1966. pp. 445-536.

21. Kojihara, A.; Kojima, A.; Onaya, T.; Takemura, Y. and Yamada, T.: Placental transport of thyrotropin releasing factor in the rat. Endocrinology, in press.

22. Miyai, et al., J. Clin. Endocrinol. and Metab. 29:1438, 1969.

23. Fisher and Oddie: J.Clin.Endocrinol.and Metab. 27:1637-1654,1967.

24. Fisher, D.A.: Hyperthyroidism in the pregnant women and the neonate. J. Clin. Endocrinol. and Metab. 27:1637-1654, 1967.

25. Logothetopoulos, J. and Scott, R.F.: Active iodide transport across the placenta of the guinea-pig, rabbit, and rat. *J. Physiol.* (Lond.) 132:365-371, 1956

HYPOTHALAMO-PITUITARY INTERRELATIONSHIPS IN THYROID PATHOLOGY, WITH SPECIAL REFERENCE TO CRETINISM

C. Beckers

Centre de Médecine Nucléaire et Laboratoire de Pathologie Générale, School of Medicine, University of Louvain, Belgium

The neurohumoral control of thyrotropin (TSH) secretion has been largely documented in recent years, especially since the recognition of the presence of a substance contained in hypothalamic extracts which stimulates secretion of TSH from the adenohypophysis (1). Studies on the purification of this substance led to the identification of three amino acids: histidine, glutamic acid and proline (2,3). Later it was demonstrated that the sequence Glu-His-Pro became active after acetylation of this tripeptide (4). The acetylation step apparently caused formation of pyroGlu at the N terminus of the tripeptide (4,5). Further studies indicated that the structure of "thyrotropin-releasing hormone" (TRH) was 1-(pyro)Glu-1-His-1-Pro-NH_2 (the term pyroGlu, or PCA, refers to 2-pyrrolidone-5-carboxylyl). Further studies showed that the synthetic substance was identical to the natural product of porcine or ovine origin (4-10), or at least that the synthetic PCA-His-Pro-NH_2 corresponded to the minimal active core of natural TRH.

The availability of synthetic TRH has offered new possibilities for investigation of the control mechanisms of the thyroid. After briefly reviewing present knowledge of the role of TRH in thyroid physiology and physiopathology, the effects of TRH in cretins will be discussed and compared to the results reported in dwarfed children with or without hypothyroidism and in dwarfs suffering from various abnormalities of the central nervous system.

EFFECTS OF TRH IN NORMAL SUBJECTS

Similar results have been obtained by different groups of investigators using synthetic TRH in man (11-23). Whatever the route of administration (24), TRH stimulates TSH release from the pituitary, the most rapid and the highest response being generally observed after the intravenous injection of 200-400 µg of TRH (Fig. 1). Radioimmunoassayable HTSH (17,21,25,26) rapidly increases in the circulation after giving intravenously 200-400 µg of TRH. The peak value was obtained after 20-30 minutes. The effect of an oral dose (10 mg) of TRH is delayed, the maximal level of TSH being observed only after 120-180 minutes (Fig. 1).

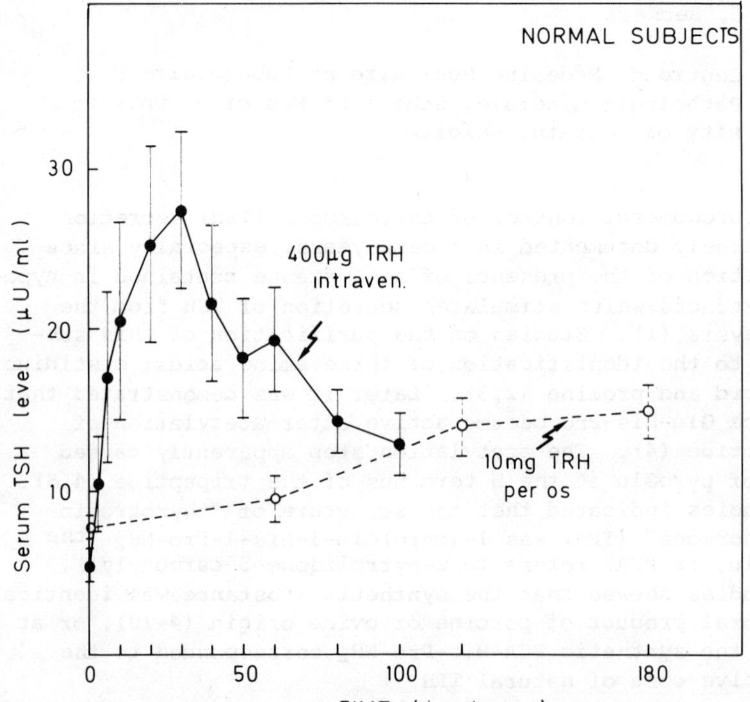

Fig. 1. Response of TSH to TRH given intravenously (400 µg) or orally (10 mg) in normal subjects (21).

In order to interpret the TSH response to TRH, it should be stressed that the magnitude of the TSH response is dependent on the level of the circulating thyroid hormones (21-22, 27-29). This is well known in situations where thyroid secretion is either increased, as in thyrotoxicosis, or decreased as in myxedema. In the first case, no TSH response to TRH is observed, while in the second situation, the TSH response is impressively enhanced.

Such observations are not only correct for hypothyroid or hyperthyroid states as compared to normal conditions, but also in subjects with a level of circulating thyroid hormones within the normal range. Indeed, this can be nicely demonstrated in normal subjects receiving TRH orally in order to get a more progressive and sustained stimulation of the pituitary. As shown in Fig. 2, the lower the level of blood T_4, the higher the maximal TSH response to TRH (21-22). Inversely, the higher the TSH concentration before TRH administration, the higher the maximal TSH response to the drug, and vice versa (Fig. 2)

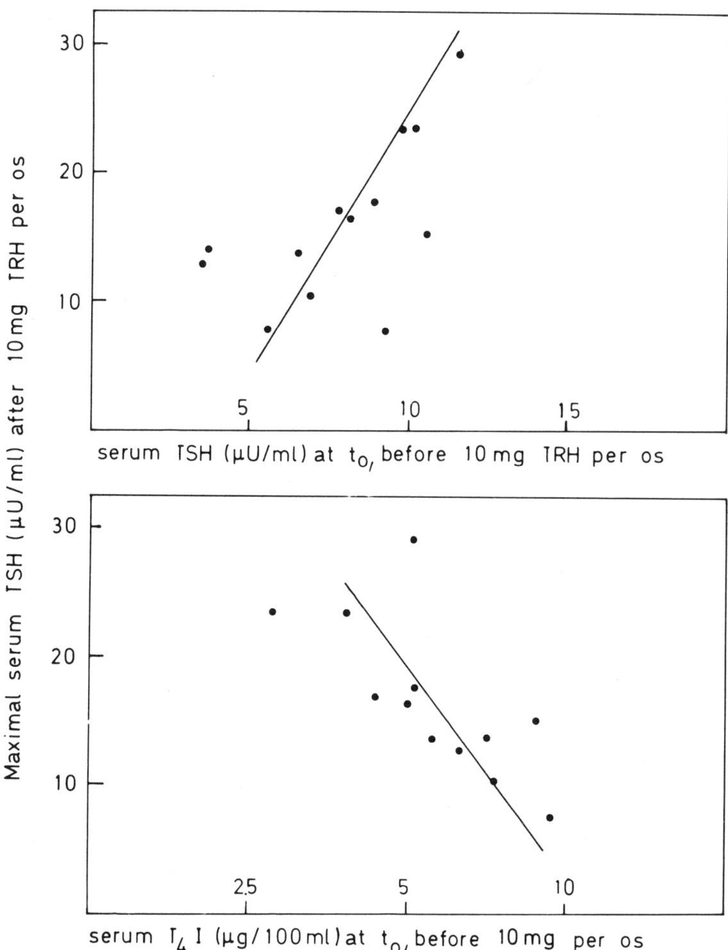

Fig. 2. Importance of the baseline serum TSH and T_4 on the maximal response to TRH (10 mg) given orally (21).

It is important to keep these observations in mind in order to understand the significance of the TSH response: in all cases investigated with TRH, the exact level of circulating T_4 and T_3 should be determined before drawing any definite conclusion as to the state of hyper- or hyporesponsiveness to the hypothalamic stimulus. We need a way to "normalize" the TSH response to the T_4-T_3 levels, just as other metabolic parameters are expressed per square meter of body surface or per kilo of body weight. The relationship between the TSH response to TRH and the concentration of the circulating thyroid hormones is probably related to the mechanisms responsible for the inactivation of TRH (30-31).

TRANSPLACENTIAL PASSAGE OF TRH: FETOMATERNAL INTERRELATIONSHIPS

The functional development of the fetal pituitary-thyroid axis has been the object of several studies in different species and in man. As recently pointed out by d'Angelo *et al.* (32), the functional development of the rat fetal pituitary-thyroid axis has been investigated often, but much less is known of the role of the hypothalamus in the functional maturation of this system. The same may be said for the rabbit (33). In rats it has been shown that TRH can cross the placental barrier and activates the thyroid activity of the fetus (32). Bioassay studies have clearly demonstrated that TRH stimulates in vivo and in vitro the release of TSH from the fetal hypophysis (32). In the rabbit TRH activity in hypothalamic heterografts or extracts first appears in 14-day-old animals (33). It is not known if endogenous TRH is present in the fetal hypothalamus. It seems likely that in the rabbit and rat the functional maturation of the hypothalamo-hypophysial-thyroid system occurs in the perinatal period.

In man, measurements of serum TSH levels were obtained by Fisher and Odell in maternal and fetal blood during labor and delivery and the early postnatal and neonatal periods (34). Mean TSH concentration is significantly higher in cord blood than maternal blood. By 30 minutes after delivery, there is a high rate of TSH secretion, followed by a fall of serum TSH and then a more chronic TSH hypersecretion which persists throughout the first 24-48 hr of extrauterine life. From the studies of the effect of cooling, it may be concluded that the acute release of TSH involves a potent stimulus other than cooling itself, possibly TRH.

CLINICAL STUDIES OF THE HYPOTHALAMO-PITUITARY RELATIONSHIPS

The possibility of measuring TSH by radioimmunoassay and the availability of TRH for clinical investigation has enabled exploration of the hypothalamo-hypophyseal-thyroid system in several pathological conditions. The entity of hypothalamic hypothyroidism has thus been fully documented (35). Patients with primary hypothyroidism or low levels of circulating thyroid hormones have an increased pituitary TSH reserve, while a decreased or suppressed response is observed in secondary hypothyroidism, in active thyrotoxicosis, and in patients with autonomous thyroid adenomas (11-23) (Fig. 3).

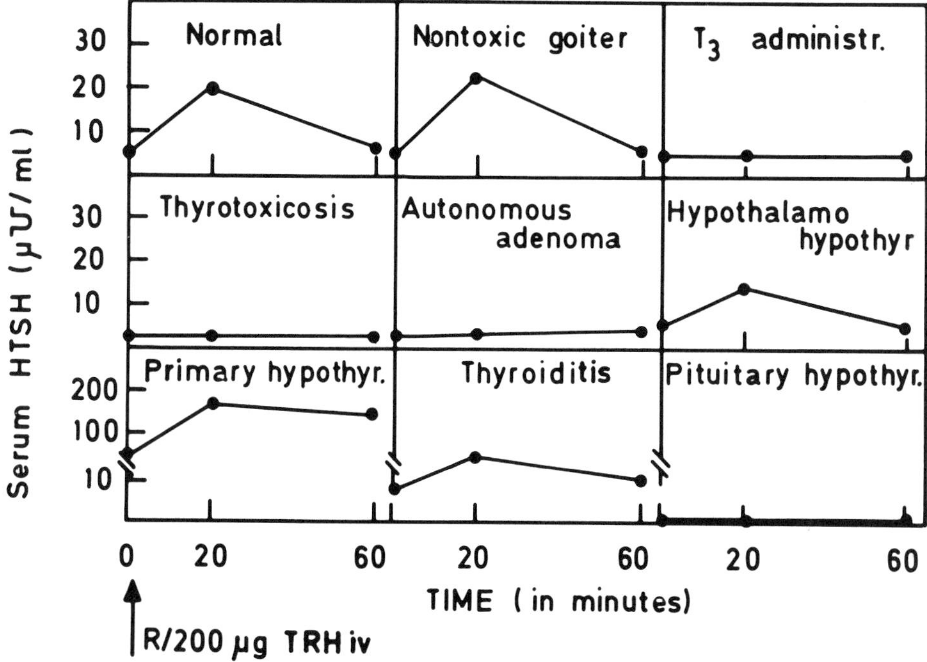

Fig. 3. General pattern to TRH given intravenously (200 μg) in various thyroid conditions.

In sporadic nontoxic goiter the TSH level and the TSH response to TRH is normal, provided the plasma T_4 and T_3 levels are normal (36-38). TSH production rate is normal in nontoxic goiter (39-40). Similar conclusions can be drawn from the results of plasma TSH levels reported in endemic goiter (37). No data have yet been reported with TRH. Such an investigation would be most interesting since similarly to the glucose tolerance test for early detection of diabetes, the TRH stimulation is the test of choice to demonstrate a mild state of hypothyroidism. In most of the studies on endemic goiter, the peripheral thyroid state is never completely clear since the information is generally limited to protein-bound iodine or the thyroxine levels, even if in some instances a preferential secretion of T_3 is suspected (41).

In cretinism, either endemic or sporadic and associated with low levels of circulating thyroid hormones, the serum TSH level is elevated (42-44). These cretins should show an increased TSH response to TRH related to the concentration of serum T_4 and T_3. The T_3 suppression tests performed in four endemic cretins of the Uele endemic (Zaire Republic) rather suggested a normal response of the hypothalamo-pituitary axis but no TSH determinations were performed (45).

There is no general consensus on the exact definition of cretinism as related to endemic goiter and iodine deficiency and the various abnormalities of the central nervous system and dwarfism (46-47). The results of a recent study look promising (48). In dwarfs it was shown that one can encounter some instances of isolated growth hormone deficiency associated with a normal plasma TSH and a normal TSH response to TRH, while others with undetectable baseline levels of TSH may have normal, delayed or suppressed TSH response to TRH. No doubt the TRH test may help to distinguish among different forms of dwarfed cretins or defective patients who may have other deficiencies of the different hypothalamic releasing hormones and in whom the role of hypothyroidism is not definitively settled.

SUMMARY

Little is known of the hypothalamo-pituitary interrelationships during fetal life. In animals, TRH can cross the placental barrier from the mother to the fetus but the functional maturation of the hypothalamo-hypophyseal-thyroid systems seems merely to occur in the perinatal period. Hypothyroid cretins are hyperresponsive to TRH stimulus. Various patterns in the pituitary response to TRH have been observed in dwarfed persons. Studies with TRH would be most interesting in understanding the pathophysiology underlying the disturbances observed in dwarfed cretins and in the defective patients living in areas of endemic goiter.

ACKNOWLEDGEMENTS

The present work has been partly supported by the Fonds de la Recherche Scientifique Médicale, Belgium. Figures 1 and 2 reprinted by kind permission of European Journal of Clinical Investigation. HTSH and anti-TSH antibodies have been kindly provided by the National Pituitary Agency (USA), the TRH by Hoffman-La Roche (Switzerland) and the TSH standard by the Medical Research Council (England).

DISCUSSION BY PARTICIPANTS

MOSIER: To what extent does the hypothyroid state affect the response of TSH and TRF?

BECKERS: Apparently, thyroid hormones control an enzyme present in the plasma, which is able to inactivate TRH. If the level of thyroid hormone is low, the inactivating mechanism is not working and one gets an enhanced response to TRH, probably as a result of a longer biological half-life of TRH in the circulation.

STANBURY: Another loop.

PITTMAN: There is yet another one T_4 and T_3 apparently act mainly at the pituitary and not at the hypothalamic level to modulate the loop. As Dr. Beckers showed, hyperthyroid individuals, with a high level of circulating thyroid hormone, have an impaired or absent response to TRF. Hypothyroid individuals have an exaggerated response. With assay animals given thyroid hormone and then TRF, one can block the TRF response. This is true only if he gives the thyroid hormone a half-hour or an hour before the TRF. Given five minutes before TRF, it fails to block. Another bit of evidence is that actinomycin will block the T_4 blockade. This implies that something is synthesized within the pituitary in response to T_4 and T_3 which blocks the TRF action (49).

REFERENCES

1. Guillemin, R.; Yamazaki, E.; Jutisz, M. and Sakiz, E.: Présence dans un extrait de tissus hypothalamiques d'une susbstance stimulant la sécrétion de l'hormone hypophysaire thyréotrope (TSH). Prèmiere purification par filtration sur gel Sephadex. C.R. Acad. Sci. 255:1018, 1962.

2. Schally, A.V.; Bowers, C.Y.; Redding, T.W. and Barrett, J.F.: Isolation of thyrotropin releasing factor (TRF) from porcine hypothalamus. Biochem. Biophys. Res. Commun. 25: 165, 1966.

3. Schally, A.V.; Redding, T.W.; Bowers, C.Y. and Barrett, J.F.: Isolation and properties of porcine thyrotropin-releasing hormone. J. Biol. Chem. 244:4077, 1969.

4. Burgus, R.; Dunn, T.F.; Desiderio, D.; Guillemin, R. and Vale, W.: Dérivés polypeptidiques de synthèse doués d'activité hypophysiotrope TRF. Nouvelles observations. C.R. Acad. Sci. 269: 226, 1969.

5. Burgus, R.; Dunn, T.F.; Desiderio, D. and Guillemin, R.: Structure moléculaire du facteur hypothalamique hypophysiotrope TRF d'origine ovine: mise en évidence par spectrométrie de masse de la séquence PCA-His-Pro NH_2. C.R. Acad. Sci. 269:1870, 1969.

6. Folkers, K.; Enzmann, F.; Boler, J.; Bowers, C.Y. and Schally, A.V.: Discovery of modification of the synthetic tripeptide-sequence of the thyrotropin releasing hormone having activity. Biochem. Biophys. Res. Commun. 37:123, 1969.

7. Nair, R.M.G.; Barrett, J.F.; Bowers, C.Y. and Schally, A.V.: Structure of porcine thyrotropin releasing hormone. Biochemistry 9:1103, 1970.

8. Burgus, R.; Dunn, T.F.; Desiderio, D.; Ward, D.N.; Vales, W. and Guillemin, R.: Characterization of ovine hypothalamic hypophysiotropic TSH-releasing factor (TRF) Nature (Lond) 226: 321, 1970.

9. Schally, A.V.; Arimura, A., Bowers, C.Y.; Wakabayashi, I.; Kastin, A.J.; Redding, T.W.; Mittler, J.C.; Nair, R.M.G.; Pizzolato, P.and Segal, A.J.: Purification of hypothalamic re-releasing hormone of human origin. Endocrinology 31:29, 1970.

10. Burgus, R.; Dunn, T.F.; Desiderio, D.M.; Ward, D.N.; Vale, W.; Guillemin, R.; Felix, A.M.; Gielessen, D. and Studer, R.O.: Biological activity of synthetic polypeptide derivaties related to the structure of hypothalamic TRF. Endocrinology 86:573, 1970.

11. Fleischer, N.; Burgus, R.; Vale, W.; Dunn, T. and Guillemin, R.: Preliminary observations on the effect of synthetic thyrotropin-releasing factor of plasma thyrotropin levels in man. J. Clin. Endocrinol. Metab.31:109, 1970.

12. Hall, R.; Amos, J. and Garry, R.: Thyroid stimulating hormone response to synthetic thyrotropin-releasing hormone in man. Br. Med. J. 2:279, 1970

13. Hershman, J.M. and Pittman, J.A.: Response to synthetic thyrotropin-releasing hormone in man. J. Clin. Endocrinol. Metab. 31:457, 1970.

14. Beckers, C.; Maskens, A. and Cornette, C.: Réactivité hypophysaire à la stimulation par la TRH synthétique chez l'homme. Ann. Endocrinol. 32:214, 1971.

15. Karlberg, B.S.; Almqvist, S. and Werner, S.: Effect of synthetic pyroglutamyl-histidyl-proline-amide on serum levels of thyrotropin, cortisol, growth hormone, insulin and PBI in normal subjects and patients with pituitary and thyroid disorders. Acta Endocrinol. 67:288, 1971.

16. Beckers, C.; Cornette, C. and Maskens, A.: Program 53rd Meeting Ann. Endocr. Soc. San Francisco, p. 168, 1971.

17. Beckers, C.; Maskens, A. and Cornette, C.: Réactivité hypophysaire à la stimulation par la TRH synthétique chez l'homme. Ann. Endocrinol. 32:214, 1971.

18. Ormston, B.J.; Garry, R.; Cryer, R.J.; Besser, G.M. and Hale, R.: Thyrotropin-releasing hormone as a thyroid function test. Lancet 2:10, 1971.

19. Haigler, E.D.Jr.; Pittman, J.A.; Hershman, J.M. and Baugh, C.M.: Direct evaluation of pituitary thyrotropin reserve utilizing synthetic thyrotropin-releasing hormone. J. Clin. Endocrinol. Metab. 33:573, 1971.

20. Ormston, B.J., Kilborn, J.R.; Garry, R.; Amos, J. and Hall, R.: Further observations on the effect of synthetic thyrotrophin-releasing hormone in Man. Br. Med. J. 2:199, 1971.

21. Beckers, C.; Maskens, A. and Cornette, C.: Thyrotropin response to synthetic thyrotropin-releasing hormone in normal subjects and in patients with nontoxic goiter. Eur. J. Clin. Invest., in press.

22. Beckers, C.; Maskens, A. and Cornette, C.: Intérêt de la thyrotropin-releasing hormone (TRH) en physiopathologie thyroïdienne. Ann. Endocr., in press.

23. Gual, C.; Kastin, A.J. and Schally, A.V.: Clinical experience with hypothalamic-releasing hormones. I : Thyrotropin-releasing hormone (TRH). Recent Progr. Horm. Res., in press.

24. Redding, T.W. and Schally, A.V.: A study on the mode of administration of thyrotropin-releasing hormone (TRH) in mice. Neuroendocrinology 6:329, 1971.

25. Odell, W.D.; Wilber, J.F. and Utiger, R.D.: Studies of thyrotropin physiology by means of radioimmunoassay. Recent Progr. Horm. Res. 232:47, 1967.

26. Beckers, C. and Cornette, C.: Dosage radioimmunologique de la thyréostimuline en pathologie thyroïdienne. Ann. Endocr. 30:291, 1969.

27. Averill, R.L.W.: Depression of thyrotropin-releasing factor induction of thyrotropin release by thryxine in small doses. Endocrinology 85:67, 1969

28. Suematsu, H.; Matsuda, K.; Shizume, K. and Nakao, K.: Thyroid response to acute reduction of circulating thyroid hormone level. Endocrinology 84:1161, 1969.

29. Suematsu, H.; Matsuda, K.; Shizume, K. and Nakao, K.: Effect of plasmapheresis on thyroid hormone secretion. Endocrinology 86:1281, 1970.

30. Redding, T.W. and Schally, A.V.: Studies on the thyrotropin-releasing hormone (TRH) activity in peripheral blood. Proc. Soc. Exp. Biol. Med. 131:420, 1969.

31. Vale, W.W.; Burgus, R.; Dunn, T.F. and Guillemin, R.: Plasma inactivation of thyrotropin-releasing factor (TRF) and related peptides. Its inhibition by various means and by the synthetic dipeptide PCA-His-OME. Hormones 2:193, 1971.

32. d'Angelo, S.A.; Wall, N.R. and Bowers, C.Y.: Maternal-fetal endocrine interrelations: demonstration of TSH release from the fetal hypophysis in pregnant rats administered synthetic TRH. Proc. Soc. Exp. Biol. Med. 137:175, 1971

33. Slebodzniski, A.; Mach, Z. and Walinowska, W.: The development of thyroid-stimulating hormone releasing factor activity in the neonatal rabbit. J. Endocrinol. 49:559, 1971.

34. Fisher, D.A. and Odell, W.D.: Acute release of thyrotropin in the newborn. J. Clin. Invest. 48:1670, 1969.

35. Pittman, J. A.; Haigher, E.D.; Hershman, J.M. and Pittman, C.S.; Hypothalamic hypothyroidism. New Engl. J. Med. 285: 844, 1971.

36. Wahner, W.H.; Mayberry, W.E.; Gaitan, E. and Gaitan, J.E.: Endemic goiter in the Canca Valley. III. Role of serum TSH in goitrogenesis. J. Clin. Endocrinol. Metab. 32:491, 1971.

37. Delange, F.; Hershman, J.M. and Ermans, A.M.: Relationship between the serum thyrotropin level, the revalence of goiter and the pattern of iodine metabolism in Idjwi Island. J. Clin. Endocrinol. Metab. 33:261, 1971.

38. Beckers, C.: Pathophysiology of nontoxic goiter. In: Endemic Goiter. Report of the meeting of the PAHO Scientific Group on Research in Endemic Goiter held in Mexico, 1968 (J.B. Stanbury, ed.). PAHO Scientific Publication No. 193, Washington, 1969. p. 30.

39. Beckers, C. and Cornette, C.: TSH production rate in non-toxic goiter. J. Clin. Endocrinol. Metab. 32:852, 1971.

40. Beckers, C.; Machiels, J.; Soyez, C. and Cornette, C.: Metabolic clearance rate and production rate of thyroid-stimulating hormone in man. Horm. Metab. Res. 3:34, 1971.

41. Buttfield, I.H.; Hetzel, B.S. and Odell, W.D.: Effect of iodized oil on serum TSH determined by immunoassay in endemic goitre subjects. J. Clin. Endocrinol. Metab. 28:1664, 1964.

42. Bowers, C.Y.; Schally, A.V.; Hawley, W.D.: Gual, C. and Parlow, A.: Effect of thyrotropin releasing factor in man. J. Clin. Endocrinol. Metab. 28:978, 1968.

43. Delange, F. and Ermans, A.M.: Further studies on endemic cretinism in Central Africa. Horm. Metab. Res. 3:431, 1971.

44. Job, J.C.; Milhand, G.; Binet, E.; Rivaille, P. and Moukthar, M.S.: Effet de l'hormone de libération de la thyréostimuline (TRH) sur le taux sanguin de thyréostimuline (TSH) chez l'enfant: enfants normaux, enfants atteints d'hypopituitarisme, de goitre. Eur. J. Clin. Biol. Res. 16:537, 1971.

45. Dumont, J.; Ermans, A.M. and Bastenie, P.A.: Thyroid function in a goiter endemic. V. Mechanism of thyroid failure in the endemic cretins. J. Clin. Endocrinol. Metab. 23:847, 1963.

46. Querido, A.: Endemic cretinism: a search for a tenable definition. In: Endemic Goiter. Report of the meeting of the PAHO Scientific Group on Research in Endemic Goiter held in Mexico, 1968 (J.B. Stanbury, ed.). PAHO Scientific Publication No. 193, Washington, 1969. p. 85

47. Dumont, J.E.; Delange, F. and Ermans, A.M.: Endemic cretinism: a search for a tenable definition. In: Endemic Goiter. Report of the meeting of the PAHO Scientific Group on Research in Endemic Goiter held in Mexico, 1968 (J.B. Stanbury, ed.). PAHO Scientific Publication No. 193, Washington, 1969. p. 91.

48. Comston, B.H.; Grumbach, M.M. and Kaplan, S.L.: Effect of thyrotropin-releasing factor on serum thyroid stimulating hormone. An approach to distinguish hypothalamic forms of idiopathic hypopituitary dwarfism. J. Clin. Invest. 50:229, 1971.

49. Pittman, J.A. and J.M. Hershman: Physiology of the Thyroid Feedback Loop. In: Recent Advances in Endocrinology. Proceedings of the Seventh Pan-American Congress of Endocrinology, São Paulo, Brazil, 16-21 August, 1970. Excerpta Medica Int. Congr. Ser. 238:69-90, 1970.

HYPOTHALAMIC HYPOTHYROIDISM: ITS POSSIBLE RELATIONSHIP TO ENDEMIC GOITER

J. A. Pittman, Jr.

Georgetown University School of Medicine
and Department of Medicine and Surgery,
Veterans Administration, Washington, D.C.

The impact of thyroid deficiency on the developing central nervous system is described elsewhere in this volume. Whether this damage extends to the hypothalamus and involves the complex innervation and function of the nuclei of this structure is not presently known, but in this context it seems appropriate to review what is presently known about hypothyroidism resulting from failure of normal hypothalamic control of the cells of the pituitary involved in thyrotropin secretion.

The original patient with hypothalamic hypothyroidism was described in 1971 (1). In 1970, when he was referred, he was a 19-year old peanut farmer from Southern Alabama with short stature, dry skin and sluggishness. He was apparently normal until age 12 years, when he received two severe blows to the head with loss of consciousness. Shortly thereafter, polyuria and polydipsia developed, and a diagnosis of diabetes insipidus was made. He was successfully treated for this. Growth rate slowed at that time, and about age 17 dryness of the skin appeared.

On examination he appeared mildly hypothyroid. Visual fields were normal as were x-rays of the skull. Thyroid function tests gave markedly hypothyroid results, with T_4-iodine of 1.6 mg per 100 ml, normal thyroxin-binding globulin capacity, low-normal T_3-resin uptake, and a thyroid radioiodine uptake of less than one percent at four, six and 24 hours. This rose to 9.5 percent at 24 hours after administration of TSH, and at this time the thyroid scan appeared normal. Antithyroglobulin antibodies were not detected. Serum TSH concentration was undetectable on four occasions (i.e., less than 1.2 microunits per ml).

Urinary excretions of 17-hydroxycorticosteroids, 17-ketosteroids, and gonadotropins were normal, and plasma cortisol concentration rose normally in response to insulin hypoglycemia. Serum and urine osmolalities confirmed the diagnosis of diabetes insipidus. Plasma growth hormone was undetectable during insulin hypoglycemia or arginine infusion even after estrogen priming. Thus, the patient appeared to lack growth hormone, vasopressin and TSH, though ACTH was intact as were gonadotropins. Sexual maturation had arrived some time after the age of 15 years, as would be consistent with growth hormone lack.

Because of the history of trauma and diabetes insipidus, he was given thyrotropin releasing factor (TRF), 500 mg intravenously. Serum TSH rose promptly from zero to 3.8 microunits per ml at 15 min, 10 at 30 min, 10 at 45 min, and eight at 60 min after TRF. Two other TRF tests gave similar results. Thus,the pituitary was capable of secreting TSH. The evidence therefore indicated that this patient lacked three hypothalamic hormones: vasopressin, TRF and presumably growth hormone releasing factor.

The 15 recorded cases of hypothalamic hypothyroidism reported thus far appear in Table 1. The first is the one just discussed. The next nine are from the report by Costom, Grumbach and Kaplan (2). All of their patients from California were selected because of short stature and were found to lack growth hormone. They had variable deficiencies of other pituitary hormones - ACTH, gonadotropins, ADH and TSH. Though their ages ranged up into the 20's, the diagnoses of hypothyroidism had usually been made much earlier in childhood and sometimes in infancy. It is also of interest that all of these patients except one were males. Costom _et al._ gave 500 μg of TRF to each and measured the plasma TSH at frequent intervals thereafter. There was a clear response in all of the ones listed in the table. This response was compared with that found in a control series of normal individuals and another with idiopathic short stature without hypothyroidism. In the latter groups the response was brisk, occurring clearly at five min and peaking at 20 to 30 min, then falling. By contrast, the patients with idiopathic hypothyroidism, showed a delayed response with a rising curve which was still increasing two hr after the injection of TRF. Normal subjects invariably show a response within two to 10 min and have a peak at 20 to 30 min. Several of the patients in the report of Costom _et al._ showed initial rises only after 20 to 60 min and showed clearly rising curves several hours after the TRF injection. This suggests that the pituitaries in these patients were being "awakened" after having been dormant from lack of stimulation by endogenous TRF. Interpretation is complicated by the fact that these

Table 1. The reported patients with hypothalamic hypothyroidism

PT.	Age	GH	ACTH	FSH-LH	ADH	T_4 (c) µg/100ml	Pathogenesis	Ref.
	Deficiencies							
1. J.L.	19	A	P	P	A	2.4	Head trauma?	(1)
2. L.R.	20	A	A	A	P	0.5	Idiopathic	(2)
3. J.O.	15	A	A	P	P	3.1	Idiopathic	(2)
4. L.N.	9	A	A	-	P	3.7	Idiopathic	(2)
5. J.M.	20	A	A	A	P	0.8	Idiopathic	(2)
6. J.T.	12	A	P	-	P	1.7	Idiopathic	(2)
7. D.W.	24	A	P	A	P	2.3	Idiopathic	(2)
8. P.D.	14	A	A	A	P	2.1	Idiopathic	(2)
9. J.R.(a)	9	A	P	-	A	2.0	Idiopathic	(2)
10. J.P.(b)	14	A	A	-	P	0.5	Idiopathic	(2)
11. M-1	20	A	A(PpAVP)	A	P	2.0	Idiopathic	(4)
12. M-2	24	P(AVP)	A(PpAVP)	A	P	0.9	Idiopathic	(4)
13. SWR	18	?	?	A	A	1.8	Pineal germinoma	*
14. N-1	6	A	A	-	-	3.2	Idiopathic	(5)
15. N-2	12	A	A	-	-	4.3	**Craniopharyngioma**	(5)

* Courtesy Dr. Beverly Towery
(a) Female
(b) Prosencephalon dysplasia syndrome
(3) Basal serum TSH undectectable in all except
N-1 (1.6µu/ml) and N-2 (5µU/ml)
T_4 levels are given as total T_4, not T_4-iodine

patients had been treated with thyroid hormone until about three weeks before the test.

Kaplan and Grumbach are reporting on a series of patients with prosencephalon dysplasia (3). These interesting patients are characterized by various combinations of deficiencies of pituitary hormones, pendular nystagmus, malformation of the optic discs - which appear abnormally small, elliptical or otherwise misshapen - and various anatomic abnormalities of the brain, such as absence of the septum pellucidum and thinning of the optic nerves. The importance of the Kaplan-Grumbach syndrome is that it demonstrates that abnormalities of the neural structures can lead to pituitary hormone deficiencies in the absence of any evidence of an anatomic lesion of the pituitary gland itself.

The next two patients in Table 1 have been reported from the University of Maryland in Baltimore (4). One was tall and the other short. Both were hypothyroid and both showed a normal response to TRF with a brisk rise in serum TSH. The patients lacked ACTH and growth hormone by the conventional tests, metyrapone and insulin hypoglycemia. However, there was a response in each patient to intravenously administered vasopressin. After vasopressin the plasma cortisol levels rose distinctly although less than might be expected in a normal individual. Plasma growth hormone rose in the tall subject but not in the short one. If one accepts that vasopressin acts directly on the anterior pituitary gland, then these responses support the view that the deficiencies were the result of lack of hypothalamic hypophysiotropic hormones.

Patient 13, from the University of Louisville, was studied by Dr. Beverly Towery and is of interest because the cause was a pineal germinoma which apparently compressed the hypothalamus and reduced TRF secretion. The patient never received treatment for hypothyroidism other than radiation of the tumor. Following this, the hypothyroidism regressed.

The last two patients in the table are listed because they were mentioned in a report on TRF (5) and were thus the first instances of this syndrome in the literature.

There are several possible explanations for the findings in these patients. The most probable by far is that lesions of the hypothalamus, probably of many different kinds, may interfere with secretion of TRF. Other possibilities include secretion of an abnormal TRF and abnormally rapid destruction of TRF in the plasma. Another possibility is that some lesions of the pituitary are sufficiently severe to reduce spontaneous TSH secretion to levels low enough to cause hypothyroidism, but leave adequate reserve to permit a clear but perhaps blunted response to large doses of exogenous TRF. We have observed this in one patient and have heard reports of others. An additional report has recently appeared confirming this (6).

The severity of hypothyroidism appears in most cases to be less as one progresses farther up the control system. Thus, primary athyreotic hypothyroidism is frequently very severe; pituitary hypothyroidism is usually less severe although it can be quite marked; and hypothalamic hypothyroidism is usually mild. In most instances the findings described here probably reflect damage to the hypothalamus itself and, hence, justify the designation, "hypothalamic hypothyroidism." Final proof of the pathogenesis awaits development of methodology sufficiently sensitive to detect circulating TRF, and a "negative-signal test" for TRF comparable to metyrapone for ACTH or insulin hypoglycemia for growth hormone.

The potential relevance of these observations to endemic cretinism is twofold. First, it is possible that lesions of the hypothalamus may in some patients be responsible for the development of hypothyroidism and cretinism with otherwise normal pituitaries and thyroid glands. Second, patients with thyroid failure due to insufficiency of the thyroid gland itself might develop central nervous system lesions which impair the secretion of pituitary TSH. This seems quite hypothetical, but might result in failure of serum TSH to rise spontaneously in spite of thyroid failure (primary hypothyroidism). Such patients should show a TSH rise in response to exogenous TRF.

With this exception and the exception of technical errors, the only other recognized lesion which could result in a normal or low serum TSH in the presence of primary hypothyroidism would be a lesion of the pituitary. Since both hypothalamic and pituitary lesions are probably quite rare, an elevated serum TSH should be a good marker for the confirmation of hypothyroidism in a population. One certainly would not propose it as a screening test for endemic cretinism, but only for the confirmation of hypothyroidism.

SUMMARY

The occurrence and pathogenesis of hypothalamic hyperthyroidism are reviewed. These patients customarily have mild hypothyroidism, but it is hypothetically possible that if the disorder occurred as a primary event in fetal life severe hypothyroidism and retardation could result. Plasma TSH concentration is a good marker for hypothyroidism or a tendency toward hypothyroidism in the absence of pituitary or hypothalamic disease.

REFERENCES

1. Pittman, J.A.; Haigler, E.D.; Hershman, J.M. and Pittman, C.S.: Hypothalamic hypothyroidism. N. Engl. J. Med. 285:844, 1971.

2. Costom, B.H.; Grumbach, N.M. and Kaplan, S.L.: Effect of thyrotropin-releasing factor on serum thyroid-stimulating hormone: an approach to distinguishing hypothalamic from pituitary forms of idiopathic hypopituitary dwarfism. J. Clin. Invest. 50:2219, 1971.

3. Kaplan, S.L.; Grumbach, M.M. and Hoyt, W.F.: A syndrome of hypopituitary dwarfism, hypoplasia of optic nerves, and maldevelopment of prosencephalon: report of six patients. Pediatr. Res. 4:480, 1970.

4. Martin, L.G.; Martul, P.; Connor, T.B. and Wiswell, J.G.: Hypothalamic origin of idiopathic hypopituitarism. Metabolism 21: 143, 1972.

5. Job, J.G.; Milhaud, G.; Binet, E.; Rivaille, P. and Moukhtar, M.S.: Effet de l'hormone de liberation de la thyreostimuline (TRH) sur le taux sanguin de thyreostimuline (TSH) chez l'enfant: enfants normaux, enfants atteints d'hypothyroidie, d'hypopituitarisme, de goitre. Rev. Eur. Etudes Clin. et Biolog. 16:537, 1971

6. Faglia, G.; Peccoz, P.B.; Ambrosi, B.; Ferrari, C. and Neri, V.: Prolonged and exaggerated elevations in plasma thyrotropin (HTSH) after thyrotropin-releasing factor (TRF) in patients with pituitary tumors. J. Clin. Endocrinol. and Metab. 33:999, 1971.

SECTION 6
ETIOPATHOLOGY OF CRETINISM

ROLE OF THE PLACENTA AND OF PLASMA HORMONE BINDING IN THE PATHOGENESIS OF CRETINISM

Eduardo A. Pretell

Departamento de Endocrinologia

Instituto de Investigaciones de la Altura, Lima, Peru

There is virtually no published information on the role of the placenta and of the serum thyroxine binding proteins in the pathogenesis of cretinism. We present here the results of our investigations on the effects of chronic and severe dietary deficiency on hormone synthesis in the pregnant woman and the possible effects of maternal hormone levels during pregnancy on fetal thyroid function and development and possibly on the irreversible changes in the central nervous system which characterize cretinism. Our data may possibly have implications on the role of the placenta and of the thyroxine binding proteins in the pathogenesis of cretinism.

There is no doubt that endemic cretinism is found only where endemic goiter is severe and where the problem has been present for a long time. The prevalence of cretinism in general seems to be related to the severity of the iodine deficiency. Even so, the hypothesis that iodine deficiency is the sole responsible factor in the pathogenesis of cretinism has been vigorously challenged, and it has been established that in some areas comparable states of iodine deficiency may be accompanied by clinical findings including cretinism in some regions and not in others. This has been reported by Delange from the Kivu region of the Zaire Republic. On the other hand, iodine prophylaxis uniformly has prevented cretinism. Finally, it may be noted that there are regions where iodine deficiency is severe and endemic goiter is common and yet only occasionally cretins are encountered. Accordingly, it is

*Transcript of tape recording of Dr. Pretell's remarks. This paper has not been edited by Dr. Pretell.

necessary to address the central question, which is, "Under what circumstances does iodine deficiency in the pregnant woman result in a cretinous child? "

First it is necessary to describe the typical cretins of the Peruvian Andean region. They are mainly of the neurological type, rather than the myxedematous, but in physical characteristics they show a wide spectrum. They may be mentally deficient with goiter and with normal stature, or they may be mentally deficient, have normal stature, and be deaf-mutes with large goiters. On the other hand, there may be severe limitation in linear growth. Motor abnormalities are found and strabismus is common.

The suggestion has been made that when low maternal thyroxine values are found in a population group, a number of mentally deficient children may be expected. Accordingly, we have measured the plasma concentrations of thyroxine in our pregnant women. We found that a significant number of iodine-deficient pregnant women had thyroxine values which were in the range between 1.8 and 2.0 μg per 100 ml. One might expect a deleterious effect on the fetuses of such subjects during gestation. These low values did not appear amongst pregnant women in our series treated previously with ethiodol. In order to rule out the possibility that low thyroxine values in pregnant women might be caused by impairment in thyroxine binding proteins, the binding proteins have been measured. Both iodine-treated and iodine-deficient pregnant women showed similar values in the endogenous distribution of thyroxine among the binding proteins in the serum as well as in the thyroxine binding capacity. These values were in accord with those found in patients in non-endemic areas.

The question of special interest relates to the effect of low T_4 values in iodine-deficient pregnant women on fetal hormone levels. It appeared that thyroxine levels in the iodine-deficient pregnant women were significantly lower than in the iodine-treated group. In spite of these differences the total thyroxine in the plasma of the iodine-deficient neonates was not significantly different from the group born to iodine-treated mothers. Nevertheless, in spite of mean values which were not different it might be that individual cases might occur with low values. Thus, in one instance a child born to a cretinous mother who had a thyroxine level of 1.8, had a normal concentration of T_4 in the cord blood. Thus, occasionally in individual patients, a cretinous mother may have a low plasma thyroxine and yet the fetus may have entirely normal levels of thyroxine.

Through the courtesy of Dr. Robert Utiger, TSH has been measured on maternal and cord blood of some of our patients. Mean values were not significantly different between children born to iodine-treated and iodine-deficient mothers, but the results in the iodine-deficient children were more scattered. It is interesting that in a cretinous mother we have found a value of 50 milliunits of TSH per ml and yet the value of the fetus was within the normal range. We found a negative correlation when comparing TSH vs T_4 values in maternal and cord blood. Thus, in summary, it appears that the plasma of patients with endemic goiter generally have a normal content of TSH, but there are individuals with high levels which correspond to the lowest value of T_4. Thyroxine binding globulin and thyroxine binding prealbumin increase normally during pregnancy, just as they do in non-endemic areas. Depending principally on the lack of iodine, T_4 values are lower than in the iodine-treated mothers in the same population. In the fetus TSH is also normal, as are TBPA and TBG. The cord blood shows similar values in total T_4, but because of the lower maternal values in TBPA and TBG in some instances the free thyroxine is significantly higher in the fetal than in the maternal circulation. If one speculates about the placental transfer of thyroid hormone and if he accepts what has already been published to the effect that free thyroxine is the only species capable of crossing the placental barrier, then the possibility must be entertained that free thyroxine will pass more easily from the fetal to the maternal side.

It has been shown by others that during the first 24 to 48 hr of postnatal life, TSH rises significantly and is back to normal by the 48th hr. Thyroxine, on the other hand, increases from birth through the first week and even for longer periods of time. It was, therefore, of interest to measure TSH and thyroxine levels during the first days of postnatal life in order to see what effect iodine deficiency and repletion might have on these functions in our region. Most of the children from whom we were able to obtain samples showed the normal increase in thyroxine levels with the exception of two very obvious cases. These two did not increase. One was from the iodine-treated group and the other from the iodine-deficient group.

We have been unable to detect any correlation between maternal T_4 levels and the developmental quotient. The same lack of correlation applies to bone age and to birth length, since all children were in the normal range for length.

From our observations several conclusions can be drawn. In the first place, dietary iodine deficiency results in low T_4 values in the pregnant woman in a significant number of instances, but these low maternal T_4 values do not necessarily result in low fetal values. Nevertheless, in individual cases very low maternal values may be responsible for low values in the fetus. Unfortunately, at this time it is not possible to form rigid conclusions until one can take into account T_3 values, and these are not yet generally available. One may not speak of maternal or fetal hypothyroidism based solely on T_4 levels. The possibility exists that in the patient with severe maternal hypothyroidism and low T_4 values the unsaturated thyroxine binding protein existing in the maternal circulation would create a situation in which it might be possible for significant fetal to maternal flux of thyroid hormone to occur, with deleterious effect on the fetus. Finally, it may be said that it is possible that,even though the fetal gland is receiving marginally an adequate amount of iodine from the placenta,a metabolic defect theoretically might be sufficient to make thyroid disease manifest.

SUMMARY

The complex interrelationships existing between mother and fetus with respect to thyroid function in endemic cretinism remain to be fully defined. The normal rise in thyroxine binding globulin may be attenuated or fail to occur in the iodine-deficient subject. It is possible that this will have a deleterious effect on the developing fetus. On the other hand, normal plasma concentrations of T_4 may be found in cord blood while maternal blood is normal or low in thyroxine content. This situation could result in a flow of T_4 from fetus to the mother, which conceivably could be deleterious. It is obvious that more physiological data are required before the maternal and environment factors can be defined in the pathogenesis of endemic cretinism.

DISCUSSION BY PARTICIPANTS

HERSHMAN: There were some unusual data in the comparison of TSH in the neonate with that of the mother. They might be explained by the timing of the serum samples obtained from the neonates. One of the consistent findings in a number of studies done in the United States was that levels of TSH in cord blood obtained at birth were always greater than maternal levels. It looked in your data as if the levels were slightly lower in the neonates. Fisher and Odell showed that secretion increases very rapidly after birth (1).

PRETELL: We were aware of this factor and were careful to take blood samples immediately after delivery. We discarded those cases in which we knew the blood was taken some hours later. Except for the iodine-treated blood, the mean value for the neonates is higher than the mother's. We have discussed this with Utiger and it is similar to his findings.

HERSHMAN: The consistent relationship is that the sample for a baby is higher than the mother's.

PRETELL: We did them as matched samples. The majority showed a tendency to be higher in the fetus.

BECKERS: In normal pregnant women, stable T_3 concentration appears to be increased. For a valid conclusion of your investigation, it is essential that stable T_3 values be known. It should be expected that in these pregnant and iodine-deficient women, the T_3 levels are elevated. That is necessarily going to modify the TSH levels.

QUERIOD: We have some data on stable T_3 in iodine-deficient people from Kenya (to be published), also during pregnancy. The T_3 determinations (Table) were done by Dr.Benotti with a modified Sterling method.

Table: T_3 in iodine-deficient subjects (Kenya)

Normal Cases	Neck Uptake 24 hr% dose	Average 24 hr I excr. in µg.	PBI µg/100 ml	T_3 ng/100 ml
5	85%	14	1.9 - 3.1	167
5	75%	22	4.6 - 5.5	200

To our astonishment there was in these normal individuals no compensatory rise in serum stable T_3 when the PBI was low. In pregnant women with PBI's from 2.5 - 5.1, and who also had urinary iodine excretions below 15 µg/24 hr, the stable T_3 averaged 190 ng/100 ml, so that even the expected rise in pregnancy was absent, just as previously has been reported for T_4 in iodine-deficient subjects. The four pregnant women with PBI's from 7.8 - 10.8 µg per 100 ml, and normal iodine excretions, on the contrary, doubled their stable T_4 values.

PRETELL: With this method of Benotti, your T_3 values would only have validity in this group in which the T_4 or the PBI is low. As T_4 increases in this method, it strongly influences the T_3 results.

QUERIDO: I think that this criterion has been fulfilled both in the non-pregnant and pregnant cases. The low PBI sera gave the same stable T_3 as the normal PBI sera. The interesting point is that, in this area, cretinism was absent.

PRETELL: At what stage of pregnancy were these taken?

QUERIDO: They were all later than three months.

BALÁZS: How is it possible that the thyroid functions are

apparently normal in the fetus, although iodine, which is a substrate in the synthesis of thyroid hormones, is not available in sufficient amounts?

PRETELL: We do not know what the normal requirements for fetal iodine are. The gland is very active and the turnover of thyroid hormone seems to be very high. We do not know quantitatively what the amounts are for the fetal gland. The extrathyroidal hormone space is very small in that organism.

BALÁZS: Is the implication not that the fetus is able to extract enough iodine from the maternal organism to maintain a normal thyroid function?

COSTA: The placenta might be a large deposit of iodine. Extremes of 2.7 and 148 μg of iodine per 100 gm wet tissue have been measured by us in 54 subjects. Parenteral administration of organic iodine compounds was accompanied by a sharp rise in total placental iodine values.

PHAROAH: It is just the women who have the low T_4s that are going to be avid for iodine. These are just the ones whose fetuses might be deficient in iodide. Just showing low T_4s does not mean that this is the cause of cretinism in the infant.

KOENIG: We talked this morning about the active transport of iodine through the placenta. That would be interesting in this context.

COSTA: We have given ^{132}I to pregnant women in order to study the position of the fetus. With this isotope the dose of radiation given to the fetus is one-twentieth of the dose given with roentgenological diagnostic techniques. Twenty minutes after intravenous iodine injection to the mother, iodine collects in the placenta and concentrates in the fetal thyroid. By this technique it was possible to ascertain (after the third month), if the fetus was alive, and to establish its position.

REFERENCES

1. Fisher, D.A.; and Odell, W.D.: Acute release of thyrotropin in the newborn. _J. Clin. Invest._ 48:1670-1677, 1969.

POSSIBLE ROLE OF CYANIDE AND THIOCYANATE IN THE ETIOLOGY OF ENDEMIC CRETINISM

A.M. Ermans, F. Delange, M. Van Der Velden, and J. Kinthaert

Department of Radioisotopes, St. Peter Hospital
University of Brussels, Belgium and CEMUBAC Medical Team

The existence of an abnormal prevalence of mentally defective subjects in many areas of endemic goiter has led to the idea that common etiological factors are responsible for both endemic cretinism and endemic goiter. The factor most often cited is iodine deficiency; the major role played by this factor in the pathogenesis of endemic goiter is undeniable (1,2). However, an increasing number of findings suggest that iodine deficiency constitutes only a permissive factor and not the sole etiological factor responsible for endemic goiter (3,4).

The role of dietary goitrogenic factors has been advanced in the pathogenesis of numerous endemics (5,6,7), but their role has never been proved. Careful investigations carried out by Delange et al. (3,4) leave little room for doubt as to the role of such substances. By studying systematically a large number of communities scattered throughout Idjwi Island in the Kivu (Republic of Zaire), these authors have shown that the whole population of the island is subjected to a severe and uniform iodine deficiency, but that a very high prevalence of endemic goiter is present only in the inhabitants of one particular region, whereas in another part of the island goiter prevalence is barely above normal. Subsequent studies led to the conclusion that the environmental factor responsible for goiter in this population was probably related to the consumption of cassava (8). This root vegetable is eaten in large quantities by all the population, but in even larger amounts in the goitrous area than in the non-goitrous area of the island (9). Cassava does not seem to contain any of the goitrogens found in Brassicaceae, which are considered as the most frequent source of natural goitrogens. Its anti-thyroid activity seems to result from the fact that it contains high quantities of a cyanogenetic glucoside, linamarin, which liberates cyanide on hydrolysis. After ingestion by humans or animals, this cyanide is detoxified in the form of thiocyanate, whose anti-thyroid action is well known.

A large number of subjects afflicted with cretinism have also been observed on Idjwi by Delange (3); these cretins, of the myxedematous type, are found solely in the goitrous area of the island, where they represent one percent of the population (10). This very particular epidemiologic distribution suggests that, on Idjwi at least, the iodine deficiency on its own can no more account for the prevalence of cretinism than it can for that of endemic goiter. It is possible that - as in the case of goiter - the difference of prevalence of cretinism on Idjwi could be due to the ingestion of cassava or to the action of a factor liberated during its catabolism. Such a hypothesis has no more than potential interest at the present time; it has some backing, however, in the fact that the two principal metabolites of linamarin, namely cyanide and thiocyanate ions, are capable of causing major disturbances in the two systems most often involved in endemic cretinism, i.e. the central nervous system and thyroid function. It seemed pertinent, therefore, to examine the quantities of cyanide and thiocyanate furnished by various foods eaten by man, and also to recall the principal characteristics of their metabolism and the mechanisms of their action in human beings and in animals. Special attention has been paid in this review to the influence of a chronic thiocyanate overloading on thyroid function, and also on the kinetics and distribution of thiocyanate itself. Our findings in this field may explain some of the conflicting observations reported hitherto, which have given rise to doubt concerning the role of certain goitrogenic factors.

SOURCES OF CYANIDE AND CYANOGENETIC GLUCOSIDES IN FOOD

Cyanide intake in men and animals is essentially due to ingestion of vegetables containing cyanogenetic glucosides. The commonest glucosides in the vegetable kingdom are amygdalin, identified in bitter almond and in the kernel of various fruits, dhurrin, a closely-related compound found in sorghum, and linamarin, which is found in pulses, linseed and cassava (12). Cyanogenetic glucosides are compounds which liberate hydrogen cyanide, one or more molecules of sugar, and an aldehyde or ketone on treatment with dilute acid or appropriate hydrolytic enzymes.

The structure of linamarin, for instance, is represented by the following formula:

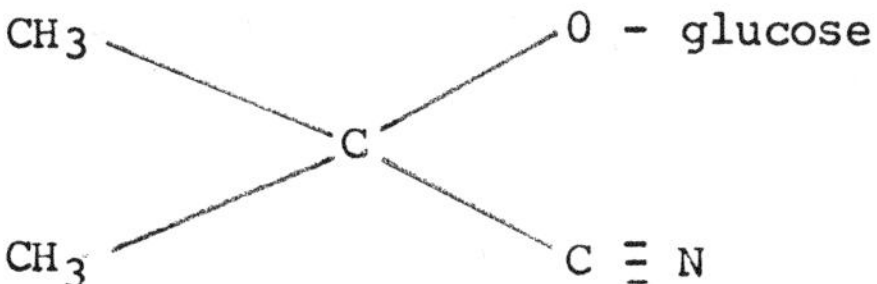

The cyanogenetic glucosides most frequently consumed by man are found in cassava, sweet potatoes, maize, millet, bamboo, sugar cane, peas, beans and the kernel of different fruits (Table 1).

Table 1. Alimentary sources of cyanide and thiocyanate

CYANIDE (Cyanogenetic Glucosides)	THIOCYANATE (Thioglucosides)
- Cassava	- Cabbage, Kale, Brussel sprouts, Cauliflower, Broccoli, Kohlrabi
- Lima beans	- Turnips
- Sorghum	- Rutabagas
- Linseed	- White and black mustard
- Kernel of fruits	- Rape and rapeseed
- Sweet Potatoes	- Horseradish
- Maize	- Garden cress
- Millets	
- Bamboo shoots	
- (Tobacco smoke) --------	Detoxification of CN^- —

The cyanide content of certain plants, such as linseed, which is an important cattle food, may cause animal poisoning. Maximum yields reported for certain vegetables may reach 100 to 300 mg per 100 gm; this is true of bitter cassava (13), sorghum (12) and lima beans (14-16). Much higher values have been found in the tips of immature bamboo shoots consumed in many eastern countries (12).

Cassava (Manihot utilissima) constitutes one of the staple foods of most Central African populations and also those of other countries. On Idjwi Island in the Kivu, consumption of cassava flour has been estimated at about 100 gm per person per day in the goitrous region (9). According to the data of Osuntokun, consumption in Nigeria is much higher (17). The cyanide content is generally considered to be greater in the bitter varieties of cassava than in the sweet varieties; but there is in fact no clear differentiation between the two strains (18). The type of soil undoubtedly plays a predominant role in the amount of linamarin contained in the plant (18). In cassava roots, the quantities of cyanide are markedly higher in the cortex than in the flesh (18-19). Figure 1 gives a series of data concerning the cyanide content of the various types of cassava eaten in the Kivu. These varieties have not been identified botanically, but they are distinguished by the local populations because of their different degrees of toxicity. The cyanide content of cassava flour, for instance, is very low or even nonexistent (Fig.1). In the Kivu this flour is prepared after lengthy

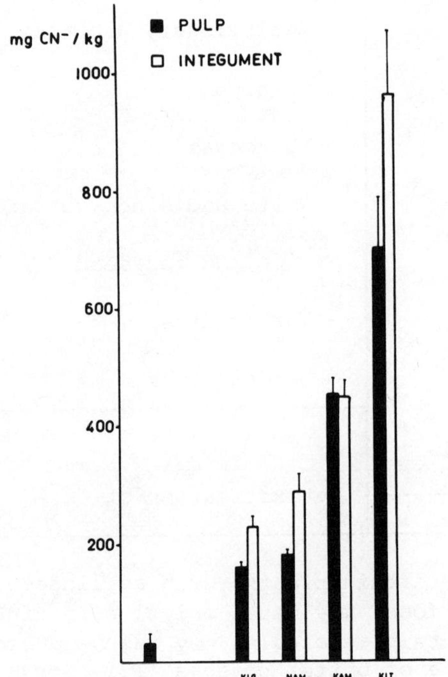

Fig. 1. Cyanide content in the flour and in fresh roots of cassava for four distinct varieties usually consumed in Idjwi Island.

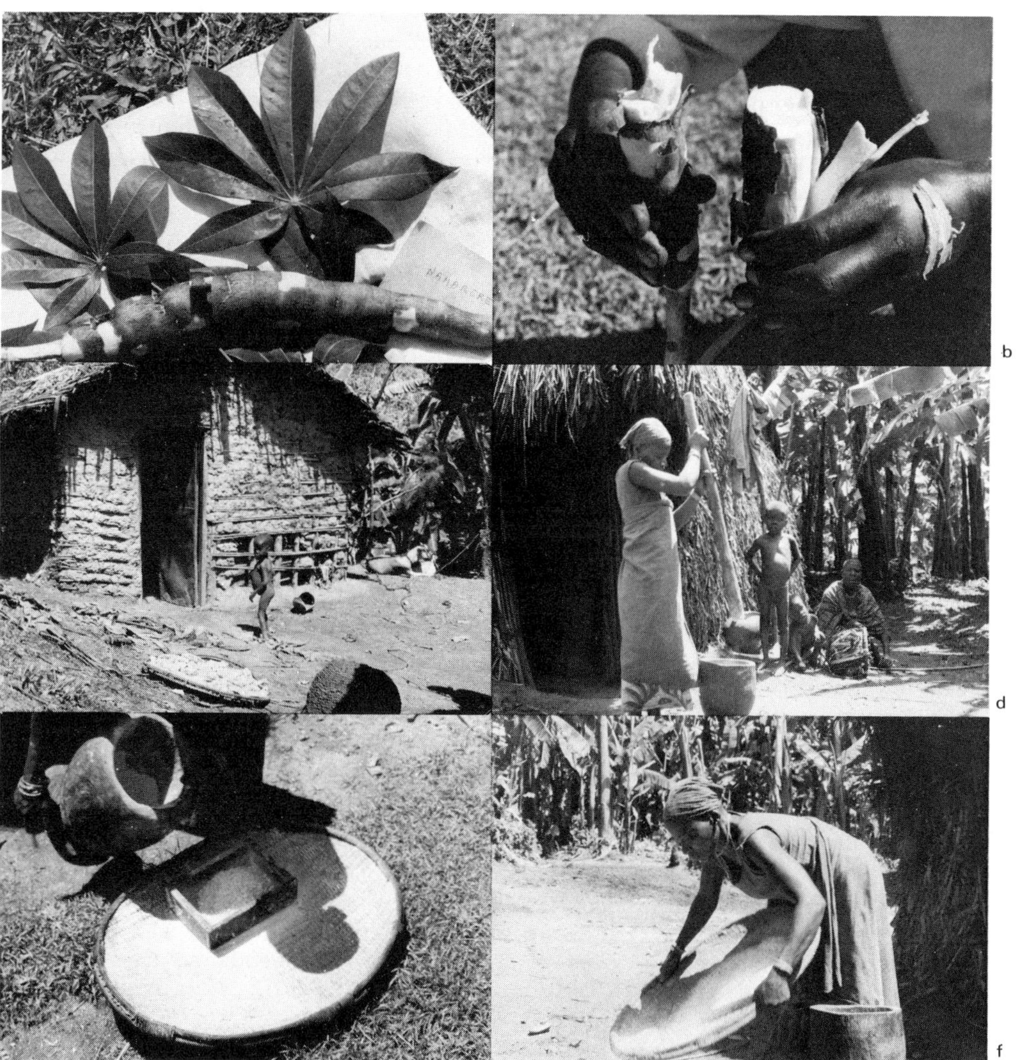

Fig. 2. Preparation of cassava on Idjwi Island (Kivu)

a) Fresh roots and leaves of the most common variety.
b) Roots are peeled and often eaten raw.
c) Roots are sieved in the sun which allows evaporation of HCN.
d) Roots are ground in a mortar.
e) Flour is first of all roughly sieved.
f) Finest flour is separated from the course grains by winnowing between two wicker trays.

exposure of the roots to sunlight (Fig. 2). In other regions of Central Africa, the roots are left to soak in running water for a long time before cooking. It is significant that in various parts of the tropics the long-established local traditions relating to the preparation of cassava serve in effect to reduce the HCN (12). Recent observations made by one of the authors (AE) indicate that fresh cassava roots are eaten peeled and raw in relatively large quantities, particularly by infants and children; these quantities may attain 200 to 300 gm per day. Cases of poisoning, sometimes fatal, have been reported, particularly after ingestion of lima beans (15) or as a result of handling of immature bamboo shoots (12).

SOURCES OF THIOCYANATE AND THIOGLUCOSIDES IN FOOD

The small quantities of thiocyanate usually observed in body fluids come from cyanide produced by protein metabolism or introduced by tobacco smoke (20,21). Apart from increases due to a greater intake of cyanide, the chief cause of a high thiocyanate content in the organism is the catabolism of thioglucosides contained in vegetables, mainly of the cruciferous family.

Interest in these foods was originally aroused because of their goitrogenic action (22,23). Although the problem has long been underestimated, it has lately acquired considerable economic importance in view of the fact that oil seed meals prepared from rape and related crucifers are used on a large scale to feed cattle and poultry (24). Present chemical knowledge of thioglucosides and derived products shows quite definitely that these substances have distinct goitrogenic properties. This question has been discussed in several thoroughgoing studies (23-29).

The Brassicaceae most commonly eaten by man are cabbage and related plants, turnips, rutabaga and mustard seed (Table 1). The concentration in thiogluosides is highest in ripe seeds so the most frequently observed thioglucosides are sinigrin, sinalbin, progoitrin, glucobrassicin and neo-glucobrassicin. Most of these thioglucosides are hydrolyzed into isothiocyanate, nitriles or thiocyanate. The general formula is given in Fig. 3. It is possible that each of these substances is capable of exerting goitrogenic action, but for most of them and particularly for glucobrassicin it has been proved that the goitrogenic action can be explained by the formation of thiocyanate resulting from hydrolysis (30-33). For other thioglucosides, however, it seems to be due to the presence of goitrin, iso-thiocyanate or other substances (23, 34-37). The ingestion of most of these vegetables by man or animals is accompanied by a rapid increase in the level of thiocyanate in the blood, and then in the urine; these levels fall swiftly as soon as ingestion ceases (31,38).

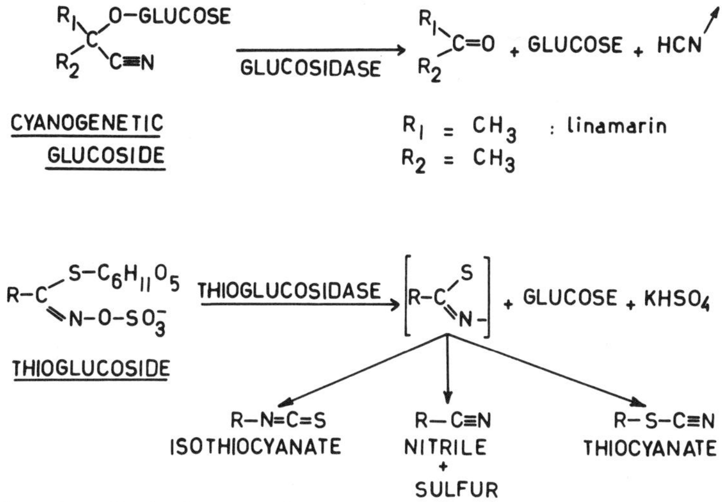

$$\begin{array}{c} R_1 \quad O\text{-GLUCOSE} \\ C \\ R_2 \quad C\equiv N \end{array} \xrightarrow[\text{GLUCOSIDASE}]{} \begin{array}{c} R_1 \\ C=O \\ R_2 \end{array} + \text{GLUCOSE} + HCN\uparrow$$

CYANOGENETIC GLUCOSIDE

$R_1 = CH_3$: linamarin
$R_2 = CH_3$

$$R\text{-}C\begin{array}{l} S\text{-}C_6H_{11}O_5 \\ N\text{-}O\text{-}SO_3^- \end{array} \xrightarrow{\text{THIOGLUCOSIDASE}} \left[R\text{-}C\begin{array}{l} S \\ N\text{-} \end{array} \right] + \text{GLUCOSE} + KHSO_4$$

THIOGLUCOSIDE

R–N=C=S ISOTHIOCYANATE | R–C≡N NITRILE + SULFUR | R–S–C≡N THIOCYANATE

Fig. 3. Hydrolysis of a cyanogenetic glucoside and of a thioglucoside.

METABOLIC PATHWAYS OF CYANOGENETIC GLUCOSIDES AND THIOGLUCOSIDES

CYANOGENETIC GLUCOSIDES

Autohydrolysis. Spontaneous release of hydrogen cyanide from the plant depends on the presence of a specific glucosidase and water. The enzymes are extracellular and gain access to the glucoside after physical disruption of the cell. They are readily destroyed by heat. Not only may autohydrolysis occur before the glucosidase has been destroyed, but after it has been inactivated by heating; contact with fresh glucosidase may still lead to the decomposition of the glucoside, which is heat-stable.

Metabolic Pathways of Inorganic Cyanide in the Body. Ingested cyanide is rapidly absorbed from the upper gastrointestinal tract. In the body the principal metabolic pathway (Fig. 4) is by reaction with thiosulfate to form thiocyanate and sulfite, the reaction being catalyzed by thiosulfate - cyanide sulfurtransferase [Rhodanese (39)]. This enzyme is wide-spread in living tissues, reaching its highest concentration in the liver, kidney, thyroid, adrenal and pancreas. Organic cyanides or nitriles only give rise to thiocyanate in the body if they are first broken down to cyanide ions. The resulting thiocyanate is excreted in the urine or slowly oxidized to sulfate.

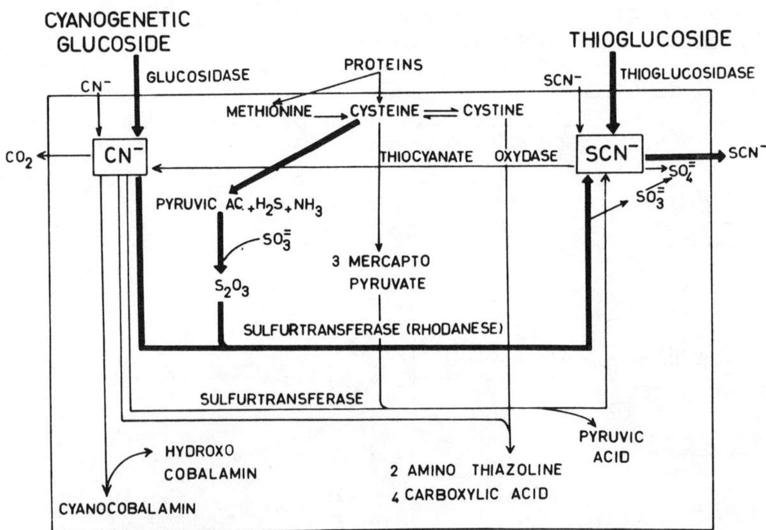

Fig. 4. Principal metabolic pathways of the thioglucosides, cyanogenetic glucosides, cyanide and thiocyanate.

In a second pathway to thiocyanate (Fig. 4), cyanide reacts with 3 mercapto-pyruvate, aided by 3 mercapto-pyruvate-cyanide sulfurtransferase to form thiocyanate and pyruvic acid (40). These reactions require the presence of adequate amounts of cystine as a sulfur donor. Otherwise cystine may react more directly with cyanide to produce 2 amino 4 thiazoline carboxylic acid (41). There are no doubt other pathways. Isotope studies indicate that some of the carbon of ingested cyanide is lost as carbon dioxide (42).

Finally, it is well known that hydroxocobalamin (vitamin B_{12}) takes up cyanide as cyanocobalamin and readily liberates it on exposure to light (43). This could be merely a secondary effect of the presence of cyanide in the body, but there is some evidence that hydroxocobalamin may play a more active role in cyanide detoxication.

We have so far considered only the possibility of hydrolysis before the food is eaten. The question remains as to whether the whole intact plant, or the intact glucoside itself, may be toxic after ingestion. In spite of negative findings, the ultimate fate of the ingested cyanogenetic glucoside remains unknown and it may quite possibly lead to an appreciable increase in the body's cyanide or thiocyanate pool. Microbial flora might play a part in the decomposition of the glucoside (44). Experimental data obtained in rats fed with fresh cassava roots (Fig. 5) are in agreement with this view.

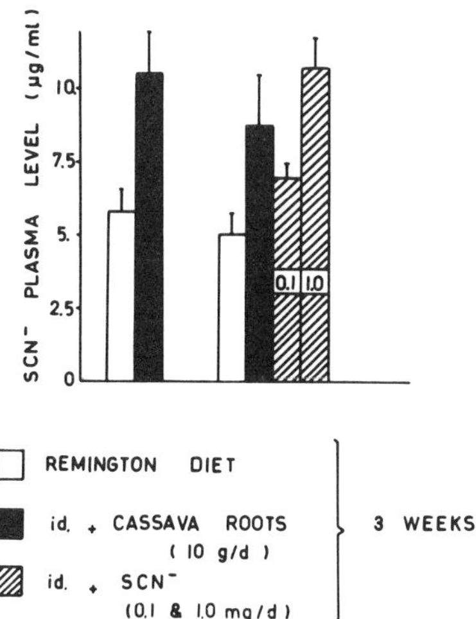

Fig. 5. Thiocyanate level in plasma in rats fed for 4 weeks with a Remington diet with or without supplementation with fresh cassava roots (10gm/day) or with thiocyanate (0.1 or 1.0 mg/day).

THIOGLUCOSIDES

Autohydrolysis. Thioglucosides are hydrolyzed when the wet, unheated plant material is crushed. The hydrolysis is catalyzed by an enzyme, thioglucosidase, in the plant material (44,45). Hydrolysis liberates glucose, acid sulfate ion and, depending on conditions of hydrolysis, isothiocyanates, thiocyanates or nitriles. These nitriles give rise to thiocyanate if they are first broken down to cyanide.

Metabolic Pathways of Thiocyanate in the Body. Goldstein and Rieders (46) demonstrated in red blood cells an endogenous oxidase, thiocyanate oxidase, which converts thiocyanate to free cyanide.

Thiocyanate is slowly oxidized to sulfate, but this does not appear to be an important factor in body tissues. Greer and Deeney (35) showed that goitrin accumulated in the blood and urine after ingestion of progoitrin without thioglucosidase. An antithryoid effect was also observed. Both Greer (28) and Oginsky and co-workers (47) demonstrated that thioglucosidases from microorganisms that are often found in the digestive tract act on progoitrin to yield goitrin. But hydrolysis by the thioglucosidase produced by microflora of the intestine, as tested in vivo by Greer and co-workers was slower and more erratic than by the thioglucosidase accompanying progoitrin in a plant.

Later Michajlowski and Langer (30) showed that unhydrolyzed glucobrassicin fed to rats, without the active thioglucosidase, had no goitrogenic action. The antithyroidal activity of glucobrassicin (with myrosinase) is practically identical to that of the equivalent amount of thiocyanate (30). The various metabolic pathways of the cyanogenetic glucoside and thioglucosides are summarized in Fig. 4; thiocyanate appears as the main end product of the catabolism of a large number of goitrogenic foodstuffs.

ACTION OF CYANIDE AND CYANOGENETIC GLUCOSIDES

In man the lethal dose of HCN is around 0.5 to 3.5 mg per kg of body weight when absorbed orally (48). As mentioned earlier, numerous cases of fatal cyanhydric poisoning have been reported in man and animals after ingestion of foods containing cyanogenetic glucosides (16).

The toxicity of cyanide has been investigated experimentally after chronic poisoning with sublethal doses. Particular attention has focused on impairment of the nervous system. Pathological modifications are exceptional (12,49,50); the main effect is demyelination of nerve figers. Lesions of the optic nerve have also been reported (50,51); they are identical to those observed in tobacco amblyopia which occurs in vitamin B_{12} deficiency. This finding led certain authors (52-54) to postulate that this situation could reflect the conversion of hydroxocobalamin into cyanocobalamin following cyanide poisoning.

Interest in chronic cyanide poisoning has been further stimulated by the finding that in patients suffering from a chronic degenerative neuropathy which is common in parts of Nigeria, there is an increased concentration of thiocyanate in the plasma and urine (17,54-56). The disease is associated with longstanding consumption of large amounts of cassava. Hospitalization of such patients is accompanied by a drop in the plasma concentration but this trend is reversed when a return is made to normal diet. It is of special interest that this situation is associated with a very low level of cystein + cystine in the plasma (56); the authors suggest that this was due to the utilization of these aminoacids for the detoxication of the cyanide derived from cassava. The prevalence of neurological abnormalities in this tropical disease is reported in Table 2. These data are compared to the corresponding findings concerning nervous cretins studied in New Guinea (57). It is particularly interesting to note that in both syndromes deafness, and sometimes deaf-mutism, is associated with major neurological signs (ataxic gait, hypertonia, exaggerated reflexes). Yet the two syndromes differ essentially in the fact that the degenerative neuropathy of Nigeria appears

Table 2. Neurologic Abnormalities in Tropical Neuropathy and in Neurologic Cretinism

REGION	NIGERIA	WESTERN NEW GUINEA
AUTHORS	OSUNTOKUN *et al.* 1970 - 71	CHOUFOER *et al.* 1965
DIAGNOSIS	ATAXIC NEUROPATHY	ENDEMIC CRETINISM
PREVALENCE	2.2%	5.5%
(Nerve) Deafness	41%	Most
Motor Defects	30%	Most
Ataxic Gait	61%	40%
Hyperreflexia	19%	Most
Extensor Plantar Reflex	7%	15%
Optic Atrophy	81%	(Not reported)
Posterior Column Sensory Loss	83%	(Not reported)
Age of Maximal Prevalence	40 - 49 Y	18%
Mental Retardation	(Not reported)	100%

late in life whereas the neurological signs of cretinism are considered to be present at birth. There is no mental retardation in the neuropathy, and there has been no report so far of any lesion of the optic nerve in cretinism.

Figure 5 shows that addition of cassava roots to a Remington diet in rats induces after three weeks a marked increase in the plasma level of thiocyanate (19). This finding is based on two distinct series of investigations; in the second one, the results were compared with the ones obtained by supplementing the Remington diet with a daily dose of 0.1 and 1.0 mg of thiocyanate. The findings are in agreement with previous data of Osuntokun (84).

The goitrogenic action of cassava was reported for the first time in the rat by Eckpechi (85,86); its action was attributed to the presence in cassava roots of a substance which would act like the thionamide group of antithyroid drugs. Studies performed in man on Idjwi Island by the authors of this chapter rather suggest a thiocyanate-like action (8,9). Indeed ingestion of cassava grown in the goitrous area of this island induces a prompt drop of thyroid uptake of radioiodine, associated with a corresponding rise in urinary excretion of ^{131}I (Fig. 6) and concomitantly of stable iodine.

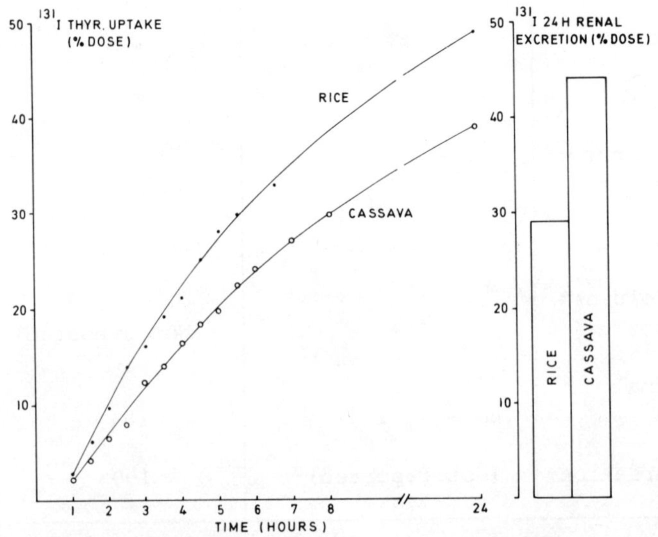

Fig. 6. Distribution in the thyroid gland and in urine of two successive tracer doses of ^{131}I given per os to one of the authors (F.D.) after the absorption of a large meal of rice and after a meal of boiled cassava flour.

Estimation of thiocyanate concentration in the inhabitants of the island revealed a marked increase in comparison with the levels observed in Belgian controls (9). However, the range of concentration was found to be the same in both the goitrous and non-goitrous areas; on the other hand, urinary excretion of thiocyanate was significantly higher in the goitrous area (9).

ACTION OF THIOCYANATE

The antithyroid properties of potassium thiocyanate were first observed by Barker (58-59), who found that several patients being treated with thiocyanate for hypertension developed signs of myxedema associated with enlargement of the thyroid gland. This effect could be rapidly reversed by the administration of small doses of thyroid powder or iodide.

It was shown in 1946 that thiocyanate markedly inhibits the accumulation of iodide by the thyroid gland (60,61). At about the same time Vanderlaan and Vanderlaan (62) showed that in rats, in which organic binding of iodine was blocked by thiouracil, thiocyanate decreased the ability of the thyroid gland to maintain a concentration of iodide above that of the blood. This action of thiocyanate on iodide uptake was interpreted as a specific inhibitory effect on the iodide-concentrating mechanism of the thyroid gland.

On the other hand, in vivo and in vitro studies by Raben (63) suggest that, in addition, thiocyanate might inhibit the iodination process. According to Woolman (64), no appreciable effect on the rate of incorporation of iodide into protein-bound ^{131}I would occur at low concentrations of serum thiocyanate. The marked decrease in the binding rate observed for higher thiocyanate concentrations could be due to inhibition of iodinating enzymes but also to a decrease of the radioiodide concentration at the binding site which could be related to an increase it its exit rate. Data of Scranton *et al.* (65) are in agreement with this view.

Further biochemical studies have clearly emphasized the direct interference of thiocyanate in the organic binding of iodine in the thyroid gland (67-69).

Iodide/thiocyanate competition has been studied in various extrathyroidal tissues which also have the ability to concentrate iodide, i.e.: salivary glands, stomach, mammary glands and placenta (69). All attempts made to inhibit extrathyroidal I^- transport with SCN^- and or ClO_4^- have so far been successful. Considerable variations were observed, however, depending on the organs and the species studied (69). Concentrations of iodide and thiocyanate in saliva and gastric juice are greater than their respective concentrations in plasma (70-71).

The mammary gland concentrates iodide into milk in rats (72); thiocyanate is also concentrated in the milk but only during the latter part of lactation, when the milk/plasma ratio reached an average of 5.3; the corresponding ratio averaged 0.69 in human lactating subjects (21).

In studies of the transfer of thiocyanate to milk, Piironen and Virtanen (73) noticed that the iodine content of the milk was consistently lowered by thiocyanate feeding but rose to high levels as soon as the thiocyanate was stopped. Apparently thiocyanate feeding inhibits iodine absorption by the mammary gland as well as by the thyroid. Thus the mammary gland conserves the iodine for the lactating animal but lowers the iodine content of the milk for her young. Such an effect has also been mentioned by Garner et al. (74) and by Miller et al. (75). Reviewing the problem, Van Etten (24) concludes that "a lactating mammal ingesting thiocyanate ions could possibly cause goiter in her young or in those drinking large amounts of her milk by lowering its iodine content ."

The transmittal of thiocyanate or other goitrogens to man from cow's milk has been extensively investigated (27,76-79). The data obtained by different authors are so conflicting that at the present time the question of its possible influence in the development of endemic goiter remains unanswered.

Studies by Funderburk and Van Middleworth contributed important data about the modifications of the distribution of thiocyanate in various experimental conditions (21,80-82). SCN production is decreased in fasting rats; however the observed SCN concentration in plasma rises because of a decrease of the destruction rate of SCN and of its volume of distribution. On the other hand, large doses of thiocyanate have a much faster rate of disappearance than does endogenous thiocyanate at normal concentration.

EFFECT OF PROLONGED ACTION OF SCN AND CYANOGENETIC GLUCOSIDES ON THYROID FUNCTION IN THE RAT

Few experimental data are available on the long term influence of continuous administration of thiocyanate or its precursors. It is interesting to investigate such experimental conditions, because they can simulate the possible influence of goitrogenic foods consumed more or less regularly by man. A series of investigations was undertaken with this in view by various members of our laboratory; the results of these investigations are reported briefly.

The basic experimental protocol consisted in estimating various parameters of iodine and thiocyanate metabolism in male White Star rats subjected to a low-iodine diet (Remington), supplemented with varying doses of thiocyanates over a period of four to six weeks. The same estimations were made in rats subjected to a similar diet with the addition of 10 gm of fresh cassava roots per day. Some investigations were conducted after continuous supplementation with 10 µg of iodide per day. Findings concerning iodine metabolism after the administration of these

Table 3: Action of long-term intake of SCN⁻ and of fresh cassava roots on the thyroid size and the organic iodine metabolism, in rats.

PARAMETER	IODINE SUPPLY	CONTROLS	SCN 1 mg/d	SCN 2 mg/d	SCN 5 mg/d	CASSAVA 10 g/d
Thyroid Weight (mg/100g)	5 μg/d	10.7	12.7*	12.8	11.9	13.7**
	No	13.4	11.2	14.7	-	14.2
Thyroid Iodine content (μg)	5 μg/d	11.9	10.5	7.9**	7.6**	9.2**
	No	1.0	0.7	0.6*	-	0.5*
Plasma $PB^{127}I$ (μg/100ml)	5 μg/d	2.6	2.3	2.2	2.3	2.3
	No	1.8	1.3*	1.2**	-	1.1**

Value statistically different from the controls value: *P <.01; **P <.001

different diets are represented in Table 3. In the iodine supplemented rats the daily dose of 0.1 to 5.0 mg of thiocyanate caused a progressive depletion of the iodine content of the thyroid; the level of plasma $PB^{127}I$ remained unchanged. A goitrogenic effect was only observed for the highest doses.

In the iodine-deficient rats, the iodine content of the thyroid was already reduced by a factor of 10, in the absence of any administration of thiocyanate. Chronic overloading with thiocyanate brought about an even greater reduction of the iodine content. All the deficient animals showed marked hyperplasia of the thyroid, but chronic overloading with thiocyanate did not increase the hyperplasia. On the other hand it reduced significantly the level of $PB^{127}I$ in the serum. It is interesting to note that the administration of cassava modified these various parameters in exactly the same way as the administration of thiocyanate did.

Table 4. Distribution of ^{125}I-labeled iodoaminoacids in iodine-deficient rats[1]; influence of chronic SCN administration and of manioc[2].

TREATMENT	MIT^x/DIT^x Ratio	I^x - T4 (%)[3]	I^x - T3 (%)
10 $\mu g^{127}I/d$	.50 ± .05	22 ± 10	4 ± 1
Controls	.89 ± .10	21 ± 8	9 ± 1
0.1 SCN/d	.94 ± .10	24 ± 5	7 ± 1
1.0 SCN/d	1.31 ± .14	18 ± 4	10 ± 1
2.0 SCN/d	1.62 ± .15	11 ± 6	11 ± 2
10.0 SCN/d	2.00 ± 2.4	6 ± 2	13 ± 3
Manioc carrots	1.63 ± .15	11 ± 6	9 ± 3

1 Remington diet.
2 10 μcuries of carrier-free ^{125}I were injected intraperitoneally before starting SCN or manioc administration. Both treatments were maintained during four weeks until sacrifice.
3 Percentage of the whole ^{125}I content of the thyroid tissue.

Table 4 shows the changes observed in hormonogenesis in the iodine-deprived rats in this series of investigations. These observations were made one month after the administration of a single dose of iodine-125 to deprived rats. The MIT/DIT ratio was close to one,i.e. a similar value to that observed by the majority of authors (87,88).

The administration of thiocyanate increased this ratio markedly once the daily dose exceeded one mg per day, the increase being the more marked as the thiocyanate dose was augmented. Simultaneously, a reverse change in the gland's thyroxin content was observed; the T_3 content remained unchanged. Here again, the administration of cassava gave rise to changes identical to those caused by thiocyanate. For the cassava dose used, the changes corresponded approximately to the administration of 2 mg of SCN per day.

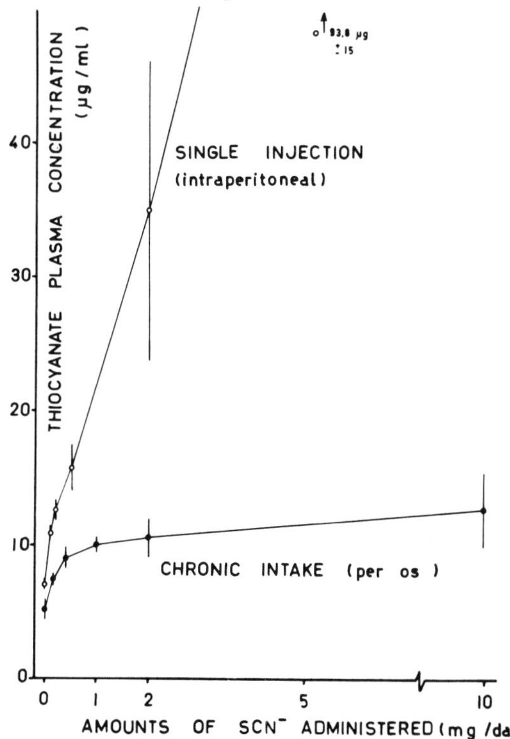

Fig. 7. Thiocyanate levels in serum of rats fed with a Remington diet after the administration of thiocyanate with doses ranging from 0.1 to 5.0 mg. A single intraperitoneal dose of thiocyanate is administered in "acute experiments"; in "chronic experiments", the same dose is mixed every day with the Remington diet for four weeks.

Figure 7 shows the levels of blood thiocyanate observed in the same experimental conditions. Unexpectedly, it was found that although these levels rose distinctly for the lower doses, the subsequent increase for higher doses was only slight. This finding is just the opposite to what was observed after single injections of similar quantities of SCN. In these cases SCN concentrations in the blood were very high.

Thyroid uptake of radioiodine in animals subjected to chronic thiocyanate overloading is reported in Table 5. Whatever the dose of thiocyanate used, binding of ^{131}I was not diminished; on the contrary, it was significantly higher.

The question thus arose as to why the administration of high doses of thiocyanate could cause such a considerable depletion of iodine reserves without entailing any block of the gland's iodide pump or any marked rise in the plasma level of thiocyanate. This situation is explained at least in part by major modifications occasioned by the thiocyanate in the kidney. On the one hand, the quantities of thiocyanate collected in the urine during overloading indicated almost complete recovery of the dose administered (Table 5). Secondly, renal clearance increased dramatically in direct proportion to the quantity of thiocyanate administered. Finally, when ^{35}S labelled thiocyanate was injected into the rats submitted to thiocyanate overloading, a considerable increase in the disposal rate of labelled thiocyanate in the plasma was observed; this acceleration became more marked as the loading dose was augmented. The absorption of cassava entailed a similar acceleration of plasma turnover of thiocyanate; the acceleration was identical to that observed for a daily dose of one to two mg of thiocyanate. Measurements of renal clearance of iodine under the same experimental conditions showed a significant increase for the animals receiving the highest doses of thiocyanate. These findings seem explainable, assuming thiocyanate/iodide competition in the kidney, by a saturation of tubular reabsorption by thiocyanate. The existence of an iodide carrier playing some role in tubular reabsorption of iodine was suggested by Halmi _et al._ (83); such a carrier could be inhibited by iodine and perchlorate. The increase of iodine leakage from the kidney due to saturation of tubular reabsorption caused by thiocyanate could offer a plausible explanation of the iodine depletion observed in these animals.

Nevertheless, in view of the marked increase of thiocyanate turnover in the blood, we could not exclude the possibility of transitory inhibition of the iodide pump. Table 5 gives the results of investigations conducted according to the original schedule, with the difference that the feeding period of the animals

Table 5. Action of long-term intake of thiocyanate on iodide and SCN distribution and kinetics, in rats.

ADMINISTRATION OF THE DIET	PARAMETERS - UNITS	CONTROLS	SUPPLEMENT SCN/DAY (mg)			
			.2	1	2	5
AD LIBITUM	^{131}I thyroid uptake (%D) at 4 hrs	8.5	11.8**	11.2**	10.2	13.3**
	Iodide renal clearance (10^{-2}ml/mn)	3.3	5.1**	5.0*	4.9	6.0**
	SCN renal excretion (mg/day)	0.06	0.21	0.81	1.91	4.15
	^{35}SCN plasma disposal rate (10^{-2}/hr)	0.3	1.5	5.1	7.4	-
RESTRICTED TO 6 HRS/DAY	SCN plasma concentration (μg/ml)	4.6		13.4**		27.1**
	Iodide thyroid clearance (10^{-2}/hr)	1.54		1.37		1.16**
	Iodide renal clearance (10^{-2}ml/mn)	6.7		8.2		9.3**
	^{131}I thyroid uptake (% Dose) at 4 hrs.	5.4		5.6		4.3
	SCN renal clearance (10^{-2}ml/mn)	0.4		4.2**		15.0**

Value statistically different from the controls value: *P <.01; **P <.001

was reduced to six hours per day. The measurements were made during the actual absorption period. For the 5 mg dose, the results show that on the one hand the plasma concentration of thiocyanate attained a much higher level (27.1 μg per ml) and on the other hand partial decrease of iodide thyroid clearance occurred.

SUMMARY

With regard to the possible intervention of the thiocyanate ion in the pathogenesis of endemic goiter and cretinism, these investigations lead to the following conclusions:

1. Continuous intake of cassava is capable of causing changes in iodine and thiocyanate metabolism which are both qualitatively and quantitatively identical to those obtained by prolonged administration of thiocyanate.

2. Ingestion of thiocyanate or cassava entails marked depletion of iodine stores; depletion is fairly moderate in non-deprived rats, but very severe in iodine-deprived rats; during iodine deprivation, the two substances cause major changes in intrathyroidal metabolism which iodine deficiency alone is incapable of causing.

3. Chronic ingestion of thiocyanate does not necessarily cause blocking of the thyroidal iodide pump; iodine uptake by the gland seems, on the contrary, to be increased, probably due to thyrotropic stimulation triggered by iodine depletion. But this does not preclude transitory inhibition during the phase of thiocyanate absorption.

4. Chronic administration of thiocyanate or its precursors even in increasing doses does not necessarily entail a very marked rise of SCN concentration in the blood. Evidence of increased ingestion is only obtained by measurements of urinary excretion or estimation of plasma turnover.

5. A schema which may explain the goitrogenic action of cassava and thiocyanate on the basis of the present experimental data appears in Fig. 8. In particular, this interpretation is compatible with the concept that iodine deficiency plays a permissive role, and explains why this etiological mechanism can be completely reversed by stepping up iodine intake.

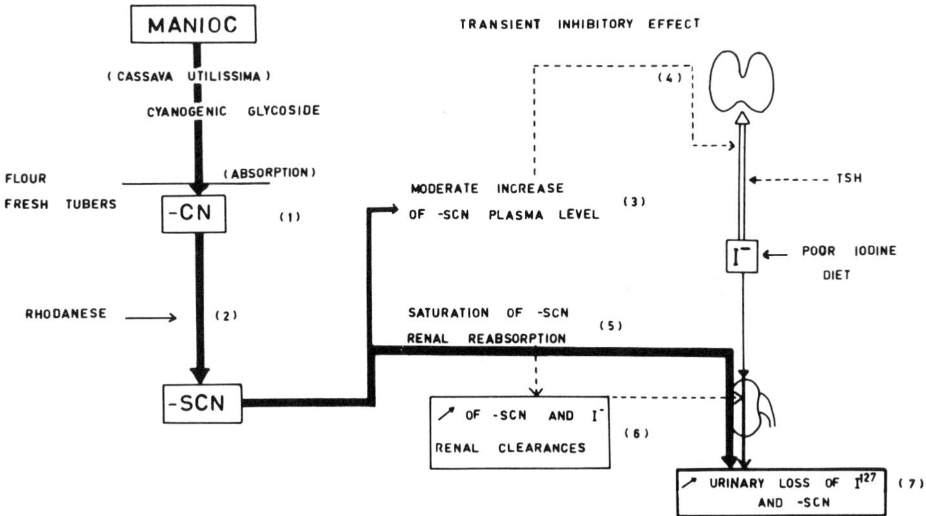

Fig. 8. Possible mechanism of the goitrogenic action of a cyanide, thiocyanate and of alimentary foodstuffs containing cyanogenetic glucosides or thio-glucosides

6. The investigations reveal the difficulty of verifying the role of thiocyanate-like goitrogens in the mechanisms of goiter development in man. More especially, they show that such a role cannot be assessed by using as criteria the classic observations made after the administration of thiocyanate to man or animals. Further studies are therefore essential to find out the real role of these substances in the pathogenesis of endemic goiter. A series of findings made on Idjwi in the Kivu already seem to fit in with certain of these experimental results.

7. And finally, in view of the severity of the metabolic changes induced by the association of iodine deficiency with ingestion of thiocyanate-like compounds, the question arises as to whether the action of these factors on the fetal thyroid could not give rise to transitory or permanent lesions responsible for the development of cretinism. This hypothesis seems to constitute a basis for further studies in this field.

ACKNOWLEDGEMENTS

Supported by grants of the "Fonds de la Recherche Médicale Scientifique" (Brussels), of the Institut Belge de la Nutrition et de l'Alimentation, and by the contract Euratom - ULB - Pisa Universities.

DISCUSSION BY PARTICIPANTS

STANBURY: Do you have any ideas on the possible role of thiocyanate given postpartem in inhibiting transfer of iodine through the milk?

ERMANS: First of all, it has been shown in cows that the iodine content of milk was markedly decreased after ingestion of vegetable food-stuffs containing thiocyanate precursors. Thus the lactating cows keep iodine for themselves without giving it to their young (73). Another point to be considered is the transfer of thiocyanate by milk from the mother to the young. Funderburk and Van Middlesworth (21) reported that the thiocyanate ratio between milk and serum reached 5.3 during the last phase of lactation in rats; however for women, this ratio averaged only 0.69.

DEGROOT: Would goitrogenesis be a "prophylaxis" against the effect of thiocyanate, because thiocyanate could be metabolized more rapidly by the hyperplastic thyroid? Secondly, would cysteine or methionine deficiency be important here? Large amounts of these essential amino acids are being used up to metabolize the cyanide.

ERMANS: It has been shown that TSH markedly increases the accumulation and the oxidation rate of thiocyanate in the thyroid (68). In this regard, we have observed that in TSH stimulated rats, the SCN^- level, after SCN^- overloading, was significantly lower than in non-stimulated animals. This means that the degree of stimulation of the thyroid gland plays a determining role in the kinetics and the distribution of the SCN^-, just as it does for iodide.

On the other hand, the conversion of cyanide into thiocyanate requires large amounts of cysteine, as a sulfur donor. It may be calculated that the conversion of each mg of cyanate needs about six mg of this sulfur-containing aninoacid. When the protein supply is low, availability of the sulfur donors could be critical for an adequate detoxification of cyanide.

DEGROOT: Maybe that is why they can't grow goiters there.

STANBURY: That is one of the theories that we are looking into.

PITTMAN: Is there any iodine in the cassava?

ERMANS: We were unable to detect any amount.

COSTA: You say that Idjwi island is subjected as a whole to uniform iodine deficiency, and that there is considerable overlapping of the thyroidal uptake and of the daily urinary elimination values in the North and in the Southwest of the island. How can you postulate as a cause of the striking difference in the prevalence of goiter between the two regions a partial inhibition of iodine uptake by the thyroid and an increase of its renal excretion in the North of the island?

FIERRO: There is endemic cretinism in the north of Idjwi and in both north and south there is extreme iodine deficiency. What about the cassava in the region where there is no endemic cretinism?

ERMANS: This is the weak point of our study. We were unable to detect a dramatic difference in the cyanide content of the cassava in the two regions. We suspect that the consumption of cassava, and more specifically of fresh cassava, is higher in the North than in the South, but we have not demonstrated it.

DELANGE: Maybe Dr. DeGroot's remark made the important point: with the same quantity of cyanide, more thiocyanate would be made in the goitrous area because of a higher content of sulfur aminoacids in the food. Actually, the sulfur aminoacid intake is higher in the North than in the South. This is just a hypothesis, but the people in the South perhaps are protected from goiter because they have a low sulfur aminoacid intake.

PHAROAH: Kamchatnov and Gurevich [quoted in (89)] have reported that manganese is a goitrogen.

BALAZS: You mentioned that in adults in Nigeria deafness may result from the action of goitrogens. If this is so, one does not need to postulate that the neurological defect leading to deafness in the endemic cretin occurs during an early period of the development of the CNS.

ERMANS: I don't think that this defect is related to any antithyroid activity of cassava, but to a direct action of cyanide on the central nervous system.

BALAZS: It is rather unlikely that free cyanide concentrations can be chronically maintained at a relatively high level in the body without causing death.

ERMANS: Ostuntokun et al. (56) found that plasma levels of cysteine of these patients are very low; their nutritional situation is apparently much worse than that of our subjects in the Kivu. Detoxification of cyanide might be inadequate or imcomplete in such conditions. It must be noted that the Nigerian authors do not describe any goiter in the subjects suffering from this particular neuropathy.

REFERENCES

1. Stanbury, J.B., Brownell, G.L., Riggs, D.S., Perinetti, H., Itoiz, J. and Del Castillo, E.B.: Endemic Goiter. The Adaptation of Man to Iodine Deficiency. Cambridge, Mass., Harvard University Press, 1954.

2. Ermans, A.M., Dumont, J.E. and Bastenie, P.A.: Thyroid function in a goiter endemic. II. Non hormonal iodine escape from the goitrous gland. J. Clin. Endocrinol. Metab. 23:550-560, 1963.

3. Delange, F.: Le goître endémique à l'Ile d'Idjwi (Lac Kivu Republique du Congo). Données preliminaires. Ann. Endocrinol. (Paris) 27:256-261, 1966.

4. Delange, F., Thilly, C. and Ermans, A.M.: Iodine deficiency, a permissive condition in the development of endemic goiter. J. Clin. Endocrinol. Metab. 28:114-116, 1968.

5. Silink, K.: Goitrogens in foods and endemic goiter. In: Naturally Occurring Goitrogens and Thyroid Function. (J. Podoba and P. Langer, eds.) Slovak Academy of Sciences, Bratislavia, 1964, pp. 241-246.

6. Tillez, M., Gianetti, A., Covarrubias, E. and Barzelatto, J.: Endemic goiter in Pedegroso (Chile). Experimental goitrogenic activity of "Pinon". In: Endemic Goiter. Report of the meeting of the PAHO Scientific Group on Research in Endemic Goiter held in Mexico, 1968. (J.B. Stanbury, ed.). PAHO Scientific Publication No. 193, Washington, 1969. pp. 245-251.

7. Michajlovskij, N. and Langer, P.: The relation between thiocyanate formation and the goitrogenic effects of foods. I. The preformed thiocyanate content of some foods. Z. Physiol. Chem. 312:26-30, 1958.

8. Delange, F. and Ermans, A.M.: Role of a dietary goitrogen in the etiology of endemic goiter on Idjwi Island. Am. J. Clin. Nutr. 24:1354-1360, 1971.

9. Ermans, A.M., Thilly, C., Vis, H.L. and Delange, F.: Permissive nature of iodine deficiency in the development of endemic goiter. In: Endemic Goiter. Report of the meeting of the PAHO Scientific Group on Research in Endemic Goiter held in Mexico, 1968 (J.B. Stanbury, ed.). PAHO Scientific Publication No. 193, Washington, 1969. pp. 101-117.

10. Delange, F. and Ermans, A.M.: Further studies on endemic cretinism in Central Africa. Horm. Metab. Res. 3:431-437, 1971.

11. Delange, F., Ermans, A.M., Vis, H.L. and Stanbury, J.B.: Endemic cretinism in Idjwi Island (Kivu Lake, Republic of the Congo). In: Endemic Cretinism (B.S. Hetzel and P.O. D. Pharoah, eds.). Institute of Human Biology Monographs No. 2, Papua, New Guinea, 1971.

12. Montgomery, R.D.: Cyanogens in toxic constituents of plant foodstuffs. In: Toxic Constituents of Plant Foodstuffs (I.E. Liener, ed.). Academic Press, New York, 1969. pp. 143-155.

13. Collens, A.E.: Bitter and sweet cassava-hydrocyanic acid contents. Bull. Dept. Agr. Trinidad Tobago.14:54, 1915.

14. Guignard, L.: Sur les quantités d'acide cyanhydrique fournies par le Phaseolus lunatus L. cultivé sous le climat de Paris. Bull. Sci. Pharmacol. 14:556-557, 1907.

15. Viehoever, A.: Edible and poisonous beans of the lima type (Phaseolus lunatus L.):comparative study, including other similar beans. Thailand Sci. Bull. 2:1-99, 1940.

16. Montgomery, R.D.: Observations on the cyanide content and toxicity of tropical pulses. West Indian Med. J. 13:1-11, 1964.

17. Osuntokun, B.O.: Chronic cyanide intoxication and a degenerative neuropathy in Nigerians. Thesis, University of Ibadan, 1969.

18. Oyenuga, V.A. and Amazigo, E.O.: A note on the hydrocyanic acid content of cassava (Manihot utilissima Pohl). West Afr. J. Biol. Chem. 1:39-43, 1957.

19. Van Der Velde, M., Kinthaert, J. and Ermans, A.M.: Unpublished data.

20. Osborne, J.S., Adamek, S. and Hobbs, M.E.: Some components of the gas phase of cigarette smoke. Anal. Chem. 28:211-215, 1956.

21. Funderburk, C.F. and Van Middlesworth, L.: Effect of lactation and perchlorate on thiocyanate metabolism. Am. J. Physiol. 213:1371-1377, 1967.

22. Chesney, A.M., Clawson, T.A. and Webster, B.: Endemic goitre in rabbits. I. Incidence and characteristics. Bull. Johns Hopkins Hosp. 43:261-277, 1928.

23. Greer, M.A.: Nutrition and goiter. Physiol. Rev. 30: 513-548, 1950.

24. Van Etten, C.H.: Goitrogens. In: Toxic Constituents of Plant Foodstuffs (I.E. Liener, ed.). Academic Press, New York, 1969. pp. 103-134.

25. Greer, M.A.: Goitrogenic substances in food. Am. J. Clin. Nutr. 5:440-444, 1957.

26. Kjaer, A.: Naturally derived isothiocyanates (mustard oils) and their parent glucosides. In: The Chemistry of Organic Natural Products (L. Zechmeister, ed.). Springer-Verlag, Vienna, 1960. pp. 122-176.

27. Clements, F.W.: Naturally occurring goitrogens. Br. Med. Bull. 16:133-137, 1960.

28. Greer, M.A.: The natural occurrence of goitrogenic agents. Recent Progr. Horm. Res. 18:187-219, 1962.

29. Roy, A.B. and Trudinger, T.A.: The Biochemistry of Inorganic Compounds of Sulphur. Cambridge University Press: 317-322, 1970.

30. Michajlovskij, N. and Langer, P.: Identity of the goitrogenic effect of glucobrassicin and the equivalent amount of thiocyanate in rats. Endocrinol. Exp. 1:229-236, 1967.

31. Langer, P. and Michajlovskij, N.: The relation between thiocyanate formation and the goitrogenic effect of foods. II. The thiocyanate content of foods, the chief cause of thiocyanate excretion in urine of man and animals. Z. Physiol. Chem. 312:31-36, 1958.

32. Langer, P.: Studies concerning the relationship between thiocyanate formation and goitrogenic effects of foods. IV. Concerning the relation between the thiocyanate content of different plant foods and their inhibiting influence on radioactive iodine uptake in the guinea pig thyroid. Z. Physiol. Chem. 323:194-198, 1961.

33. Langer, P. and Stolc, V.: The relation between thiocyanate formation and goitrogenic effects of foods. V. Comparison of the effect of white cabbage and thiocyanate on the rat thyroid gland. Z. Physiol. Chem. 335:216-220, 1964.

34. Greer, M.A.: Isolation from rutabaga seed of progoitrin, the precursor of the naturally occurring antithyroid compound goitrin (L-5-vinyl-2-thiooxazolidone). J. Am. Chem. Soc. 78:1260-1261, 1956.

35. Greer, M.A. and Deeney, J.M.: Antithyroid activity elicited by the ingestion of pure progoitrin, a naturally occurring thioglucoside of the turnip family. J. Clin. Invest. 38:1465-1474, 1959.

36. Jirousek, L.: On the antithyroidal substances in cabbage and other Brassica plants. Naturwissenschaften 43:328-329, 1956.

37. Langer, P.: The relation between thiocyanate formation and goitrogenic effect of foods. VI. Thiocyanogenic activity of allylisothiocyanate, one of the most frequently occurring mustard oils in plants. Z. Physiol. Chem. 339:33-35, 1964.

38. Langer, P.: Serum thiocyanate level in large sections of the population as an index of the presence of naturally occurring goitrogens in the organism. In: Naturally Occurring Goitrogens and Thyroid Function (J. Podoba and P Langer, eds.). Slovak Academy of Sciences, Bratislava, 1964. pp. 281-295.

39. Lang, K.: Die Rhodanbildung in Tierkörpor. Biochem. Z. 259:243-256, 1933.

40. Fiedler, H. and Wood, J.L.: Specificity studies on the B-mercapto-pyruvate-cyanide transsulfuration system. J. Biol. Chem. 222:387-397, 1956.

41. Wood, J.L. and Cooley, S.L.: Detoxication of cyanide by cystine. J. Biol. Chem. 218:449-457, 1956.

42. Boxer, G.E. and Rickards, J.C.: Determination of thiocyanate in body fluids. Arch. Biochem. Biophys. 39:292-300, 1952.

43. Wokes, F., Baxter, N., Horsford, J. and Preston, B.: Effect of light on vitamin B_{12}. Biochem. J. 53:XIX-XX, 1951.

44. Winkler, W.O.: Study of methods for glucosidal HCN in lima beans. J. Assoc. Offic. Agr. Chem. 41:282-287, 1958.

45. Gmelin, R. and Virtanen, A.I.: The enzymatic formation of thiocyanate (SCN^-) from a precursor(s) in Brassica species. Acta Chem. Scand. 14:507-510, 1960.

46. Goldstein, F. and Rieders, F.: Conversion of thiocyanate to cyanide by erythrocytic enzyme. Am. J. Physiol. 173: 287-290, 1953.

47. Oginsky, E.L., Stein, A.E. and Greer, M.A.: Myrosinase activity in bacteria as demonstrated by the conversion of progoitrin to goitrin. Proc. Soc. Exp. Biol. Med. 119:360-364, 1965.

48. Halstrom, F. and Moller, K.D.: Content of cyanide in human organs from cases of poisoning with cyanide taken by mouth, with contribution to toxicology of cyanides. Acta Pharmacol. Toxicol. 1:18-28, 1945.

49. Wilson, J.: Leber's hereditary optic atrophy: a possible defect of cyanide metabolism. Clin. Sci. 29:505-515, 1965.

50. Ferraro, A.: Experimental toxic encephalomyelopathy: Diffuse sclerosis following subcutaneous injections of potassium cyanide. Arch. Neurol. Psychiatr. 29:1364-1367, 1933.

51. Hurst, E.W.: Experimental demyelination of the central nervous system. Aust. J. Exp. Biol. Med. Sci. 18:201-223, 1940.

52. Wokes, F.: Tobacco amblyopia. Lancet 2:526-527, 1958.

53. Smith, A.D.M., Duckett, S. and Waters, A.H.: Neuropathological changes in chronic cyanide intoxication. Nature (Lond.) 200:179-181, 1963.

54. Monekasso, G.L. and Wilson, J.: Plasma thiocyanate and vitamin B_{12} in Nigerian patients with degenerative neurological disease. Lancet 1:1062-1064, 1966.

55. Osuntokun, B.O., Singh, S.P. and Martinson, F.D.: Deafness in tropical nutritional ataxia neuropathy. Trop. Geogr. Med. 22:281-288, 1960.

56. Osuntokun, B.O., Durowoju, J.E., McFarlane, H. and Nilson, J.: Plasma amino-acids in the Nigerian nutritional ataxic neuropathy. Br. Med. J. 2:647-649, 1968.

57. Choufoer, J.C., Van Rhijn, M. and Querido, A.: Endemic goiter in western Guinea. II. Clinical pictures, incidence and pathogenesis of endemic cretinism. J. Clin. Endocrinol. Metab. 25:385-402, 1965.

58. Barker, M.H.: The blood cyanates in the treatment of hypertension. J. Am. Med. Assoc. 106:762-767, 1936.

59. Barker, M.H., Lindberg, A. and Wald, M.H.: Further experiences with thiocyanates. Clinical and experimental observations. J. Am. Med. Assoc. 117:1591-1594, 1941.

60. Vanderlaan, W.P. and Bissell, A.: Effects of propylthiouracil and of potassium thiocyanate on the uptake of iodine by the thyroid gland of the rat. Endocrinology 39:157-160, 1946.

61. Wolff, J., Chaikoff, I.L., Taurog, A. and Rubin, L.: The disturbance in iodine metabolism produced by thiocyanate: the mechanism of its goitrogenic action with radioactive iodine as indicator. Endocrinology 39:140-148, 1946.

62. Vanderlaan, J.E. and Vanderlaan, W.P.: The iodide concentrating mechanism of the rat thyroid and its inhibition by thiocyanate. Endocrinology 40:403-416, 1947.

63. Raben, M.S.: The paradoxical effect of thiocyanate and of thyrotropin on the organic binding of iodine by the thyroid in the presence of large amounts of iodide. Endocrinology 45:296, 1949.

64. Wollman, S.H.: Inhibition by thiocyanate of accumulation of radioiodine by thyroid gland. Am. J. Physiol. 203:517-524, 1962.

65. Scranton, J.R., Nissen, W.M. and Halmi, N.S.: The kinetics of the inhibition of thyroidal iodide accumulation by thiocyanate: a reexamination. Endocrinology 85:603-607, 1969.

66. Maloof, F. and Soodak, M.: The oxidation of thiocyanate by a cytoplasmic particulate fraction of thyroid tissue. J. Biol. Chem. 239:1995-2001, 1964.

67. Sanchez-Martin, J.A. and Mitchell, M.L.: Effect of thyrotropin upon the intrathyroidal metabolism of thiocyante. Endocrinology 67:325-331, 1960.

68. Ohtaki, S. and Rosenberg, I.N.: Prompt stimulation by TSH of thyroid oxidation of thiocyanate. Endocrinology 88:566-573, 1971.

69. Halmi, N.S.: Thyroidal iodide transport. Vitam. Horm. 19:133-163, 1961.

70. Logothetopoulos, J.H. and Myant, N.B.: Concentration of radioiodide and ^{35}S-labelled thiocyanate by the stomach of the hamster. J. Physiol. 133:213-219, 1956.

71. Logothetopoulos, J.H. and Myant, N.B.: Concentration of radioiodide and S^{35}-labelled thiocyanate by the salivary glands. J. Physiol. 134:189-194, 1956.

72. Honour, A.J., Myant, N.B., and Rowlands, E.N.: Secretion of radioiodine in digestive juices and milk in man. Clin. Sci. 11:447-462, 1952.

73. Piironen, E. and Virtanen, A.I.: The effect of thiocyanate in nutrition on the iodine content of cow's milk. Z. Ernachrungswiss. 3:140-147, 1963.

74. Garner, R.J., Sansom, B.F. and Jones, H.G.: Fission products and the dairy cow. III. Transfer of ^{131}I to milk following single and daily dosing. J. Agr. Sci. 55:283-286, 1960.

75. Miller, J.K., Swanson, E.W. and Cragle, R.G.: Effect of feeding thiocyanate to dairy cows on absorption and clearance of intramammary iodine. J. Dairy Sci. 48:1118-1121, 1965.

76. Clements, F.W. and Wishart, J.W.: A thyroid-blocking agent in the etiology of endemic goiter. Metabolism 5:623-639, 1956.

77. Virtanen, A.I., Kreula, M. and Kiesvaara, M.: The transfer of L-5-vinyl-2-thiooxazolidone (oxazolidinethione) to milk. Acta Chem. Scand. 12:580-581, 1958.

78. Virtanen, A.I., Kreula, M. and Kiesvaara, M.: Investigations on the alleged goitrogenic properties of cow's milk. Z. Ernachrungswiss Suppl. 3:23-37, 1963.

79. Peltola, P.: Goitrogenic effect of cow's milk from the goiter district of Finland. Acta Endocrinol. 34:121-128, 1960.

80. Funderburk, C.F.: Studies on the physiological occurrence and metabolism of thiocyanate. Thesis, University of Tennessee, 1966.

81. Funderburk, C.F. and Van Middlesworth, L.: Thiocyanate physiologically present in fed and fasted rats. Am. J. Physiol. 215:147, 1968.

82. Funderburk, C.F. and Van Middlesworth, L.: The effect of SCN concentration on SCN distribution and excretion. Proc. Soc. Exp. Biol. Med. 136:1249, 1971.

83. Halmi, N.S., King, L.T., Widner, R.R., Hass, A.C. and Stuelke, R.G.: Renal excretion of radioiodine in rats. Am. J. Physiol. 193:379-385, 1958.

84. Osuntokun, B.O.: Cassava diet and cyanide metabolism in wistar rats. Br. J. Nutr. 24:797-800, 1970.

85. Ekpechi, O.L., Dimitriadou, A. and Fraser, R.: Goitrogenic activity of cassava (a staple Nigerian food). Nature (Lond.) 210:1137-1138, 1966.

86. Ekpechi, O.L.: Pathogenesis of endemic goiter in eastern Nigeria. Br. J. Nutr. 21:537-545, 1967.

87. Rosenberg, L.L., Goldman, M., La Roche, G. and Dimick, M.K.: Thyroid function in rats and chickens. Equilibration of injected iodine with existing thyroidal iodine in Long-Evans rats and White Leghorn chickens. Endocrinology 74:212-225, 1964.

88. Barnaby, C.F., Davidson, A.M. and Plaskett, L.G.: Intrathyroidal iodine metabolism in the rat. The influence of diet and the administration of thyroid-stimulating hormone. Biochem. J. 95:811-818, 1965.

89. Kelly, F.C. and Snedden, W.W.: The prevalence and distribution of endemic goitre. In: Endemic Goitre. WHO Monogr. Ser. No. 44:27-233, 1960.

CRETINISM AND THE FETAL-MATERNAL RELATIONSHIP

John B. Stanbury

Unit of Experimental Medicine, Department of Nutrition and Food Science, Massachusetts Institute of Technology Cambridge, Massachusetts

In searching for the pathogenesis of the various manifestations of endemic cretinism it is necessary to explore the roles of the maternal, fetal and placental endocrine systems and of auxiliary factors in shaping embryonic development. Many of the clinical features of the endemic cretin are not found or are rarely found in the sporadic cretin, and disturbances common to both have been found in familial goitrous cretinism. Thus, deaf-mutism often accompanies endemic cretinism, is rarely found in the sporadic cretin, and is required for the diagnosis of Pendred's syndrome, a disorder often marked by mild congenital hypothyroidism but usually not by intellectual retardation. Neurological disorders such as squint and spasticity are often (but not always) found in the endemic but are less common and severe in the sporadic cretin. Testimony suggests that a diagnosis of sporadic cretinism can often be made with comparative certainty at birth or shortly thereafter, while it seems to be difficult to do so in the endemic cretin. This last point might not hold up under close examination: the first diagnosis is usually made in a hospital setting, while the diagnostic opportunities are less favorable for the latter.

Optimal maturation depends upon a programmed unfolding of structural change and biochemical competence which to some degree in man are dependent upon a supply of thyroid hormones. Presumably these hormones come in part from the maternal thyroid and in part from the developing fetal gland. Hypothetically control could be exerted through neural centers of both mother and fetus; the placenta might act only as a diffusion barrier, or might transport hormone actively in response to undefined stimuli.

Finally, the availability of iodide and possibly of other nutritional factors may be decisive in fetal maturation. In the paragraphs which follow some aspects and anomalies of thyroid function in embryogensis will be examined.

THE CONTRIBUTION OF THE FETAL THYROID

Accumulation of iodide by the human fetal thyroid begins about the tenth to twelfth week. At about the same time thyroxine can be demonstrated in fetal plasma. Greenberg et al. (1) demonstrated a low but detectable concentration of T_4 in a fetus of approximately 11 weeks but not in one slightly smaller (Fig. 1).

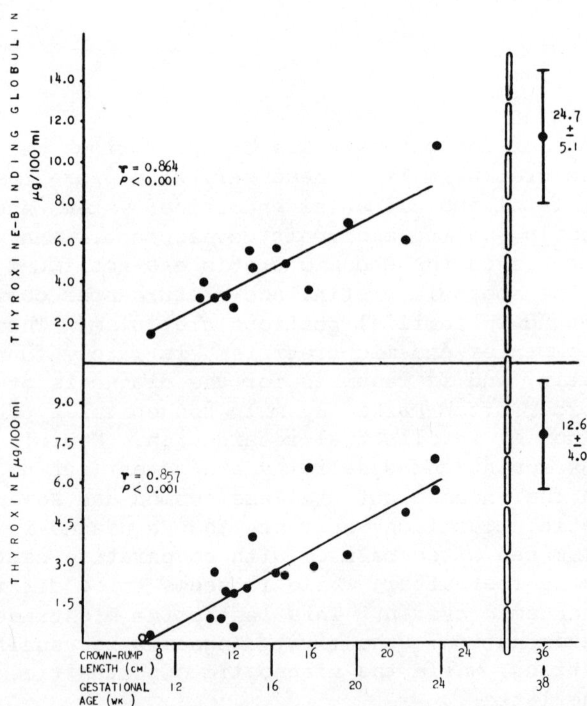

Fig. 1. (Top) The thyroxine-binding globulin concentration in fetal plasma as a function of gestational age.
(Bottom) Thyroxine concentration of fetal plasma as a function of gestational age. [From Greenberg et al. (1)].

Thereafter, there was a linear rise in fetal serum T_4 concentration, reaching approximately six μg per 100 ml by the 24th week and approximately twice that value at term. There was a corresponding rise in thyroxine-binding globulin. Free T_4 values reached the term level at about the 24th week (Fig. 2). The

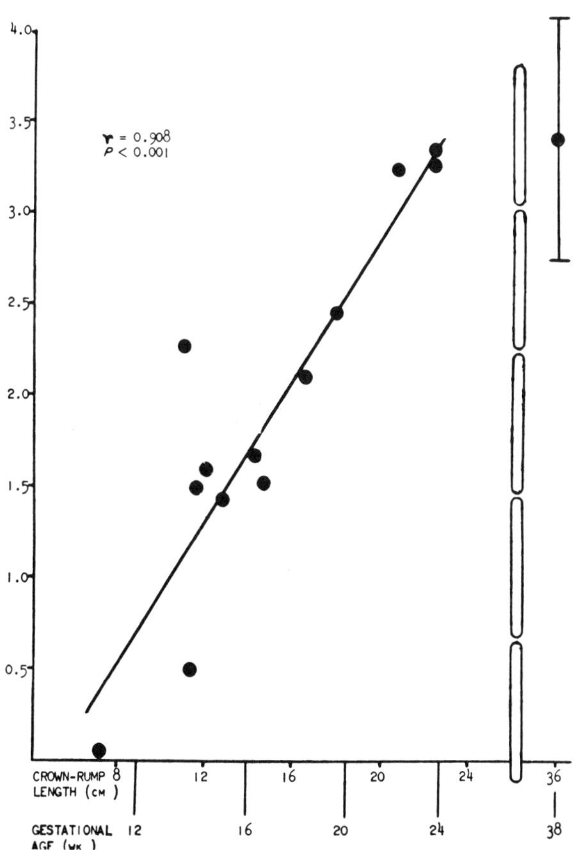

Fig.2. Free thyroxine in fetal plasma (ordinate) as a function of gestational age. [From Greenberg et al. (1)].

studies of Greenberg et al. give no information regarding the possibility that the fetus younger than 11 weeks receives a supply of T_3 from the maternal circulation. T_3 crosses the placenta late in fetal life, but there is no information on this point in early gestation (2,3).

Shepard (4) obtained corresponding information from human fetal thyroids incubated in vitro. He found that cell cultures from embryos taken at the 68 mm stage (74 days) synthesized iodotyrosines and iodothyronines, but not at earlier stages of development. Initiation of synthesis corresponded to evidence of the beginning of follicle and colloidal formation. Thus, it is clear that the human fetal thyroid synthesizes thyroid hormone by the 11th week, and that the concentration of T_4 rises in the fetal plasma from this point until term. Secretion of thyroxine by the fetal thyroid of animals is well established (5,6).

MATERNAL HORMONE CONTRIBUTION

What is not so clear is what fraction of fetal hormone derives from the maternal circulation. Pickering (7,8) on monkeys (Macaca mulatta) showed that at least some of the fetal hormone comes from the maternal side. He injected the animals with labeled T_4 and observed that at all fetal ages the specific activity of T_4 in the fetal plasma was higher than in the thyroid. This proved that the T_4 in the fetal plasma was at least in part maternal in origin rather than from the thyroid of the fetus. These findings, while important, provide no quantitative information on the relative contributions of mother and fetus to fetal T_4. Several studies have demonstrated transplacental transfer of T_4 late in pregnancy but the transfer is slow (3,9,10). Grumbach and Werner (3) found that the ratio of maternal to fetal ^{131}I-T_4 approached a steady state only after several days and in their patients never fell to one. T_3 seemed to cross the placenta more rapidly. Whether the slow placental transfer can meet fetal needs will depend on the transfer rate and the fetal degradative rate, and neither has been established. Clinical evidence (v.i.) indicates that transplacental transfer is often adequate for normal growth of the athyreotic fetus. The situation may be quite different in the sheep, where there appears to be no placental transfer of thyroid hormone at all (11). The T_4 content of amniotic fluid is much lower than that of the maternal or fetal plasma (0.7-2.0 μg per 100 ml; mean 1.26), and is little altered from the 16th week to term (12). The value reflects maternal T_4 concentration and may possibly have prognostic value for the fetus.

FETAL REQUIREMENTS FOR THYROID HORMONES

The observations already described indicate that the normal human fetus develops in a milieu containing a rising concentration of thyroxine (and presumably T_3). Experimental data related to the developmental importance of the hormones is scanty and derived from observations on rats and monkeys. It should be kept in mind that the nervous system of the newborn rat is at a much earlier stage of development than is the human neonate.

Hamburgh (13,14,15) has induced "hypothyroidism" in fetal rats by administering 0.2 percent PTU in the drinking water beginning with the 15th day of pregnancy. There appeared to be no difference between the newborn rats and control animals treated in the same way but also given T_4. If these rats were then treated with T_4 they developed normally, but if not, neural, intellectual and bony retardation rapidly became evident. These experiments appear to show that in the rat thyroid hormone only becomes significant at a critical stage in development beginning at the time of birth. Evidence was not presented that these animals were in fact hypothyroid in utero. Nievel *et al.* (16) found no difference in the polysome profiles of brains of rats at age 10 and 30 days which were given 150-200 μc ^{131}I at birth when compared to controls. This suggests that protein synthesis was normal in the brains of these animals, but the hypothyroid state was indicated only by "histo-pathological and behavioral changes", without further proof being offered.

Eayrs (17,18,19) has found that thyroidectomy at birth in rats leads to behavioral deficits later (simple maze learning, escape-avoidance), but that these deficits are reversible even if replacement therapy is delayed for as long as five months. When the animals were subjected to more complex tests, differences became apparent and a critical phase in neural development was identified which extended over the first 12 days or so of postnatal life. This corresponds roughly to the fourth and sixth month of human fetal life.

Changes in the rat induced by hypothyroidism include alterations in the brain case, diminished brain vascularity, impaired myelination and reduction in size, complexity and packing of brain cells, especially those of the cortex. Hamburgh (19) has proposed the interesting concept that the role of thyroid hormone in the early development of the CNS is that of switching the proliferative phase of neural cell growth to a phase of differentiation, and thus that the essence of the thyroid effect is its timing: permanent defects may occur in neural organization if thyroid hormone is present in too great or too little concentration during a highly critical phase when the shift from proliferation to differentiation is usually proceeding at a maximal rate. This hypothesis fits with the observation that the DNA content of rat brain may be higher than that of controls if the animal is made hypothyroid from birth.

Based on the assumption that the transplacental transfer of hormone may not be sufficient by itself for attainment of normal development in man by term, Beierwaltes et al. (20) gave high doses of thyroid to patients who had previously given birth to cretins. The patients were four women who had each previously given birth to at least one cretin. Three of six children born during the program were normal and the other three were cretins, although evidently two were not so retarded as their cretinous sibs.

Pickering (7) on the other hand has conjectured that fetal plasma concentration of T_4 is the factor governing placental transfer of T_4 to the fetus, and that transfer is independent of maternal plasma T_4 concentration. He observed that doubling or tripling plasma T_4 on the maternal side resulted in no change in fetal plasma T_4. While this is an attractive concept, the factor or factors controlling the rate of transport of T_4 across the placenta are unidentified. Pickering's data suggest that the placenta may be only a diffusion barrier. After administration of labeled T_4 the concentration remains much higher in the maternal than in the fetal circulation.

THE FACTOR OF PROTEIN BINDING

At the tenth or eleventh week of human fetal life approximately half the small amount of T_4 in the serum is bound to TBG, and most of the rest is bound to albumin and TBPA (1). Free T_4 at this stage is barely detectible, but rises rapidly to reach term levels by the 20th week. TBG rises linearly from a level of approximately 2 μg T_4 capacity per 100 ml at 11 weeks to reach term values at about term. Meanwhile, maternal TBG rises early in pregnancy, but occasions little or no change in the plasma concentration of free T_4. The rise of fetal plasma T_4 with age can be attributed to the parallel rise in TBG. One might suggest that the low levels of T_4 and free T_4 in the very young fetus merely reflect rapid utilization of hormone by fetal tissues. If so, the specific activity of T_4 should be relatively high in the plasma of the young fetus when labeled T_4 is injected into the mother. Pickering's data (7) are scanty on this point, but such as they are, are consistent. Recent disclosure of the paramount role of T_3 in metabolism necessitate a complete new look at maternal-fetal thyroid relationships.

THYROTROPIN

There are no significant changes in maternal plasma thyrotropin concentration during pregnancy, and no evidence that TSH crosses the placenta. The physiological role of placental thyrotropin is presently unknown; it has not been detected in the fetal circulation. TSH was detected in the smallest (11 wk) fetus examined by Greenberg et al. (1). The concentrations increased to term levels by the 24th week, but were somewhat lower than in paired maternal samples. The rise in TSH correlated with the rise in free T_4, but TSH reached term levels somewhat earlier. These findings are open to several interpretations. They could mean that fetal TSH is driving the thyroid through the customary negative feedback loop, or that at this stage in development the sign of the loop is positive. At birth in the rat and in man the sign of the loop appears to be negative, because in both thyroid hyperplasia may occur if PTU is given during gestation. There is no information on fetal or neonatal TSH in cretinism. The nearest approach is a very high level observed in a hypothyroid endemic cretin at age 12 months (21).

IODIDE

Iodide crosses the placenta of guinea pig, rabbit, and rat (22,23,24), and transport is blocked by SCN^- and ClO_4^-. In the guinea pig and rabbit concentration ratio of fetal to maternal plasma may be as high as two to five. There seems to be no information on whether there is any placental mechanism for adapting to changes in iodide supply. If none, the fetus would be at a particular disadvantage during iodide deficiency as the clearance by the maternal thyroid increases. The fact that the fetal thyroid undergoes hypertrophy when PTU is administered suggests that the fetal thyroid might be able to improve its supply of iodide by taking better advantage of available iodide during iodide deficiency.

CLINICAL CONTRIBUTIONS

IS HUMAN FETAL DEVELOPMENT DEPENDENT ON MATERNAL THYROID HORMONE?

This question can be approached from two directions: what happens to the fetus when there is no maternal hormone, and what happens when maternal hormone is normal and there is no fetal thyroid. There are several convincing case reports of normal infants born to myxedematous mothers. The instances are understandably rare because of the low fertility in myxedema. Parkin and Green (25) reported a 34 year old patient with typical juvenile myxedema dating from about age 12. Her BMR was minus 42 percent and cholesterol 430 mg per 100 ml. She exhibited a usual response to thyroid. Four years earlier she had delivered a child who was said to have developed normally. Their only patient actually observed with pregnancy complicating myxedema delivered a large stillborn child. Thus the birth of a normal child to a myxedematous mother in this series is based only on history.

Hodges et al. (26) reported a patient with myxedema of long standing diagnosed and treated for the first time a month before delivery of her sixth child. Her first two children had died during the first year. The third and fifth were retarded. The fourth had minor congenital defects. The sixth was reported as apparently normal at seven weeks. All had retarded bone age. The PBI of the mother at eight months of pregnancy was 2.8 μg per 100 ml. She improved dramatically on thyroid therapy.

Echt and Doss (27) reported a 35 yr woman who had a thyroidectomy at age 19. She took no medication during pregnancy and was delivered of a 3 3/16 lb female child who was said to have developed normally. The mother's PBI was 1.6 μg per 100 ml and that of the newborn child 3.0 μg per 100 ml. Chatfield (28) reported a normal child born of a myxedematous mother who began medication at the 20th week. Perhaps the most convincing case report is that of Lachelin (29). The mother, age 43, developed symptoms of myxedema after a thyroidectomy for a cyst approximately 20 years earlier. Subsequently she had six successful term pregnancies. The diagnosis of myxedema was made in the 37th week of her seventh pregnancy and confirmed by a PBI of 1.6 μg per 100 ml, a tendon reflex time of 600 microseconds (normal 250-370), low T waves in an ECG, and rapid response to medication. She was begun on T_3 and was delivered of a 3.5 kg male infant two weeks later. Dr. Lachelin has recently informed me that the infant has made satisfactory progress and seems entirely normal [cf. DISCUSSION OF PARTICIPANTS section of Balázs, this volume].

Pregnancy in myxedema is rare. Chatfield (28) was able to collect only 26 reports of live births, the first being that of Townsend in 1897 from Boston (30), who described a 38 yr typical cretin who delivered a premature infant which died in a few hours. In most instances the patients have begun replacement therapy during pregnancy and produced normal infants, or prematurity or varied congenital anomalies have resulted. Deafmutism is not reported among this group. If one accepts those instances in which a normal child was born of a mother who was myxedematous during pregnancy, then it can be said that the fetus is able to generate sufficient thyroid hormone to ensure normal development. It is possible that the congenital anomalies and the prematurity so often observed in those subjects result from reduced placental blood flow or indirect effects, rather than from a lack of fetal hormone derived from the maternal circulation. The manifest fecundity of women from severe endemic goiter regions where there is low plasma T_4 concentrations without overt clinical myxedema may be explained by relatively free transfer of T_3 which circulates in higher than normal concentration in their blood (31).

Can the fetus develop normally if it is dependent entirely upon maternal hormone? The answer may be sought among athyreotic cretins. Frequently a diagnosis can be made at birth. Suggestive findings include a lethargy, weak cry, poor suck, hypothermia, umbilical hernia, large tongue, and persistent or excessive neonatal jaundice (32). The suspected diagnosis is confirmed by measurement of plasma T_4. X-ray examination may disclose failure of calcification of epiphyses which normally occur by the 36th week, especially the distal femoral and proximal tibial epiphyses. The occurrence of epiphyseal delay clearly indicates that fetal athyreosis may be accompanied by delayed fetal maturation. Epiphyseal dysgenesis is virtually pathognomonic of cretinism (33) but is usually not observed in the early cretin until medication is begun; irregular calcification of the newly formed epiphyses then makes its appearance (20).

Whether the changes which accompany athyreosis at birth, or which appear shortly thereafter,are reversible is uncertain. Some subjects treated within the first six months achieve normal stature and intellect, but most do not. In general the end-result is correlated with the delay in starting replacement therapy. There is no published account of the results obtained when replacement medication was begun within ten days of birth and given continuously thereafter. Thus, it cannot be excluded that complete catch-up would occur if the cretinous patient could be treated sufficiently early in postnatal life and with an adequate dose.

Lowry _et al._ (32) in a survey of early diagnostic features of sporadic cretinism failed to note neurological disorders, but Smith _et al._(34) in a study of 128 sporadic cretins observed as children or later noted neurological signs in 26 out of 79 severely affected patients. These included spasticity, shuffling gait, awkwardness, jerky movements, incoordination, increased deep tendon reflexes and tremor. Squint was not mentioned.

If thyroid function in both mother and fetus is impaired by administration of an antithyroid drug such as PTU, the infant at birth may show evidence of intrauterine hypothyroidism and may have a goiter. These infants are usually carried by hyperthyroid mothers whose hyperthyroidism is controlled by the drug, and the infants usually are normal. In a recent review of women treated for thyrotoxicosis during pregnancy with antithyroid drugs and thyroid hormone no excess morbidity or mortality was noted (35), but there are a number of case reports of damage both in animals and in man as a result of prolonged administration of antithyroid drugs during pregnancy (36,37,38). One can only speculate about what might happen if a normal pregnant woman received full doses of an antithyroid drug throughout pregnancy. At least in the rat and rabbit this procedure causes lethargic young with high infant mortality (39).

The possibility has been suggested both by Blizzard et al. (40) and by Sutherland et al. (41) that antithyroid antibodies may damage both maternal and fetal thyroids. Sutherland et al. reported a woman who was hypothyroid and had high plasma levels of antithyroid antibodies. She has had six children. All were cretins at birth. Two have died. More recent studies (courtesy of Dr. R. Goldsmith) indicate limited but detectable thyroid function in the surviving children. In spite of a prescribed dose of 280 mg of thyroid daily during the last pregnancy the term PBI was only eight and a cretinous child was produced. Vigorous and early treatment of the recent children has not permitted normal development. Parker and Beierwaltes (42) detected antithyroid antibodies in cord blood of newborns whose mothers had high titers. They found no evidence of fetal thyroid damage in infants with positive tests.

PLASMA HORMONE IN PREGNANCY

Man and her colleagues (43,44) have measured thyroid function in a large number of women attending a prenatal clinic. They observed that the serum butanol-extractable iodine concentration failed to rise during pregnancy in an appreciable number - perhaps 10 percent. Among this group there was an increased incidence of abortion, prematurity and congenital defects, and among survivors an increased incidence of mental retardation. Measurements of TBG in many but not all the women in this group were normal for the pregnant state. With TBG levels which were normally elevated during pregnancy, and plasma T_4 concentrations which were normal for the non-pregnant state, the plasma free T_4 concentrations must have been low. When the hypothyroxinemic state of these women was identified and corrected by full doses of proloid and the BEI restored to normal pregnancy levels the outcome of the pregnancies was similar to that in normal subjects. Man et al. interpret their findings to mean that the thyroids of some women fail to respond to pregnancy, that the fetus is reared with limited maternal thyroid hormone, and that this is correctable by administration of proloid. Man's findings are provocative, and if they stand up under statistical analyses (and they appear to do so) and are confirmed, they indicate either that the reduction in placental transfer of hormone following a fall in maternal plasma free T_4 frequently has deleterious consequences for the fetus, or that the same factor which prevents the normal rise in T_4 is also damaging to the fetus.

The relationship between maternal and fetal thyroid function in iodine deficiency has been examined by Pretell et al. (45). The most interesting finding was that maternal plasma T_4 levels were lower in pregnant women than in those whose iodine deficiency had been corrected. Maternal TBG and TBPA concentrations were normal at term. Thus, the maternal plasma free T_4 must have been low in these subjects. In two instances very low cord blood T_4 levels corresponded to low maternal plasma T_4 levels. TSH levels were normal in cord and maternal plasmas, but there was a tendency for levels to be higher in those subjects with iodine replacement. No evidence of fetal or neonatal hypothyroidism was found. In Pretell's iodine deficient patients the free T_4 content of cord blood tended to be lower than normal.

When pregnancy occurs there is a physiological rise in TBG. For free T_4 to remain constant it is necessary that additional T_4 be secreted by the thyroid in order to fill the increased number of binding sites on the new TBG. In the type of patients described by Man et al. and the iodine deficient subjects of Pretell et al.,this increased secretion of T_4 evidently fails to occur. A deleterious effect of this failure is suggested by Man et al. and, if accompanied by iodine deficiency,might be an important contributing cause to fetal retardation.

SUMMARY

1) Thyroid hormone is required for normal human fetal and postnatal development. Fetal hormone is derived in part from the maternal circulation and in part from the fetal thyroid.

2) When the fetal thyroid fails to function, most, and in some instances all, fetal needs apparently can be met by hormone from the maternal circulation. Delayed bone maturation at birth is a result of insufficient hormone during late fetal life. In most cases very early thyroid replacement medication will probably enable full catch-up of these athyreotic neonates.

3) In the rare instances when a patient with myxedema becomes pregnant a normal child may be produced, but abortion is frequent and congenital abnormalities have often been reported.

4) Certain women with ample iodine intake and many with limited access to iodide fail to show the normal rise in plasma hormone during pregnancy. The progeny of these women may be at increased risk for cretinism, especially if the dietary iodine is very low.

ACKNOWLEDGEMENTS

Supported by USPH Grant #AM 10992. Figures 1 and 2 published by permission of the authors and *The Journal of Clinical Investigation*.

DISCUSSION

DEGROOT: You mentioned that some of the patients had low PBIs and gave birth to ostensibly normal children, but the newborns also had low PBIs. That suggests that there is an obligatory requirement for maternal hormone on the fetal side.

STANBURY: Yes, although the evidence is very sketchy. There are not many cases in the literature. The best case is from Lachelin (29). One case did suggest that some of the hormone needs to come from the mother, but that even so the fetus may develop adequately without permanent retardation.

GARDNER: The diagnosis of cretinism in the newborn reported by Carr, Beierwaltes *et al.* (46) is open to criticism. The mother received 24 grains of thyroid per day from the 22nd week of pregnancy until term. The diagnosis of cretinism was made on this premature infant on the basis of the impaired ^{131}I uptake after TSH on the ninth day of life. I think there is a good possibility that massive treatment may have suppressed the fetal thyroid. This is a difficult case to interpret.

STANBURY: I agree.

GARDNER: Your comment on fetal growth is quite appropriate. Barton Childs and I studied the birth weights of 90 of the Wilkins-Fleischmann cretins from the Johns Hopkins series and a control series (47). The cretins had a birth weight somewhat greater than the controls. On a distribution curve there was a bimodal pattern for the cretins, with one peak superimposed on the control distribution and another higher peak. We did not measure birth length. Finally, I would have to say that the diagnosis of sporadic athyreotic cretinism is only rarely made in newborns. This is one of the great challenges for screening programs. It is not an uncommon disease, and if it is treated early, one may be able to avoid mental retardation.

KOENIG: This bimodal weight distribution has also been seen by Bernheim (48) from Lyons in a series of about 50 hypothyroid children. It is my feeling from my own experience and from the literature that the few individuals with severe congenital hypothyroidism and neurological symptoms were truly athyreotic. By this I mean that we and others were not able to find any thyroid function by any means. In all the cases where the diagnosis of congenital hypothyroidism was made after the third month, we were able to find active thyroid tissue. Is it not possible that all those who were said to be athyreotic and were not able to be diagnosed at birth had enough thyroxine from their thyroid remnant to meet their limiated need without their mother's production contributing a substantial amount? In those in whom the disease was particularly severe,and they were truly athyreotic, there was no thyroxine available.

STANBURY: We do not have the information to argue that point. One would like to know what would happen to the severely-affected patients if one treated them very early.

KOENIG: We have treated some as early as ten days after birth and were not able to avoid very severe oligophrenia. In others in whom the hypothyroidism was diagnosed six months after birth, for example, and treatment was started then, there was much less oligophrenia.

DELANGE: For fifteen months in our Department, PBI has been systematically measured in any newborn who remained icteric without any apparent reason past the age of six days. We have 2,000 deliveries per year. Three cases of congenital hypothyroidism were detected. All three patients develop well under thyroid therapy.

PRETELL: I had experience with a child six months old who was diagnosed as hypothyroid because she was becoming worse and worse with many of the characteristic symptoms. She was treated with thyroid but is now retarded. The mother's second child was brought to me immediately. T_4 was measured and found low, and thyroxine treatment was started during the first days of life. She is now four years of age and is fine. In the third pregnancy, we put the mother on T_4, 300 μg. We also added a little T_3, because it is said that T_3 more easily crosses the placental barrier. The third child, a boy, had no evidence of depression at birth. We checked uptake and PBI.

HERSHMAN: In reference to Beierwaltes' case that Dr. Gardner mentioned, a woman who gave birth to cretins and possibly had suppressed thyroid function, there is experimental data in rats (49) given large doses of thyroid hormone in the perinatal period. There was suppression of the hypothalamic-pituitary-thyroid axis so that the response to a challenge with goitrogen was depressed after birth. This suggests that in this period large doses of thyroid hormone can produce permanent impairment of thyroid function.

KOENIG: I have studied some 20 patients with ectopic thyroid recently. All of their mothers were normal.

HETZEL: I would like to ask the pediatricians here what they do with a patient who has been put on thyroid as a newborn without adequate diagnosis of cretinism being made. If one sees the patient six months later, can the thyroid be discontinued or can one assume that the thyroid has not developed.

GARDNER: I have personally kept them on a reasonable dose of hormone, following their T_4 levels, until they are four or five years old. Then thyroid can be withdrawn and thyroid function tested.

HERSHMAN: What happens when you do withdraw it?

MOSIER: Some years ago De Golia and I published studies of euthyroid children and adolescents who had been put on suppressive doses of thyroid (various preparations) for different orthopedic conditions by other physicians (50). Thyroid hormone had been started as early as two years of age and continued from 20 to 125 months. We stopped thyroid abruptly and followed various parameters. The ages at stopping thyroid ranged from nine to 17 years. In all cases serum cholesterol, PBI, RAI uptake, and clinical signs all returned to normal within four months.

KOENIG: We have stopped treatment at two years in a few children we put on thyroid as soon as diagnosis was made shortly after birth. At age two or more, we were able to find the ectopic or normally-located thyroid and do the tests to determine whether they were hypothyroid. Then we put them back on thyroxine.

GARDNER: How long did it take for the ectopic thyroid to light up after you took them off thyroid?

KOENIG: We first changed them from thyroxine to T_3, then stopped T_3 and waited about ten days, Then, without giving TSH, we could find the thyroid tissue in most cases.

REFERENCES

1. Greenberg, A.H., Czernichow, P., Reba, R.C., Tyson, J. and Blizzard, R.M.: Observations on the maturation of thyroid function in early fetal life. J. Clin. Invest. 49:1790-1803, 1970.

2. Raiti, S., Holzman, G.B., Scott, R.L. and Blizzard, R.M.: Evidence for the placental transfer of tri-iodothyronine in human beings. N. Engl. J. Med. 277:456-459, 1967.

3. Grumbach, M.M. and Werner, S.C.: Transfer of thyroid hormone across the human placenta at term. J. Clin. Endocrinol. Metab. 16:1392-1395, 1956.

4. Shepard, T.H.: Onset of function in the human fetal thyroid: Biochemical and radioautographic study from organ culture. J. Clin. Endocrinol. Metab. 27:945-958, 1967.

5. Jost, A.: Action du propylthiouracile sur la thyroide du foetus de Lapin intact, decapité ou injecte de thyroxine. C. R. Soc. Biol. (Paris) 153:1900-1902, 1959.

6. Geloso, J.P., Hemon, P., Legrand, J., Legrand, C. and Jost, A.: Some aspects of thyroid physiology during the perinatal period. Gen. Comp. Endocrinol. 10:191-197, 1968.

7. Pickering, D.E.: Maternal thyroid hormone in the developing fetus. Am. J. Dis. Child. 107:567-573, 1964.

8. Pickering, D.E.: Thyroid physiology in the developing monkey fetus (Macaca mulatta). Gen. Comp. Endocrinol. 10:182-190, 1968.

9. Peterson, R.R. and Young, W.C.: The problem of placental permeability for thyrotrophin, propylthiouracil and thyroxine in the guinea pig. Endocrinology 50:218-225, 1952.

10. Myant, N.B.: The passage of thyroxine and triiodothyronine from mother to foetus in pregnant rabbits, with a note on the concentration of protein-bound iodine in foetal serum. J. Physiol. (Lond.) 142:329-342, 1958.

11. Dussault, J., Hobel, C.J. and Fisher, D.A.: Thyroxine secretion in the fetal sheep (Abstract) In: Proc. Sixth Int. Thyroid Conference (Vienna) 1970. p. 41.

12. Hollingsworth, D.R. and Austin, E.: Thyroxine derivatives in amniotic fluid. J. Pediatr. 79:923-929, 1971.

13. Hamburgh, M.: An analysis of the action of thyroid hormone on development based on in vivo and in vitro studies. Gen. Comp. Endocrinol. 10:198-213, 1968.

14. Hamburgh, M., Mendoza, L.A., Burkart, J.F. and Weil, F.: Thyroid-dependent processes in the developing nervous system. In: Hormones in Development (M. Hamburgh and E.J.W. Barrington, eds.). Appleton-Century-Crofts, New York, 1971. pp. 403-415.

15. Hamburgh, M., Lynn, E. and Weiss, E.P.: Analysis of the influence of thyroid hormone on prenatal and postnatal maturation of the rat. Anat. Rec. 150:147-162, 1964.

16. Nievel, J.G., Robinson, N. and Eayrs, J.T.: Protein synthesis in the brain of rats thyroidectomized at birth. Experientia 24:677-678, 1968.

17. Eayrs, J.T.: Effects of thyroid hormones on brain differentiation. In: Brain-Thyroid Relationships, Ciba Foundation Study Group No. 18 (M.P. Cameron and M. O'Connor, eds.). Little, Brown, Boston, 1964. pp. 60-74.

18. Eayrs, J.T.: Thyroid and central nervous development. In: Scientific Basis of Medicine. Annual Reviews, London, 1966. p. 317.

19. Eayrs, J.T.: Thyroid and developing brain: Anatomical and behavioral effects. In: Hormones in Development (M. Hamburgh and E.J.W. Barrington, eds.). Appleton-Century-Crofts, New York, 1961. pp. 345-355.

20. Beierwaltes, W.H.: Thyroid dysfunction and pregnancy. Hosp. Prac. 3:31-35, 1968.

21. Stanbury, J.B., Fierro-Benitez, R., Estrella, E., Milutinovic, P.S., Tellez, M.U. and Refetoff, S.: Endemic goiter with hypothyroidism in three generations. J. Clin. Endocrinol. Metab. 29:1596-1600, 1969.

22. Logothetopoulos, J. and Scott, R.F.: Active iodide transport across the placenta of the guinea-pig, rabbit and rat. J. Physiol. (Lond.) 132:365-371, 1956.

23. Postel, S.: Placental transfer of perchlorate and triiodothyronine in the guinea pig. Endocrinology 60:53-66, 1957.

24. Hall, P.F. and Myant, N.G.: Passage of exogenous thyroxine and of iodide beyween mother and foetus in pregnant rabbits. J. Physiol. (Lond.) 133:181-193, 1956.

25. Parkin, G. and Greene, J.A.: Pregnancy occurring in cretinism and in juvenile and adult myxedema. J. Clin. Endocrinol. 3:466-468, 1943.

26. Hodges, R.E., Hamilton, H.E. and Keettel, W.C.: Pregnancy in myxedema. Arch. Intern. Med. 90:863-868, 1952.

27. Echt, C.R. and Doss, J.F.: Myxedema in pregnancy. Report of 3 cases. Obstet. Gynecol. 22:615-620, 1963.

28. Chatfield, W.R.: Hypothyroidism in pregnancy complicated by hypothermia. J. Obstet. Gynaecol. Br. Commonw. 73:311-315, 1966.

29. Lachelin, G.C.L.: Myxoedema and pregnancy. J. Obstet. Gynaecol. Br. Commonw. 77:77-79, 1970.

30. Townsend, C.W.: A pregnant cretin. Arch. Pediatr. 14:20-21, 1897.

31. Delange, F., Camus, M. and Ermans, A.: Circulating hormones in endemic goiter, in press.

32. Lowrey, G.H., Aster, R.H., Carr, E.A., Ramon, G., Beierwaltes, W.H. and Spafford, N.R. Early diagnostic criteria of congenital hypothyroidism. Am. J. Dis. Child. 96:131-143, 1958.

33. Wilkins, L.: Epiphysial dysgenesis associated with hypothyroidism. Am. J. Dis. Child. 61:13-34, 1941.

34. Smith, D.W., Blizzard, R.M. and Wilkins, L.: The mental prognosis in hypothyroidism of infancy and childhood. A review of 128 cases. Pediatrics 19:1011-1022, 1957.

35. Herbst, A.L. and Selenkow, H.A.: Hyperthyroidism during pregnancy. N. Engl. J. Med. 273:627-632, 1965.

36. Hughes, A.M.: Cretinism in rats induced by thiouracil. Endocrinology 34:69-76, 1944.

37. Elphinstone, N.: Thiouracil in pregnancy. Lancet 1:1281-1284, 1953.

38. Morris, D.: Transient hypothyroidism in a newborn infant. Lancet 1:1284-1285, 1953.

39. Freiesleben, E. and Kjerulf-Jensen, K.: The effect of thiouracil derivatives on fetuses and infants. J. Clin. Endocrinol. 7:47-51, 1946.

40. Blizzard, R.M., Chandler, R.W., Landing, B.H., Pettit, M.D. and West, C.D.: Maternal autoimmunization to thyroid as a probable cause of athyrotic cretinism. N. Engl. J. Med. 263:327-336, 1960.

41. Sutherland, J.M., Esselborn, V.M., Burket, R.L., Skillman, T.B. and Benson, J.T.: Familial nongoitrous cretinism apparently due to maternal antithyroid antibody. N. Engl. J. Med. 263:336-340, 1960.

42. Parker, R.H. and Beierwaltes, W.H.: Thyroid antibodies during pregnancy and in the newborn. J. Clin. Endocrinol. Metab. 21:792-798, 1961.

43. Man, E.B., Holden, R.H. and Jones, W.S.: Thyroid function in human pregnancy. VII. Development and retardation of 4-year-old progeny of euthyroid and of hypothyroxinemic women. Am. J. Obstet. Gynecol. 109:12-19, 1971.

44. Man, E.B., Jones, W.S., Holden, R.H. and Mellits, E.D.: Thyroid function in human pregnancy. VIII. Retardation of progeny aged 7 years; relationships to maternal age and maternal thyroid function. Obstetrics, in press.

45. Pretell, E.A. and Stanbury, J.B.: Effect of chronic iodine deficiency on maternal and fetal thyroid hormone synthesis. In: Endemic Cretinism (B.S. Hetzel and P.O.D. Pharoah, eds.). Institute of Human Biology, Papua, New Guinea, 1971. pp. 117-124.

46. Carr, E.A., Jr.; Beierwaltes, W.H.; Raman, G.; Dodson, V.N.; Tanton, J. and Betts, J.S.: The effect of maternal thyroid function on fetal thyroid function and development. J. Clin. Endocrinol. 19:1-18, 1959.

47. Childs, B. and Gardner, L.I.: Etiologic factors in sporadic cretinism: An analysis of 90 cases. Br. Ann. Human Genetics 19:90-96, 1954.

48. Bernheim, M.; Berger, M.; Uzan, R. and Chambron, J.: Les causes du myxoedème congénital et l'aspect génetique des maladies thyroidiennes. Sem. Hop. Paris, 32:4102-4112, 1956.

49. Bakke and Lawrence: J. Lab. Clin. Med. 67:477, 1966.

50. Mosier, H.D., Jr. and De Golia, R.C.: Effect of prolonged administration of thyroid hormone on thyroid gland function of euthyroid children. J. Clin. Endocrinol. Metab. 20:1296-1301, 1960.

GENERAL DISCUSSION

IQ TESTS AND INTELLIGENCE IN ENDEMIC CRETINISM

IBBERTSON: I think it would be advantageous if we could take away a consensus on how to test intellectual function. Some of us will be going to the field in the next year or so to look at new populations.

TROWBRIDGE: I think it would be valuable to use intersensory techniques for children of school age. Dr. Klein is using these at Incap in Guatemala. Published reports on the use of such techniques are in Craviotto [a special supplement (1) on applying them to malnourished children]. For younger children, (less than six years of age), these intersensory techniques become difficult because the concept is difficult to convey to a young child. Something along the line of an adapted Stanford-Binet or other standard score would be reasonable.

FIERRO: The Leiter test is very good because it does not require verbal ability.

ROSMAN: If one were to pick a single test, I would select the Leiter test. It requires neither verbal instruction nor response. It can be used with ages two to 18. It requires no manipulative skill on the part of the testee. It is untimed. It costs about $200. It is very sturdy. The child answers by placing a block in one of several indentations in a large board, each identation corresponding to an answer. Different questions are asked by putting paper overlays on the larger board. I think it could be easily standardized for use in other countries.

FIERRO: All of our normal scholars performed on it according to their chronological age.

TROWBRIDGE: I think the important point is to see whether any test discriminates between children who one knows are clever or stupid by other criteria. I would also like to warn about hidden cultural biases. The concept of testing, of using blocks and so on, may be culture-related, just as automobiles are. The

Stanford-Binet is the most certain of the tests discussed in predicting future intelligence.

PRETELL: From the practical point of view, it is very difficult to make a longitudinal follow-up on the intelligence of these children. Not only that, but our data show a deterioration of scores with age, no matter whether the initial scores are good or not. At what age is these children's intellectual development most clearly demonstrated?

ROSMAN: I think it would be unfortunate were anyone to leave this meeting with the idea that a mental deterioration occurs in cretinism. I know of no clinical or neuropathological evidence suggesting such a decline. I think any apparent deterioration is explicable on the basis of two artifacts. If you switch from a Gesell test at age two yr to a Stanford-Binet test at age five yr and find a lower IQ, this does not necessarily mean there is a loss of intelligence; one cannot compare apples and oranges. Secondly, any child's IQ may appear to change on the Stanford-Binet because the test becomes more abstract at older chronological ages. The child who cannot make the jump from the concrete to the abstract may seem to dement. For example, a 6 yr old who achieves an IQ of 75 on the Binet, may obtain an IQ of 60 at 8 yr of age because of the more abstract nature of the questions at the 8 yr level. While cretinism is associated with mental subnormality, I do not believe there is any deterioration of intelligence.

TROWBRIDGE: Despite all these difficulties, testing needs to be done. One should pick a test and stick with it long enough to determine what the differences it shows mean.

BALÁZS: I think it may be worthwhile to consult statisticians concerning problems such as the grouping of subjects, the planning of the follow-up studies and the criteria by which observations be excluded from a statistical analysis.

ADVERSE REACTIONS TO IODINE PROPHYLAXIS AND DOSAGE

STANBURY: We are presumably trying to promote prevention of a disease. We have to be sure that our prevention does not carry with it its own risks. There certainly are instances of toxic effects of iodine. Dr. Fierro has reported three patients with thyrotoxicosis, Dr. Pretell has had one, and the Argentines have had three out of 94 (2).

QUERIDO: The problem is that thyrotoxicosis has been documented during the last five years better than it was before. The question is whether the initial few cases of thyrotoxicosis which may happen after iodine prophylaxis outweigh the advantages of reducing the goiter rate and the prevention of cretinism. I think there is no choice. In a developing country, where there are poor communications, you might overlook a case of hyperthyroidism and that is the worry. I think the advantages far outweigh the risk. However, we might be able to identify certain groups who are more at risk and observe them more carefully. Also, we might determine whether there is a relationship between dose and frequency of adverse reaction. As to the first question, I have the impression that it is the old age group that is more at risk. As to the second, I have no answer.

PRETELL: Our one case of thyrotoxicosis, out of 2,000 people treated, does not seem to be different from any other hyperthyroid patient, either by scan, by turnover, by secretion rate, and so on. I just wonder if the so-called iodine-Basedow syndrome really exists as a consequence of iodine prophylaxis.

STANBURY: There is experience in Panama (not yet published) of a striking rise in thyrotoxicosis when they instituted a salt iodization program in the past three or four years. The Argentines saw the same thing and it was talked about in Switzerland a generation ago. The puzzling thing is why the Australians haven't seen it in New Guinea.

HETZEL: I think we have not seen it in New Guinea because it depends on the length of time a population has been iodine-deficient. My thesis is that you usually do not get this disease in people under the age of 50. I think some people have autonomous glands that do not shut down when you increase their iodine intake.

KOENIG: There was a terrible argument in Switzerland over iodized salt 40 years ago. We also think in Switzerland that it is largely seen in the older patients. What we call iodine-Basedow is in patients over 40 with nodular goiter.

IBBERTSON: It is not just autonomy. We studied autonomy with T_3 suppression, using 120 μg per day. A high proportion of patients over 30 showed considerable autonomy. Yet, we haven't seen Jod-Basedow in this population, although we've followed some of them for five years.

HETZEL: In Tasmania there were more in the older ages. The incidence of thyrotoxicosis tripled, associated with increased iodine intake through iodized bread. The intake was not excessive - 150 μg per day. It was a matter of lifting a moderate deficiency to a normal intake. It occurred within six months of bread iodation. In developing countries there is not a large population over 50. It was 20 percent in Tasmania. A full report has been published (3).

STANBURY: Would the group accept that iodine should only be recommended for females up to 40 and males up to puberty?

PHAROAH: There are many people over 40 who derived great benefit from iodized oil, so you have to weigh that against the risk of Jod-Basedow.

BUTTFIELD: I support that. We first gave iodine to 60 patients in New Guinea who had large goiters. We did it for one reason - to try to get the older, influential members of the community to accept iodization. This is a very important public health point in the developing countries.

PRETELL: The Argentines claimed that when they gave iodine orally, they had thyrotoxicosis, but not when they gave it intramuscularly. The number of subjects is, of course, small.

BUTTFIELD: It appears not to be dose-dependent. On the one hand you have a low dose in Tasmania with an incidence of one in 10,000. On the other you have the total number reported at this meeting with very low incidence. It may be that you are better off with a large dose.

DELANGE: In a period of five years, we have injected 30,000 people on Idjwi, and we have seen no cases of thyrotoxicosis. Our control of the population is poor, but also the mean age of the population is 21 and there are almost no patients over 50 years.

STANBURY: Does anyone disagree with the recommendation that iodine not be given unless one is in a position to follow fairly carefully the nodular goiters in people over 40?

PRETELL: I do not think that giving a smaller dose will decrease the risk. We have demonstrated that if one gives a two ml or a 6.2 ml dose, at the beginning there is a large increase in total serum iodine and in plasma inorganic iodine. No matter what the dose, the possibility of thyrotoxicosis would be the same.

COSTA: What does one do if hyperthyroidism develops? If methimazole is continued for some months, there could be agranulocytosis instead of hyperthyroidism.

PITTMAN: Methimazole is concentrated by the thyroid, perhaps by a mechanism similar to that which concentrates iodide. The responsiveness to antithyroid drugs may be related to iodine intake (4).

BUTTFIELD: Radioiodine is a possibility for therapy in the developing countries, if necessary, because the iodine uptake goes up to a high level fairly quickly after iodized oil.

HETZEL: Could we discuss dosage recommendations in relation to the PAHO recommendations (5)?

PRETELL: We think that with the small doses given children, they should probably be re-injected before the two years recommended by PAHO. In children less than six years of age, 0.2 or 0.3 ml lasted only 15 months, at which time the urinary excretion of iodine was about 70 μg per 24 hr. When 0.5 ml was given, the difference was not significant. That reached the same level in about 18 months. In people from six to 15 years of age, one ml lasted about 24 months in keeping urinary excretion of iodine over minimum amounts. In ages over 15 years, one ml or two ml lasted about 30 months.

STANBURY: Isn't 70 μg in a child good enough for a few more months?

PRETELL: There is a risk. After 15 months there was a tendency for regression in goiter prevalence. We have seen, and Delange has seen the same thing, that when we gave two ml, we got a maximum effect at 18 months, and we still had more than 100 μg urinary excretion of iodine daily.

HETZEL: There is the problem of cost. The New Guinea administration feels strongly that one injection every five years is all they can cope with; therefore, there is a case for larger doses.

FIERRO: There is the same problem in Ecuador, too. We have decided to have an extensive injection program only once because iodized salt is gradually coming into use. We assume that in three to five years all the people will be eating iodized salt.

DELANGE: I don't agree that urinary excretion is a valid criterion for time of re-injection. The best way to check on the restoration of normal thyroid function is to estimate the level of circulating hormone.

STANBURY: The obvious thing to do is to bring blood from a fair sample of your patients to the laboratory and check their TSH concentrations. Do we agree with the PAHO recommendations (5), with the exception that re-injection every four years [instead of two years] is adequate? [There was general agreement].

INDEX